Chronicles of

Vol.

A. C. Wootton

Alpha Editions

This edition published in 2024

ISBN : 9789367243961

Design and Setting By
Alpha Editions
www.alphaedis.com
Email - info@alphaedis.com

As per information held with us this book is in Public Domain.
This book is a reproduction of an important historical work. Alpha Editions uses the best technology to reproduce historical work in the same manner it was first published to preserve its original nature. Any marks or number seen are left intentionally to preserve its true form.

Contents

PREFACE ....- 1 -
VOL. I ....- 3 -
MYTHS OF PHARMACY ....- 5 -
II PHARMACY IN THE TIME OF THE PHARAOHS ......- 31 -
III PHARMACY IN THE BIBLE ....- 40 -
IV THE PHARMACY OF HIPPOCRATES. ....- 59 -
V FROM HIPPOCRATES TO GALEN.........................- 72 -
VI ARAB PHARMACY..- 78 -
VII FROM THE ARABS TO THE EUROPEANS ....- 89 -
VIII PHARMACY IN GREAT BRITAIN. ....- 97 -
IX MAGIC AND MEDICINE....................................- 119 -
X DOGMAS AND DELUSIONS. ....- 132 -
XI MASTERS IN PHARMACY ....- 154 -
XII ROYAL AND NOBLE PHARMACISTS. ....- 210 -
XIII CHEMICAL CONTRIBUTIONS TO PHARMACY.- 233 -
XIV MEDICINES FROM THE METALS.....................- 267 -
FOOTNOTES: ....- 301 -

PREFACE

Pharmacy, or the art of selecting, extracting, preparing, and compounding medicines from vegetable, animal, and mineral substances, is an acquirement which must have been almost as ancient as man himself on the earth. In experimenting with fruits, seeds, leaves, or roots with a view to the discovery of varieties of food, our remote ancestors would occasionally find some of these, which, though not tempting to the palate, possessed this or that property the value of which would soon come to be recognised. The tradition of these virtues would be handed down from generation to generation, and would ultimately become, by various means, the heritage of the conquering and civilising races. Of the hundreds of drugs yielded by the vegetable kingdom, collected from all parts of the world, and used as remedies, in some cases for thousands of years, I do not know of a single one which can surely be traced to any historic or scientific personage. It is possible in many instances to ascertain the exact or approximate date when a particular substance was introduced to our markets, and sometimes to name the physician, explorer, merchant, or conqueror to whom we are indebted for such an addition to our materia medica; but there is always a history or a tradition behind our acquaintance with the new medicine, going back to an undetermined past.

In modern dispensatories the ever increasing accumulation of chemical, botanical, histological, and therapeutic notes has tended to crowd out the historic paragraphs which brightened the older treatises. Perhaps this result is inevitable, but it is none the less to be regretted on account of both the student and the adept in the art of pharmacy. "I have always thought," wrote Ferdinand Hoefer in the Introduction to his still valuable "History of Chemistry" (1842), "that the best method of popularising scientific studies, generally so little attractive, consists in presenting, as in a panorama, the different phases a science has passed through from its origin to its present condition." No science nor, indeed, any single item of knowledge, can be properly appreciated apart from the records of its evolution; and it is as important to be acquainted with the errors and misleading theories which have prevailed in regard to it, as with the steps by which real progress has been made.

The history of drugs, investigations into their cultivation, their commerce, their constitution, and their therapeutic effects, have been dealt with by physicians and pharmacologists of the highest eminence in both past and recent times. In Flückiger and Hanbury's "Pharmacographia" (Macmillan: 1874), earlier records were studied with the most scrupulous care, and valuable new information acquired by personal observation was presented.

No other work of a similar character was so original, so accurate, or so attractive as this. A very important systematic study of drugs, profusely illustrated by reproductions of photographs showing particularly the methods whereby they are produced and brought to our markets, by Professor Tschirch of Berne, is now in course of publication by Tauchnitz of Leipsic. In these humble "Chronicles" it has been impossible to avoid entirely occasional visits to the domain so efficiently occupied by these great authorities; but as a rule the subjects they have made their own have been regarded as outside the scope of this volume.

But the art of the apothecary, of pharmacy, as we should now say, restricted to its narrowest signification, consists particularly of the manipulation of drugs, the conversion of the raw material into the manufactured product. The records of this art and mystery likewise go back to the remotest periods of human history. In the course of ages they become associated with magic, with theology, with alchemy, with crimes and conscious frauds, with the strangest fancies, and dogmas, and delusions, and with the severest science. Deities, kings, and quacks, philosophers, priests, and poisoners, dreamers, seers, and scientific chemists, have all helped to build the fabric of pharmacy, and it is some features of their work which are imperfectly sketched in these "Chronicles."

My original intention when I began to collect the materials for this book was simply to trace back to their authors the formulas of the most popular of our medicines, and to recall those which have lost their reputation. I thought, and still think, that an explanation of the modification of processes and of the variation of the ingredients of compounds would be useful, but I have not accomplished this design. I have been tempted from it into various by-paths, and probably in them have often erred, and certainly have missed many objects of interest. I shall be grateful to any critic, better informed than myself, who will correct me where I have gone astray, or refer me to information which I ought to have given. I may not have the opportunity of utilising suggestions myself; but all that I receive will be carefully collated, and may assist some future writer.

A. C. WOOTTON.

4, SEYMOUR ROAD, FINCHLEY,
LONDON, N.

VOL. I

MYTHS OF PHARMACY

> "Deorum immortalium inventioni consecrata est Ars Medica."—CICERO, *Tusculan. Quaest.*, Lib. 3.

The earliest medical practitioners of any sort and among all peoples would almost certainly be, as we should designate them, herbalists; women in many cases. How they came to acquire knowledge of the healing properties of herbs it is futile to discuss. Old writers often guess that they got hints by watching animals. Their own curiosity, suggesting experiments, would probably be a more fruitful source of their science, and from accidents, both happy and fatal, they would gradually acquire empiric learning.

Very soon these herb experts would begin to prepare their remedies so as to make them easier to take or apply, making infusions, decoctions, and ointments. Thus the Art of Pharmacy would be introduced.

The herbalists and pharmacists among primitive tribes would accumulate facts and experience, and finding that their skill and services had a market value which enabled them to live without so much hard work as their neighbours, they would naturally surround their knowledge with mystery, and keep it to themselves or in particular families. The profession of medicine being thus started, the inevitable theories of supernatural powers causing diseases would be encouraged, because these would promote the mystery already gathering round the practice of medicine, and from them would follow incantations, exorcisms, the association of priestcraft with the healing arts, and the superstitions, credulities, and impostures which have been its constant companions, and which are still too much in evidence.

THE INVENTORS OF MEDICINE

Medicine and Magic consequently became intimately associated, and useful facts, superstitious practices, and conscious and unconscious deceptions, became blended into a mosaic which formed a fixed and revered System of Medicine. Again the supernatural powers were called in and the credit of the revelation of this Art, that is its total fabric, was attributed either to a divine being who had brought it from above, or to some gifted and inspired creature, who in consequence had been admitted into the family of the deities.

In Egypt Osiris and Isis, brother and sister, and at the same time husband and wife, were worshipped as the revealers of medical knowledge among most other sciences. Formulas credited to Isis were in existence in the time of Galen, but even that not too critical authority rejected these traditions without hesitation. In ancient Egypt, however, the priests who held in their possession all the secrets of medicine claimed Isis as the founder of their science. Some old legends explained that she acquired her knowledge of medicine from an angel named Amnael, one of the sons of God of whom we read in the book of Genesis. The science thus imparted to her was the price she exacted from him for the surrender of herself to him. The son of Isis, Horus, was identified by the Greeks with their Apollo, and to him also the discovery of medicine is attributed.

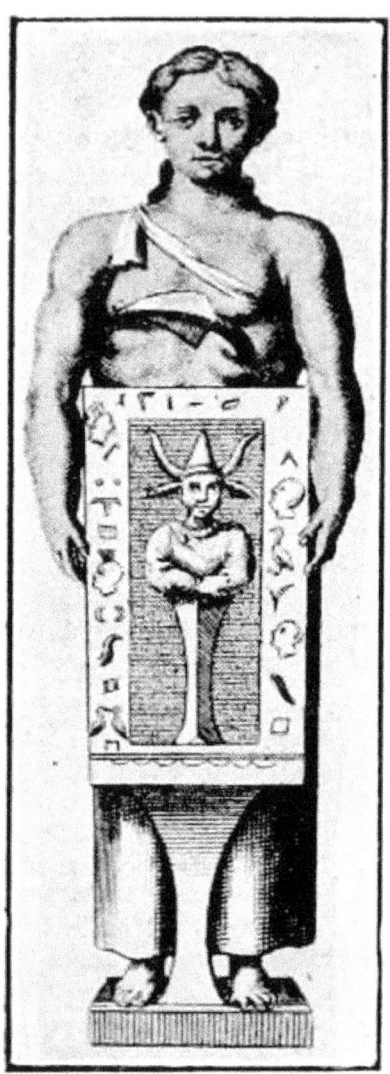

Isis.

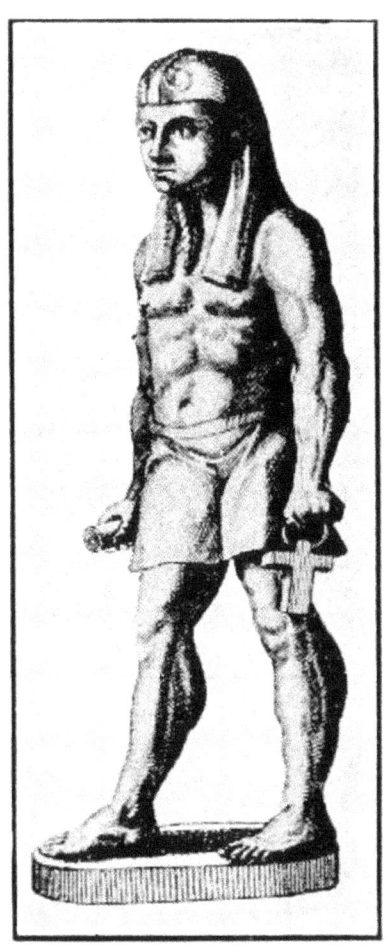

Osiris.

From the Collection of Medals and other Antiquities of Casalius (17th century).

In Leclerc's *History of Medicine*.

The legend which associated "the sons of God" with the daughters of men before the Flood, and the suggestion that they imparted a knowledge of medicine to the inhabitants of the earth, is traceable in the traditions of the Egyptians, the Assyrians, and the Persians, as well as in Jewish literature. In the 6th chapter of Genesis it is said that "they saw the daughters of men that they were fair; and they took them wives of all that they chose." From these unions came the race of giants, and the wickedness of man so "great in the earth" that the destruction of the race by the Flood resulted. The apocryphal Book of Enoch, composed, it is agreed, about 100 or 150 years before the birth of Christ, is very definite in regard to this legend, showing that it was current among the Jews at that period. We read in that Book, that "They (the angels) dwelt with them and taught them sorcery, enchantments, the properties of roots and trees, magic signs, and the art of observing the stars." Alluding to one of these angels particularly it is said "he taught them the use of the bracelets and ornaments, the art of painting, of painting the eyelashes, the uses of precious stones, and all sorts of tinctures, so that the world was corrupted."

HERMES.

With Osiris and Isis is always associated the Egyptian Thoth whom the Greeks called Hermes, and who is also identified with Mercury. He was described as the friend, or the secretary, of Osiris. Eusebius quotes an earlier author who identified Hermes with Moses; but if Moses was the inventor of medicine and all other sciences it would be hardly exact to speak of him as "learned in all the wisdom of the Egyptians." Thoth, who is also claimed as a Phoenician, as Canaan the son of Ham, and as an associate of Saturn, attained perhaps the greatest fame as an inventor of medicine. He was the presumed author of the six sacred books which the Egyptian priests were bound to follow in their treatment of the sick. One of these books was specially devoted to pharmacy.

Thoth, or Hermes, is supposed to have invented alchemy as well as medicine, the art of writing, arithmetic, laws, music, and the cultivation of the olive. According to Jamblicus, who wrote on the mysteries of Egypt in the reign of the Emperor Julian, the Egyptian priests then recognised forty-two books as the genuine works of Hermes. Six of these dealt respectively with anatomy, diseases in general, women's complaints, eye diseases, surgery, and the preparation of remedies. Jamblicus is not sure of their authenticity, and, as already stated, Galen uncompromisingly declares them to be apocryphal. Other writers are far less modest than Jamblicus in their estimates of the number of the writings of Hermes. Seleucus totals them at 20,000, and Manethon says 38,000.

The legend of Hermes apparently grew up among the Alexandrian writers of the first century. It was from them that his surname Trismegistus (thrice-great) originated. It was pretended that in the old Egyptian temples the works of Hermes were kept on papyri, and that the priests in treating diseases were bound to follow his directions implicitly. If they did, and the patient died, they were exonerated; but if they departed from the written instructions they were liable to be condemned to death, even though the patient recovered.

It is hardly necessary to say that in the preceding paragraph no attempt has been made to discuss modern researches on ancient beliefs. Greek scholars, for example, trace the Greek Hermes to an Indian source, and assume the existence of two gods of the same name.

BACCHUS, AMMON, AND ZOROASTER.

Bacchus, King of Assyria, and subsequently a deity, was claimed by some of the Eastern nations as the discoverer of medicine. He is supposed to have taught the medicinal value of the ivy, but it is more likely that he owes his medical reputation to his supposed invention of wine. Some old writers identify him with Noah. Hammon, or Ammon, or Amen, traced to Ham, the second son of Noah, has been honoured as having originated medicine in Egypt. Some attribute the name of sal ammoniac to the temple of Ammon in the Libyan oasis, on the theory that it was first produced there from the dung of camels. Gum ammoniacum is similarly supposed to have been the gum of a shrub which grew in that locality. Zoroaster, who gave the Persians their religious system, is also counted among the inventors of medicine, perhaps because he was so generally regarded as the discoverer of magic.

APOLLO.

Apollo, the reputed god of medicine among the Greeks, was the son of Jupiter and Latona. His divinity became associated with the sun, and his arrows, which often caused sudden death were, according to modern expounders of ancient myths, only the rays of the sun. Many of his attributes were similar to those which the Egyptians credited to Horus, the son of Osiris and Isis, and it is evident that the Egyptian legend was incorporated with that of the early Greeks. Besides being the god of medicine Apollo was the deity of music, poetry, and eloquence, and he was honoured as the inventor of all these arts. He evidently possessed the jealousy of the artist in an abundant degree, for after his musical competition with Pan, Apollo playing the lyre and Pan the flute, when Tmolus, the arbiter, had awarded the victory to the former, Midas ventured to disagree with that opinion, and was thereupon provided with a pair of asses' ears. Marsyas, another flute player, having challenged Apollo, was burnt alive.

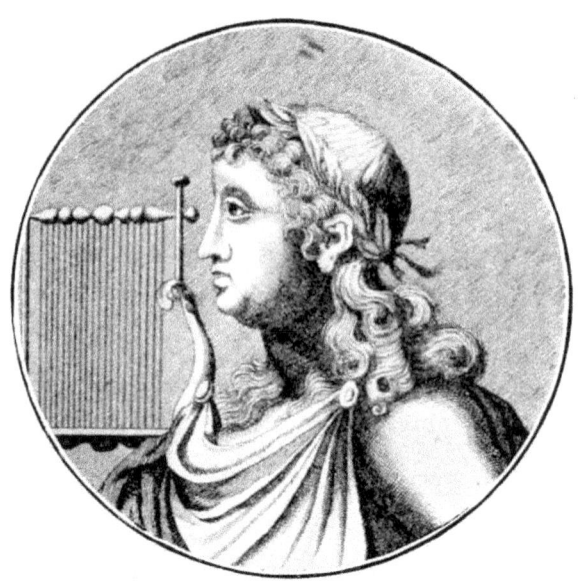

Apollo.

Peon, sometimes identified with Apollo, was the physician of Olympus. He is said to have first practised in Egypt. In the fifth book of the 'Iliad' Homer describes how he cured the wound which Diomed had given to Mars:—

> —Peon sprinkling heavenly balm around,
>
> Assuaged the glowing pangs and closed the wound.

ÆSCULAPIUS.

Æsculapius, son of Apollo and Coronis, had a more immediate connection with medicine than his father. He was taught its mysteries by Chiron the Centaur, another of the legendary inventors of the art, who also taught Achilles and others. Æsculapius became so skilful that Castor and Pollux insisted on his accompanying the expedition of the Argonauts. Ultimately he acquired the power of restoring the dead to life. But this perfection of his art was his ruin.

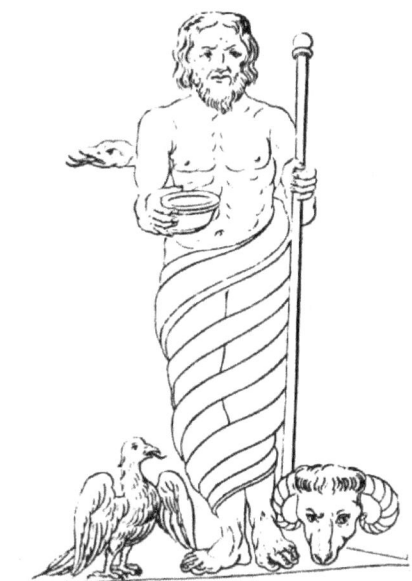
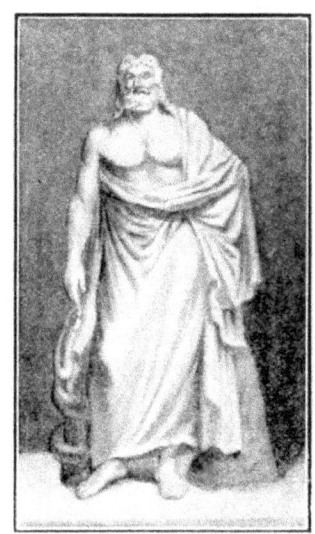

Æsculapius.

From the Casalius Collection of Medals, &c. (17th century).

From the Louvre Statue, Paris.

Pluto, alarmed for the future of his own dominions, complained to Jupiter, and the Olympian ruler slew Æsculapius with a thunderbolt. Apollo was so incensed at this cruel judgment that he killed the Cyclops who had forged the thunderbolt. For this act of rebellion Apollo was banished from Olympia and spent nine years on earth, for some time as a shepherd in the service of the king of Thessaly. It was during this period that the story of his adventure with Daphne, told by Ovid, and from which the quotation on

THE ARMS OF THE SOCIETY OF APOTHECARIES

(italicised below) is taken, occurred. Ovid relates that Apollo, meeting Cupid, jeered at his child's bows and arrows as mere playthings. In revenge Cupid forged two arrows, one of gold and the other of lead. The golden one he shot at Apollo, to excite desire; the leaden arrow, which repelled desire, was shot at Daphne. The legend ends by the nymph being metamorphosed into a laurel which Apollo thenceforth wore as a wreath. One of the incidents narrated by Ovid represents the god telling the nymph who he is. Dryden's version makes him say:

> Perhaps thou knowest not my superior state
>
> And from that ignorance proceeds thy hate.

A somewhat uncouth method of seeking to ingratiate himself with the reluctant lady. Among his attainments Apollo says:

> Invention medicina meum est, *Opiferque per orbem*
>
> *Dicor*, et herbam subjecta potentia nobis.

Dryden versifies these lines thus:

> Medicine is mine, what herbs and simples grow
>
> In fields and forests, all their powers I know,
>
> And am the great physician called below.

The arms of the Society of Apothecaries are thus described in Burke's "Encyclopædia of Heraldry," 1851:

"In shield, Apollo, the inventor of physic, with his head radiant, holding in his left hand a bow, and in his right a serpent. About the shield a helm, thereupon a mantle, and for the crest, upon a wreath of their colours, a rhinoceros, supported by two unicorns, armed and ungulated. Upon a compartment to make the achievement complete, this motto: 'Opiferque per orbem dicor.'"

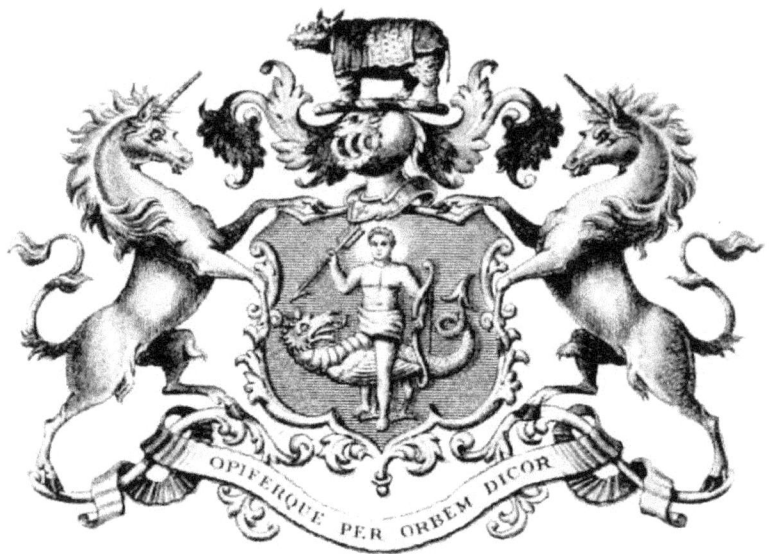

Arms of the Society of Apothecaries.

It was William Camden, the famous antiquary and "Clarenceux King at Arms" in James I.'s reign, who hunted out the middle of the above Latin quotation for the newly incorporated Society of Apothecaries.

The Sons of Æsculapius.

Æsculapius left two sons, who continued their father's profession, and three or four daughters. It is not possible to be chronologically exact with these semi-mythical personages, but according to the usual reckoning Æsculapius lived about 1250 B.C. He would have been contemporary with Gideon, a judge of Israel, about two centuries after the death of Moses, and two centuries before the reign of King David. His sons Machaon and Podalirus were immortalised in the Iliad among the Greek heroes who fought before Troy, and they exercised their surgical and medical skill on their comrades, as Homer relates. When Menelaus was wounded by an arrow shot by Pandarus, Machaon was sent for, and "sucked the blood, and sovereign balm infused, which Chiron gave, and Æsculapius used."

After the Trojan war both the brothers continued to exercise their art, and some of their cures are recorded. Their sons after them likewise practised medicine, and the earliest Æsculapian Temple is believed to have been erected in memory of his grandfather by Spyrus, the second son of Machaon, at Argos. Perhaps he only intended it as a home for patients, or it may have been as an advertisement. From then, however, the worship of Æsculapius spread, and we read of temples at Titane in the Peloponnesus, at Tricca in Thessalia, at Trithorea, at Corinth, at Epidaurus, at Cos, at Megalopolis in Arcadia, at Lar in Laconia, at Drepher, at Drope, at Corona on the Gulf of Messina, at Egrum, at Delos, at Cyllene, at Smyrna, and at Pergamos in Asia Minor. The Temple of Epidaurus was for a long time the most important, but before the time of Hippocrates that of Cos seems to have taken the lead.

The Daughters of Æsculapius

are often described as allegorical figures, Hygeia representing health, and Panacea, medicine. Hygeia especially was widely worshipped by Greeks, and when rich people recovered from an illness they often had medals struck with her figure on the reverse. Pliny says it was customary to offer her a simple cake of fine flour, to indicate the connection between simple living and good health. Panacea was likewise made a divinity. She presided over the administration of medicines. Egrea and Jaso are but little known. The former (whose name signified the light of the Sun) married a serpent and was changed into a willow, while Jaso in the only known monument on which she appears, is represented with a pot, probably of ointment, in her hand.

Prometheus.

More mythical than the story of Æsculapius, or even of Orpheus, who was also alleged to have discovered some of the secrets of medicine, is the legend of Prometheus who stole fire from heaven for the benefit of mankind. According to the older mythologists Prometheus was the same as Magog, and was the son of Japhet. Æschylus is the principal authority on his tradition. After recounting many other wonderful things he had done for humanity, the poet makes him say, "One of the greatest subtilties I have invented is that when any one falls ill, and can find no relief; can neither eat nor drink, and knows not with what to anoint himself; when for want of the necessary remedies he must perish; then I showed to men how to prepare healing medicine which should cure all maladies." Or as Dean Plumptre has rendered it:—

> If any one fell ill
> There was no help for him nor healing balm,
> Nor unguent, nor yet potion; but for want
> Of drugs they wasted till I showed to them
> The blendings of all mild medicaments
> Wherewith they ward the attacks of sickness sore.

In other words, Prometheus was the first pharmacist.

MELAMPUS.

Melampus was a shepherd to whom we owe, as legend tells us, hellebore (Gr. Melampodion) and iron as medicines. Melampus studied nature closely, and, when young, brought up by hand some young serpents, who were dutifully grateful for the cares he had bestowed on them. One day, finding him asleep, two of them crept to his ears and so effectively cleaned them with their tongues that when he woke he found he could easily make out the language of birds, and hear a thousand things which had previously been hidden from man. Thus he became a great magician. In tending his goats he observed that whenever they ate the black hellebore they were purged. Afterwards, many of the women of Argos were stricken with a disease which made them mad. They ran about the fields naked, and believed they were cows. Among the women so afflicted were the three daughters of Proetus, the king of Argos. Melampus undertook to cure the three princesses, and did so by giving them the milk of the goats after they had eaten the hellebore. His reward was one of them for his wife and a third of the kingdom. Another cure effected by Melampus was by his treatment of Iphiclus, king of Phylacea, who greatly desired to beget children. Melampus gave him rust of iron in wine, and that remedy proved successful. This was the earliest Vinum Ferri. Melampus is supposed to have lived about 1380 B.C.

GLAUCUS.

Glaucus, son of Minos, king of Crete, was playing when a child and fell into a large vat of honey, in which he was suffocated. The child being lost the king sent for Polyidus of Argos, a famous magician, and ordered him to discover his son. Polyidus having found the dead body in the honey, it occurred to Minos that so clever a man could also bring him back to life. He therefore commanded that the magician should be put into the same vat. While perplexed at the problem before him, Polyidus saw a serpent creeping towards the vat. He seized the beast and killed him. Presently another serpent came, and looked on his dead friend. The second went out of the place for a few minutes and returned with a certain herb which he applied to the dead reptile and soon restored him to life. Polyidus took the hint and used the same herb on Glaucus with an equally satisfactory result. He restored him to his father, who loaded the sorcerer with gifts. Unfortunately in telling the other details of this history the narrator has forgotten to inform us of the name of the herb which possessed such precious properties. Polyidus, according to Pausanias, was a nephew of Melampus.

CHIRON.

Chiron the Centaur was very famous for his knowledge of simples, which he learned on Mount Pelion when hunting with Diana. The Centaury owes its name to him, either because he used it as a remedy or because it was applied to his wound. His great merit was that he taught his knowledge of medicines to Æsculapius, to Hercules, to Achilles, and to various other Greek heroes. In the Iliad Homer represents Eurypylus wounded by an arrow asking Patroclus

> With lukewarm water wash the gore away
>
> With healing balms the raging smart allay
>
> Such as sage Chiron, sire of pharmacy,
>
> Once taught Achilles, and Achilles thee.
>
> (*Il.*, Bk. XI., Pope's Translation.)

Chiron was shot in the foot by Hercules by an arrow which had been dipped in the blood of the Hydra of Lerna, and the wound caused intense agony. One fable says that Chiron healed this wound by applying to it the herb which consequently bore the name of Centaury; but the more usual version is that his grief at being immortal was so keen that Hercules induced Jupiter to transfer that immortality to Prometheus, and that Chiron was placed in the sky and forms the constellation of Sagittarius. The Centaurs were a wild race inhabiting Thessaly. Probably they were skilful horse tamers and riders, and from this may have grown the fable of their form.

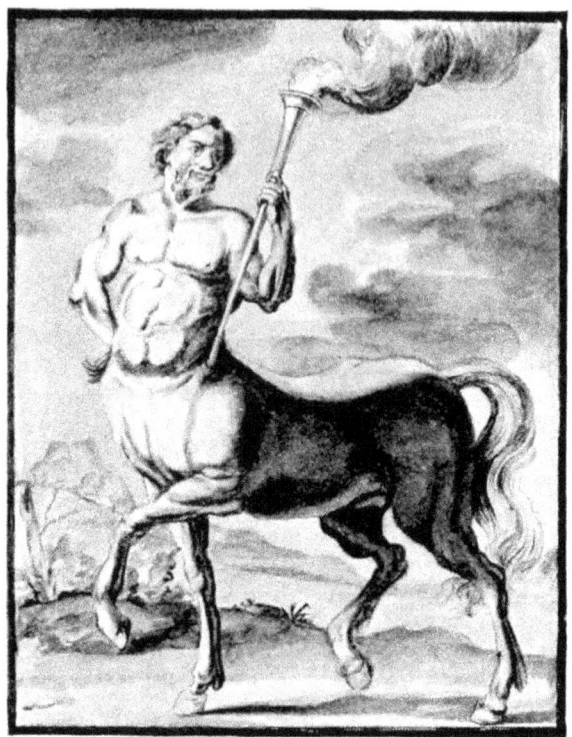

Chiron the Centaur.

ACHILLES.

Achilles carried a spear at the siege of Troy which had the benign power of healing the wounds it made. He discovered the virtues of the plant Achillea Milfoil, but Pliny leaves it doubtful whether he cured the wounds of his friend Telephas by that remedy or by verdigris ointment, which he also invented.

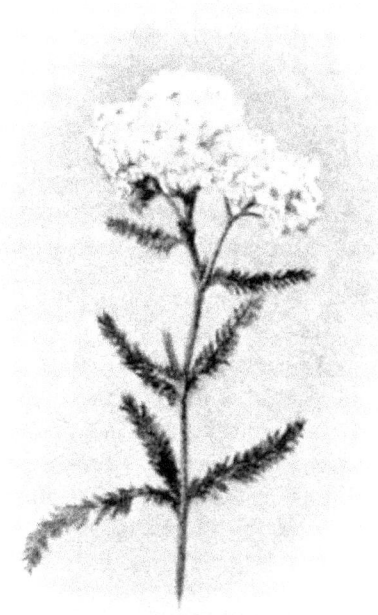

Achillea Milfoil.

ARISTES.

Aristes, king of Arcadia, was another famous pupil of Chiron. He is credited with having introduced the silphion or laser which became a popular medicine and condiment with the ancients, and which was long believed to have been their name for asafœtida, but which modern authors have doubted, alleging that silphion was the product of Thapsia silphion. Aristes is further said to have taught the art of collecting honey and of cultivating the olive.

MEDEA.

Medea of Colchis is one of the most discussed ladies of mythical history. Euripides, Ovid, and other poets represented her for the purposes of their poems as a fiend of inhuman ferocity. Some more trustworthy historians believe that she was a princess who devoted a great deal of study to the medicinal virtues of the plants which grew in her country, and that she exercised her skill on the poor and sick of her country. Certainly the marvellous murders attributed to her must have been planned by a tragic poet to whom no conditions were impossible. Diodorus declares that the Corinthians stoned her and her sons, and afterwards paid Euripides five talents to justify their crime. Medea's claim to a place in this section is the adopted theory that she discovered the poisonous properties of colchicum, which derived its name from her country. Colchis had the reputation of producing many poisonous plants; hence the Latin expression "venena Colchica."

MORPHEUS.

Morpheus was, according to the Roman poets, the son or chief minister of the god of sleep (Somnus). The god himself was represented as living in Cimmerian darkness. Morpheus derived his name from Morphe, (Gr., form or shape), from his supposed ability to mimic or assume the form of any individual he desired to pose as in dreams. Thus Ovid relates how he appeared to Alcyone in a dream as her husband, who had been shipwrecked, and narrated to her all the circumstances of the tragedy. Morpheus is represented with a poppy plant in his hand bearing a capsule with which he was supposed to touch those whom he desired to put to sleep. He also had the wings of a butterfly to indicate his lightness. Sertürner adopted the term "morphium" as the name of the opium alkaloid which he had discovered.

PYTHAGORAS.

Pythagoras, who lived in the sixth century before Christ, has been the subject of so many legends that it is difficult to separate the philosopher in him from the charlatan. He is said to have tamed wild beasts with a word, to have visited hell, to have recounted his previous stages of existence from the siege of Troy to his own life, and to have accomplished many miracles. Probably these were the myths which often gather round great men, and it is certain that from him or from his disciples in his name much exact learning, especially in mathematics, has reached us. Pythagoras was famous in many sciences. His chief contribution to pharmacy was the invention of acetum scillae. According to Pliny he wrote a treatise on squills, which he believed possessed magic virtues. Pliny also states that he attributed magic virtues to the cabbage, but it is not certain that he meant the vegetable which we call the cabbage. Aniseed was another of his magic plants. Holding aniseed in the left hand he recommended as a cure for epilepsy, and he prescribed an anisated wine and also mustard to counteract the poisonous effect of the bites of scorpions. An Antidotum Pythagoras is given in some old books, but there is no authority for supposing that this was devised by the philosopher. It was composed of orris, 18 drachms and 2 scruples; gentian, 5 drachms; ginger, 4½ drachms; black pepper, 4 drachms; honey, *q.s.*

THE PATRON SAINTS OF PHARMACY.

Cosmas and Damien, who are regarded as the patron saints of pharmacy in many Catholic countries, were two brothers, Arabs by birth, but who lived in the city of Egea, in Cilicia, where they practised medicine gratuitously. Overtaken by the Diocletian persecution in the fourth century, they were arrested and confessed their faith. Being condemned to be drowned, it is related that an angel severed their bonds so that they could gain the shore. They were then ordered to be burnt, but the fire attacked their executioners, several of whom were killed. Next they were fastened to a cross and archers shot arrows at them. The arrows, however, were turned from them and struck those who had placed them on the crosses. Finally they were beheaded, and their souls were seen mounting heavenward. For centuries their tomb at Cyrus, in Syria, was a shrine where miracles of healing were performed, and in the sixth century the Emperor Justinian, who believed he had been cured of a serious illness by their intercession, not only beautified and fortified the Syrian city, but also built a beautiful church in their honour at Constantinople. Later, their relics were removed to Rome, and Pope Felix consecrated a church to them there. Physicians and pharmacists throughout Catholic Europe celebrated their memory on September 27th for centuries.

FABLES OF PLANT MEDICINES.

The Mandrake (Atropa Mandragora) has been exceptionally famous in medical history. Its reputation for the cure of sterility is alluded to in the story of Leah and Rachel (Genesis xxx, 14–16). It is not, however, certain that the Hebrew word "dudaim" should be translated mandrake. Various Biblical scholars have questioned this which was the Septuagint rendering. Lilies, violets, truffles, citrons, and other fruits have been suggested. In Cant., vii, 14, the same plant is described as fragrant, and the odour of the mandrake is said to be disagreeable. Mandragora is described in Chinese books of medicine, and from Hippocrates down to almost modern times every writer on the art of healing treats it with reverence. Hippocrates asserts that a small dose in wine, less than would occasion delirium, will relieve the deepest depression and anxiety. The roots of the mandrake are often of a forked shape and were supposed to represent the human form, some being regarded as male and others as female. This fancy originated with Pythagoras, who conferred on the mandrake the name of anthropomorphon. It was said that when the roots were drawn from the earth they gave a human shriek. Shakespeare in *Romeo and Juliet* alludes to this superstition:

> And shrieks like mandrakes torn out of the earth
>
> That living mortals hearing them run mad.

In *Othello* again Shakespeare refers to this medicine, and particularly to its alleged narcotic properties:

> Not poppy, nor mandragora,
>
> Nor all the drowsy syrups of the world.

In *Antony and Cleopatra*, too, Cleopatra says, "Give me to drink mandragora" (that she may sleep out the great gap of time while Antony is away); and Banquo in *Macbeth*, when he asks, "Or have we eaten of the insane root that takes the reason prisoner?" is believed to allude to the mandrake.

There is a good deal of evidence that mandragora was used in ancient and mediæval times not only as a soporific, but also as an anæsthetic. Dioscorides explicitly asserts this property of the root more than once. He describes a decoction of which a cupful is to be taken for severe pains, or "before amputations, or the use of the cautery, to prevent the pain of those operations." Elsewhere he alludes to its employment in parturition, and in another passage dealing with a wine prepared from the external coat of the root, says, "The person who drinks it falls in a profound sleep, and remains deprived of sense three or four hours. Physicians apply this remedy when the necessity for amputation occurs, or for applying the cautery." Pliny refers to the narcotic powers of the mandrake, and among later writers its effects are often described. Josephus mentions a plant which he calls Baaras, which cured demoniacs, but could only be procured at great risk, or by employing a dog to uproot it, the dog being killed in the process. This Baaras is supposed to have been mandrake. Dr. Lee in his Hebrew Lexicon quotes from a Persian authority an allusion to a similar root which, taken inwardly, "renders one insensible to the pain of even cutting off a limb."

Baptista Porta describes the power of the mandrake in inducing deep sleep, and in A. G. Meissner's "Skizzen," published at Carlsruhe in 1782, there is a story of Weiss, surgeon to Augustus, King of Poland and Elector of Saxony, who surreptitiously administered a potion (of what medicine is not stated) to his royal master, and during his insensibility cut off a mortifying foot.

AMARANTH, AMBROSIA, AND ATHANASIA.

Amaranth is the name which has been given to the genus of plants of which Prince's Feather and Love-Lies-Bleeding are species. This means immortal and is the word used in the Epistle of St. Peter (v, 4), the amaranthine crown of glory, or as translated in our version "the crown of glory that fadeth not away." Milton refers to the "immortal amaranth, a flower which once in Paradise, fast by the Tree of Life began to bloom."

Ambrosia, the food of the gods, sometimes alluded to as drink, and sometimes as a sweet-smelling ointment, was also referred to by Dioscorides and Pliny as a herb, but it is not known what particular plant they meant. It was reputed to be nine times sweeter than honey. The herb Ambrose of the old herbalists was the Chenopodium Botrys, but C. Ambroisioides (the oak of Jerusalem), the wild sage, and the field parsley have also borne the name. The Ambroisia of modern botanists is a plant of the wormwood kind.

Athanasia was abbreviated by the old herbalists into Tansy, and this herb acquired the fame due to its distinguished designation. In Lucian's Dialogues of the Gods, Jupiter tells Hercules to take with him the beautiful Ganymede, whom he has stolen from earth, "and when he has drunk of Athanasia (immortality) bring him back, and he shall be our cupbearer." Naturally the ancients sought for that herb, Athanasia, which would yield immortality.

Myrrh.

Myrrha, the daughter of Cinyrus, King of Cyprus, having become pregnant, was driven from home by her father, and fled to Arabia. The story told by Ovid is that she had conceived a criminal passion for her father, and that by deception she had taken her mother's place by his side one night. Lost in the desert and overcome by remorse, she had prayed the gods to grant that she should no longer remain among the living, nor be counted with the dead. Touched with pity for her, they changed her into the tree which yields the gum which to this day bears her name.

Nepenthe.

Nepenthe, or more correctly Nepenthes, is described by Homer in the Odyssey as an Egyptian plant which Helen, the wife of Menelaus, had received from Polydamna, wife of Thonis, King of Egypt. The word is compounded of *ne*, negation, and *penthos*, pain or affliction. Helen mixed it for Telemachus in "a mirth inspiring bowl" which would

> Clear the cloudy front of wrinkled care,
>
> And dry the tearful sluices of despair.

Its effects would last all through one day. No matter what horrors surrounded,

> From morn to eve, impassive and serene
>
> The man entranced would view the dreadful scene.

Much discussion of Homer's drug has of course resulted from his description of these effects. Was it a mere poetic fancy of Homer's and was the name his invention, or was there an Egyptian drug known in his time to which the properties he describes were attributed? Plutarch, Philostratus, and some other ancient commentators suppose that the poet is only representing in a materialistic form the charm of Helen's conversation and manner. The difficulty about that interpretation is that he explicitly states that the remedy came from Egypt. Theophrastus credits the opopanax with similar properties to those which Homer claims, and Dioscorides is believed to allude to the same gum under the name of Nectarion, which he indicates to have been of Egyptian origin. This has been adopted by some old critics as the true nepenthes. Pliny asserts that Helenium was the plant which yielded the mirth-inspiring drug, but it is not clear that he means our elecampane. Borage and bugloss have also had their advocates, Galen supporting the latter. Rhazes voted for saffron. Cleopatra is assumed to have meant mandragora when she asked for some nepenthe to make her forget her sorrow while she was separated from Antony. Opium has of course been selected by many commentators, but it could hardly have furnished a mirth-inspiring bowl. Indian hemp or haschish seems to meet the requirements of the verse better than any other drug. There are also reasons for choosing hyoscyamus or stramonium. The Indian pitcher plants to which Linnaeus gave the name of nepenthes are out of the question. A learned contribution to this study may be found in the *Bulletin de Pharmacie*, Vol. V. (1813), by M. J. J. Virey.

BELLADONNA.

Atropa Belladonna is the subject of several legends. How it came by its several names it would be interesting to know. Atropa, from the eldest sister of the Fates, she who carried the scissors with which she cut the thread of life, is appropriate enough but not more to this than to any other poison plant. Belladonna—so-called because Italian ladies made a cosmetic from the berries with which to whiten their complexions; so-called because the Spanish ladies made use of the plant to dilate the pupils of their brilliant black eyes; so-called because Leucota, an Italian poisoner, used it to destroy beautiful women. These are among the explanations of the name which the old herbalists gave without troubling themselves about historical evidence. Belladonna is supposed to have been described by Dioscorides under the name of Morella furiosum lethale, and by Pliny as Strychnos manikon. It was used by Galen in cancerous affections, and its employment for this purpose was revived in the 17th century, infusions of leaves being administered both internally and externally. That it figured among the philtres of the sorcerers cannot be doubted. Like mandragora, it did not act by exciting amorous passions, but by rendering the victim helpless.

CENTAURY.

The lesser Centaury (*Erythraea Centaurium*) is alleged to owe its name to Chiron the Centaur, who is supposed to have taught medicine to Æsculapius. The story which associates Chiron with the plant has been given already.

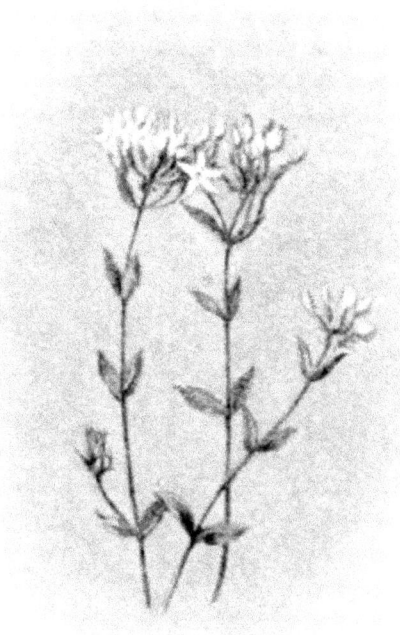

Centaury.

MINT.

Mentha was a nymph of the infernal regions beloved of Pinto. Proserpine out of jealousy caused her to be metamorphosed into the plant which thus acquired her name.

DITTANY.

Dittany, the origanum Dictamnus, was reputed to possess wonderful virtues for healing wounds. Æneas, wounded in a combat, was treated by Iapyx, who had been specially taught by Apollo, but his simples had no effect. Venus, touched by the sufferings of her son, thereupon descended from heaven in a cloud, gathered some dittany on Mount Ida, and secretly added it to the infusion with which Iapyx was vainly trying to relieve the hero. She added some ambrosial elixir, and suddenly the pain ceased, the flow of blood was arrested, the dart was easily drawn from the wound, and Æneas recovered his strength.

MYTHICAL ANIMALS.

THE PHŒNIX.

The Phœnix was largely adopted by the alchemists as their emblem, and afterwards was a frequent sign used by pharmacists. According to Herodotus this bird, which was worshipped by the Egyptians, was of about the size of an eagle, with purple and gold plumage, and a purple crest. Its eyes sparkled like stars; it lived a solitary life in the Arabian desert, and either came to Heliopolis, the city of the sun, to die and be burned in the temple of that city, or its ashes were brought there by its successor. There was only one phœnix at the same time, and it lived for 500 years. The legends vary as to its longevity, but 500 years is the period usually assigned. When the phœnix knew that its time had come, it made its own funeral pyre out of spiced woods, and the sun provided the fire. Out of the marrow of its bones came a worm, which quickly grew into a new phœnix, who, after burying its parent in Egypt, returned to Arabia.

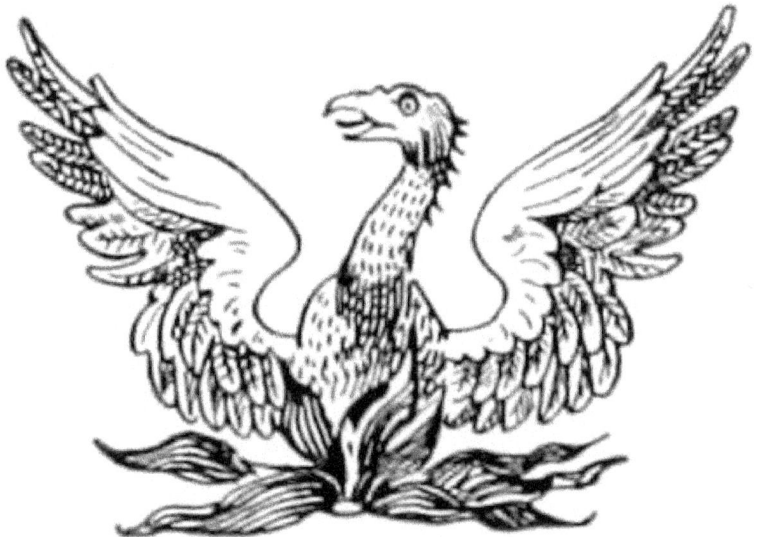

Phœnix.

The Talmud relates some curious legends of the phœnix, which the Jews believed to be immortal. One story is that when Eve had eaten the forbidden fruit she gave some to all the animals in the Garden of Eden, and that the phœnix was the only one which refused. Hence it escaped the curse of death which overtook the rest of the animal creation. Another legend is that when it was in the ark, and when all the other animals were clamouring to be fed, the phœnix was quiet. Noah, observing it, asked if it was not hungry, to which the phœnix replied, "I saw you were busy, so would not trouble you," an answer which so pleased Noah that he blessed it with eternal life. In the book of Job, xxix, 18, recalling his earlier glory, the patriarch says, "Then I said I shall die in my nest, and I shall multiply my days as the sand." Many Jewish scholars believe that the word translated sand should be phœnix, and our Revised Version gives "phœnix" as an alternative rendering. It is easy to appreciate how aptly this would express Job's idea. Some of the Hebrew commentators translate the verse in Ps. ciii, 5, "So that thy youth is renewed like the eagle," by substituting phœnix for eagle.

The Unicorn

had not quite passed into the region of fable when Pomet wrote his History of Drugs very early in the 18th century, for though he does not believe in the animal himself, he quotes from other authors not so very long antecedent to him who did. He states, however, that what was then sold as unicorn's horn was in fact the horn or tusk of the narwhal, a tooth which extends to the length of six to ten feet. The unicorn, or monoceros was referred to by Aristotle, Pliny, Aelian, and other ancient writers, and in later times it was described by various travellers who, if they had not seen it themselves, had met with persons who had.

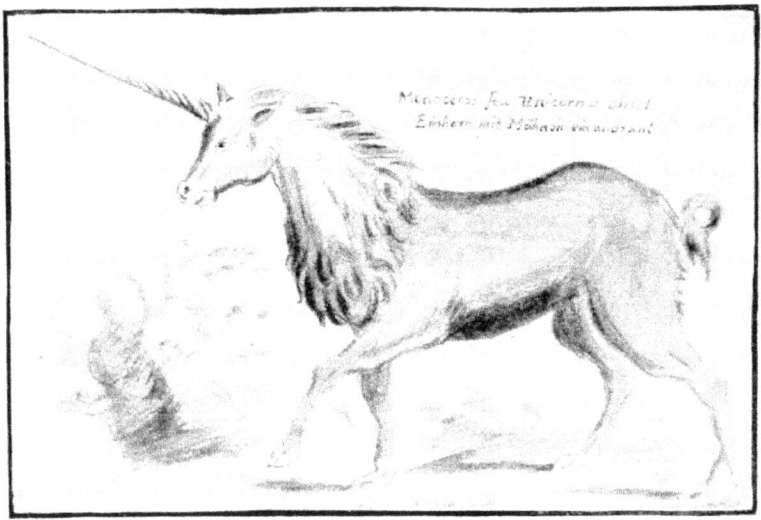

Unicorn (after Bochaut's Hierozoicon).

The details given by Aristotle are supposed to have been derived from Ctesias, whose description of the Indian wild ass is what was adopted with many embellishments for the fabulous unicorn. It is this author who first notices the marvellous alexipharmic properties so long attributed to the unicorn's horn. Drinking vessels, he says, were made of the horn, and those who used them were protected against poison, convulsions, and epilepsy, provided that either just before or just after taking the poison they drank wine or water from the cup made from the horn. In the middle ages the horn of the unicorn was esteemed a certain cure for the plague, malignant fevers, bites of serpents or of mad dogs. It was to be made into a jelly to which a little saffron and cochineal were to be added. Some writers allege that poisoned wounds could be cured by merely holding the horn of a unicorn opposite the wound. These horns are said, however, to have cost about ten times the price of gold, so that not many sufferers could avail themselves of them as a remedy.

The unicorn is mentioned several times in the Old Testament, the translators of the Authorised Version having followed the Septuagint in which the Hebrew word Re'em was rendered by the Greek term Monokeros, which corresponds with our unicorn. It is agreed that the word in the original had no reference to the fabulous animal, but that the wild ox, or ox antelope, a strong untameable beast, known in Palestine, was intended. In the Revised Version wild ox is uniformly substituted for unicorn. This animal is believed to have been the Urus mentioned by Julius Cæsar as existing in his time in the forests of Central Europe, and not entirely extinct until some 500 or 600 years ago.

The translators evidently found a difficulty in associating the unicorn with the Hebrew Re'em in Deut. xxxiii, 17, where we read of "the horns of the unicorns." In the Hebrew the horns are the plural but Re'em is singular. But the horns of the unicorn would have been a contradiction in terms.

The allusions to the unicorn in Shakespeare all seem to show unbelief in the legends. In the *Tempest* (Act 3, sc. 3) Sebastian says when music is heard in the wood, "Now I will believe that there are unicorns." In *Julius Cæsar* (Act 2, sc. 1), Decius Brutus, recounting Cæsar's superstitions, says, "He loves to hear that unicorns may be betrayed with trees"; and Timon of Athens raves about the unicorn among the legendary animal beliefs (Act 4, sc. 3). An authority on heraldry, Guillim, in 1660, however, comments thus on the scepticism of his contemporaries: "Some have made doubt whether there be any such beast as this or not. But the great esteem of his horns (in many places to be seen) may take away that needless scruple."

The unicorn was introduced into the British royal arms by James I., who substituted it for the red dragon with which Henry VII. had honoured a

Welsh contingent which helped him to win the battle of Bosworth fighting under the banner of Cadwallydr. The unicorn had been a Scotch emblem for several reigns before that of James I. (or VI.). The Scottish pound of that period was known by the name of a unicorn from the device stamped on it.

Pomet tells us that in 1553 a unicorn's horn was brought to the King of France which was valued at £20,000 sterling; and that one presented to Charles I. of England, supposed to be the largest one known, measured 7 feet long, and weighed 13 lbs. It is also related that Edward IV. gave to the Duke of Burgundy who visited him, a gold cup set with jewels, and with a piece of unicorn's horn worked into the metal. One large unicorn's horn was owned by the city of Dresden and was valued at 75,000 thalers. Occasionally a piece was sawn off to be used for medical purposes. It was a city regulation that two persons of princely rank should be present whenever this operation was performed. This was in the sixteenth century.

The unicorn was a frequent sign used by the old apothecaries. It was also adopted by goldsmiths. The arms of the Society of Apothecaries are supported by unicorns.

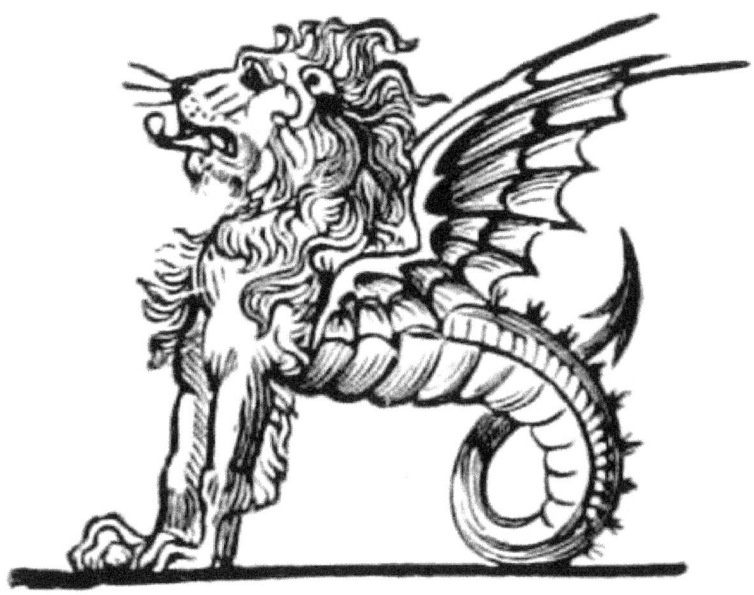

Dragon.

THE DRAGON

was only associated with pharmacy by means of the "blood" which took his name and was at one time popularly supposed to be yielded by him. I know of no evidence in support of this statement, but it is sometimes so reported.

According to Pharmacographia dragon's blood was first obtained from Socotra and taken with other merchandise by the Arabs to China. Possibly it was there that it acquired the name of dragon's blood, for the dragon has always been a much revered beast in that country. Dioscorides called this product cinnabar. I find in old books that the fruit of the calamus draconis on which the resin collects along with scales (and this is the source of our present supply), when stripped of its skin shows a design of a dragon. Lemery quoting from "Monard and several other authors," says, "When the skin is taken off from this fruit there appears underneath the figure of a dragon as it is represented by the painters, with wings expanded, a slender neck, a hairy or bristle back, long tail, and feet armed with talons. They pretend," he adds, "that this figure gave the name to tree. But I believe this circumstance fabulous because I never knew it confirmed by any traveller."

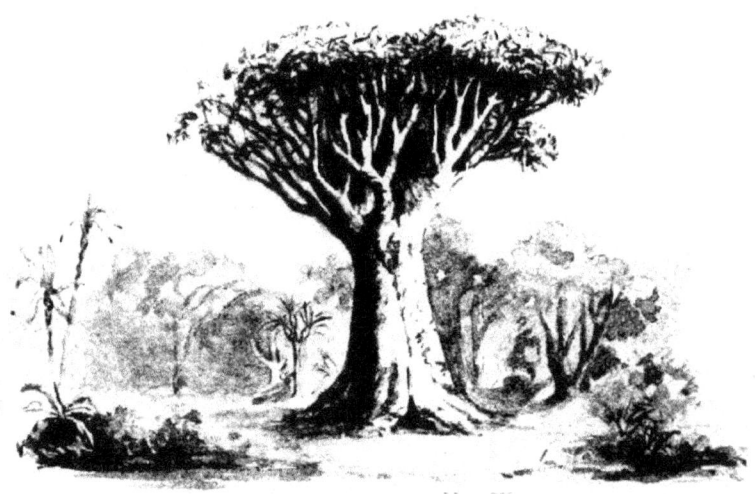

THE DRAGON TREE (*Dracona Draco*).

The tree illustrated above is at Teneriffe, and is, perhaps, the oldest tree in the world. Humboldt, in 1799, found its trunk was forty-eight feet in circumference.]

Very likely the shrewd Arabs invented the name dragon's blood to please their Chinese customers, and it may be therefore that the tree acquired its name from the resin, not the resin from the tree.

Dragon's blood was given in old pharmacy as a mild astringent, and was one of the ingredients in the styptic pills of Helvetius. It was also included in the formula for Locatelli's balsam. Now it is chiefly used as a varnish colouring, as for example in varnishes for violins. In some parts of the country it has a reputation as a charm to restore love. Maidens whose swains are unfaithful or neglectful procure a piece, wrap it in paper, and throw it on the fire, saying:

> May he no pleasure or profit see
>
> Till he come back again to me.
>
> [Cuthbert Bede in *Notes and Queries*.
>
> Series 1., Vol. II., p. 242.]

Dragons are mentioned many times in the Authorised Version of the Old Testament. In most of these instances jackals are substituted in the Revised Version, and only once, I think, the alternative of crocodiles is suggested in the margin, though in many instances it would obviously be a better rendering, as has been pointed out by many scholars.

THE SCIENCE OF MYTHOLOGY

which seeks to explain how the old myths, some poetical, many disgusting, and all impossible, originated, is a modern study which has fascinated a large number of learned scholars. The old notion that they were merely allegorical forms of representing facts and phenomena is not tenable in view of the universality of the legends among the least cultivated races. Professor Max Müller initiated a lively controversy some forty years ago by suggesting that myths were a consequence of language, a disease of language, as Mr. Andrew Lang has termed it. He traced many of the Greek myths to Aryan sources, and insisted that they had developed from the words or phrases used to describe natural phenomena. Thus, for example, he explained the myth of Apollo and Daphne (mentioned on page 9) by supposing that a phrase existed describing the Sun following, or chasing, the Dawn. He even maintained that the Sanskrit Ahana, dawn, was the derivation of Daphne. Words, of course, were invented to convey some mental conception; that conception, while it was intelligible, would (according to Max Müller's system) be developed into a story. The argument was most ingeniously worked out, but it has not proved capable of satisfying the conditions of the problem. How could it suffice, for instance, to explain the occurrence of almost identical myths treasured by the most degraded and widely separated peoples? The more likely theory is that in a very early stage of the savage mind the untrained imagination tended inevitably to associate the facts of nature with certain monstrous, obscene, and irrational forms. Perhaps the most able exposition of this view, or something like it, expounded within moderate limits, is to be found in an article on Mythology contributed to the "Encyclopædia Britannica" by Mr. Andrew Lang.

II
PHARMACY IN THE TIME OF THE PHARAOHS

> "Go up into Gilead and take balm, O virgin daughter of Egypt: in vain dost thou use many medicines; there is no healing for thee."

So wrote the prophet Jeremiah (xlvi, 11), and the passage seems to suggest that Egypt in his time was famous for its medicines. Herodotus, who narrated his travels in Egypt some two or three hundred years later, conveys the same impression, and the records of the papyri which have been deciphered within the last century confirm the opinion.

Whatever may have been the case with other arts and sciences, it does not appear that much progress was made in medicine in Egypt during the thousands of years of its history which have been more or less minutely traced. The discovery of remedies by various deities, by Isis especially, or the indication of compounds invented for the relief of the sufferings of the Sun-god Ra, before he retired to his heavenly rest, is the burden of all the documents on which our knowledge of Egyptian pharmacy is founded. It was criminal to add to or vary the perfect prescriptions thus revealed, a provision which made advance impossible to the extent to which it was enforced.

"So wisely was medicine managed in Egypt," says Herodotus, "that no doctor was permitted to practise any but his own branch." That is to say, the doctors were all specialists; some treated the eyes, others the teeth, the head, the skin, the stomach, and so forth. The doctors were all priests, and were paid by the Treasury, but they were allowed to take fees besides. Their recipes were often absurd and complicated, but there is reason to suppose that their directions in regard to diet and hygiene were sensible, and there is evidence that they paid some attention to disinfection and cleanliness.

The physicians were always priests, but all the priests were not physicians; Clement of Alexandria says those who actually practised were the lowest grade of priests. They prepared as well as prescribed medicines, but relied perhaps more on magic, amulets, and invocations than on drugs. The secrets of magic were, however, especially the property of the highest grade of priests, the sages and soothsayers. According to Celsus, the medical science of Egypt was founded on the belief that the human body was divided into thirty-six parts, each one being under the control of a separate demon or divinity. The art of medicine consisted largely in knowing the names of these demons so as to invoke the right one when an ailment had to be treated.

Symbolical names were given to many of the herbs used as medicines. The plant of Osiris was the ivy, the vervain was called Tears of Isis, saffron was the blood of Thoth, and the squill was the eye of Typhon.

Until the mystery of the Egyptian writings was unlocked, the key being found about a century ago in the decipherment of the Rosetta Stone, of which Napoleon first took possession, and which was subsequently taken from the French by the British, and is now a familiar object in the British Museum, knowledge of Egyptian science and life was limited to the information which came to us from Greek and Roman authors; and this was often fabulous. Now, however, the daily life of the subjects of the Pharaohs has been revealed in wonderful minuteness by the papyri which have been deciphered.

Among the papyri preserved in various museums a number of medical and pharmaceutical records have been found. Some medical prescriptions inscribed on a papyrus in the British Museum (No. 10,059) are said to be as old as the time of Khufu (Cheops), reckoned to have been about 3700 years B.C. Dr. E. A. Wallis Budge, the Director of the Department of Egyptian and Assyrian Antiquities in the British Museum, informs me that these prescriptions have not been translated, and that no photograph of them is available. The Papyrus itself may be of about 1400 B.C., but it refers to some medical lore of the time of Khufu, as a modern English book might quote some prescriptions of the time of Alfred the Great.

By far the most complete representation of the medicine and pharmacy of ancient Egypt is comprised in the famous Papyrus Ebers, which was discovered by Georg Ebers, Egyptologist and romancist, in the winter of 1872–3.

Ebers and a friend were spending that winter in Egypt, and during their residence at Thebes they made the acquaintance of a well-to-do Arab from Luxor who appeared to know of some ancient papyri and other relics. He first tried to pass off to them some of no particular value, but Ebers was an expert and was not to be imposed on. Ultimately the Arab brought to him a Papyrus which he stated had been discovered fourteen years previously between the knees of a mummy in the Theban Necropolis. After examination Ebers was convinced of its genuineness and bought it. His opinion was fully confirmed by all the authorities when he brought it to Germany, and the contents have proved to be of extreme value and interest in the delineation of the medical manners and customs of the ancient Egyptians.

This papyrus was wrapped in mummy cloths and packed in a metal case. It is a single roll of yellow-brown papyrus of the finest quality, about 12 inches wide and more than 22 yards long. It is divided into 108 columns each separately numbered. The numbering reaches actually 110, but there are no numbers 28 and 29, though there is no hiatus in the literary composition.

Ebers supposes there may have been some religious reason for not using the missing numbers. The writing is in black ink, but the heads of sections and weights and measures are written with red ink. The word "nefr" signifying "good" is written in the margin against many of the formulæ in a different writing and in a paler ink, evidently by someone who had used the book. It has been considered possible that this was one of the six hermetic books on medicine mentioned by Clement of Alexandria; but it is more likely to have been a popular collection of medical formulæ from various sources.

Internal evidence, satisfactory to experts, the writing, the name of a king, and particularly a calendar attached to one of the sections, establish the date of this document. The king named was Tjesor-ka-Ra, and his throne-name was Amen-hetep I., the second king of the 18th dynasty. The date assigned to the papyrus is about the year 1552 B.C., which, according to the conventional scriptural chronology, would correspond with about the 21st year of the life of Moses. If this estimation is approximately correct it follows that the prescriptions of the papyrus are considerably older than those given in the book of Exodus for the holy anointing oil and for incense, which in old works are sometimes quoted as the earliest records of "the art of the apothecary."

The papyrus begins by declaring that the writer had brought help from the King of Eternity from Heliopolis; from the Goddess Mother to Sais, she who alone could ensure protection. Speech had been given him to tell how all pains and all mortal sicknesses might be driven away. Here were chapters which would teach how to conjure away the diseases "from this my head, from this my neck, from this my arm, from this my flesh, from these my limbs. For Ra pities the sick; his teacher is Thuti" (Thoth or Hermes) "who has given him words to make this book and to save instructions to scholars and to physicians who will follow them, so that what is dark shall be unriddled. For he whom the God loveth, he maketh alive; I am one who loveth the God, and he maketh me alive."

Here are the words to speak when preparing the remedies for all parts of the body: "As it shall be a thousand times. This is the book of the healing of all sicknesses. That Isis may make free, make free. May Isis heal me as she healed Horus of all pains which his brother Set had done to him who killed his father Osiris. Oh, Isis, thou great magician, heal me and save me from all wicked, frightful, and red things, from demoniac and deadly diseases and illnesses of every kind. Oh, Ra. Oh, Osiris."

The form of words to be said when taking a remedy:—"Come remedy, come drive it out of this my heart, out of these my limbs; Oh strong magic power with the remedy." On giving an emetic the conjuration to be spoken was as follows:—"Oh, Demon, who dwellest in the body of ... son of ...; Oh, thou, whose father is called the bringer down of heads, whose name is Death, whose name is accursed for all eternity, come forth."

The following shows how the Egyptian physicians diagnosed a liver complaint: "When thou findest one with hardening of his re-het; when eating he feels a pressure in the bowels, and the stomach is swollen; feels ill while walking; look at him when lying outstretched, and if thou findest his bowels hot, and a hardening in his stomach, say to thyself, This is a liver complaint. Then make a remedy according to the secrets of botanical knowledge from the plant pa-chestat and from dates cut up. Mix it and put in water. The patient may drink it on four mornings to purge his body. If after that thou findest both sides of the bowels, namely, the right one hot and the left one cold, then say, That is bile. Look at him again, and if thou findest his bowels entirely cold then say to thyself, His liver is cleaned and purified; he has taken the medicine, the medicine has taken effect."

Superstitious notions in connection with medicine are not more apparent in the Ebers Papyrus than they are in any English herbal of three or four hundred years ago. The majority of the drugs prescribed are of vegetable origin, but there is a fair proportion of animal products, and as in comparatively modern pharmacopœias these seem to have been valued as remedies in the ratio of their nastiness. Lizards' blood, teeth of swine, putrid meat, stinking fat, moisture from pigs' ears, milk from a lying-in woman; the excreta of adults, of children, of donkeys, antelopes, dogs, cats, and other animals, and the dirt left by flies on the walls, are among the remedies met with in the papyrus.

Among the drugs named in the papyrus and identified are oil, wine, beer (sweet and bitter), beer froth, yeast, vinegar, turpentine, various gums and resins, figs, sebestens, myrrh, mastic, frankincense, opium, wormwood, aloes, cummin, peppermint, cassia, carraway, coriander, anise, fennel, saffron, sycamore and cyprus woods, lotus flowers, linseed, juniper berries, henbane, and mandragora.

There are certain substances, evidently metals by the suffixes, but they have not been exactly identified. Neither gold, silver, nor tin is included. One is supposed to be sulphur, another, electrum (a combination of gold and silver), and another alluded to as "excrement divine," remains mysterious. Iron, lead, magnesia, lime, soda, nitre and vermilion are among the mineral products which were then used in medicine.

It need hardly be said that scores of drugs named have only been guessed at, and in regard to a number of them, it has not been possible to get as far as this.

Most of the prescriptions are fairly simple, but there are exceptions. There is a poultice with thirty-five ingredients. Here is a specimen of rather complicated pharmacy. It is ordered for what seems to have been a common complaint of the stomach called setyt. Seeds of the sweet woodruff, seeds of mene, and the plant called A'am, were to be reduced to powder and mixed. Then seven stones had to be heated at a fire. On these, one by one, some of the powder was to be sprinkled while the stone was hot; it was then covered with a new pot in the bottom of which a hole had been made. A reed was fitted to the hole and the vapour inhaled. "Afterwards eat some fat," says the writer.

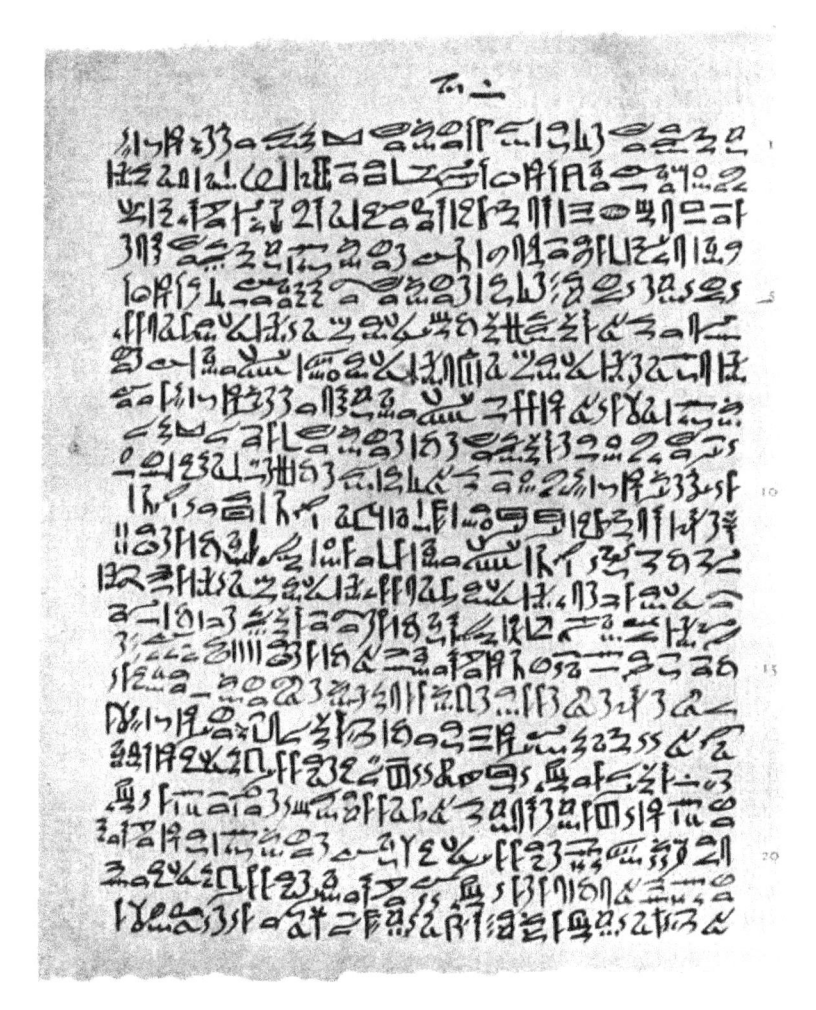

Reduced Facsimile of a page of the Papyrus Ebers.

The Papyrus Ebers has been reproduced by photography in facsimile, and published in two magnificent volumes by Mr. Wilhelm Engelmann, of Leipzig. Mr. Engelmann has kindly permitted me to copy one of the pages from his work for this book. The above is a reduced reproduction of page 47 of the Papyrus. The photograph was taken at the British Museum.

The first line of this page is the end of the instructions for applying a mixture of powders rubbed down with date wine to wounds and skin diseases to heal them. That compound was made by the god Seb, the god of the earth, for the god Ra. Then follows a complicated prescription devised by the goddess Nut, the goddess of heaven, also for the god Ra, and like the last to apply to wounds. It prescribes brickdust, pebble, soda, and sea-salt, to be boiled in oils with some groats and other vegetable matter. Isis next supplies a formula to relieve Ra of pains in the head. It contains opium, coriander, absinth, juniper berries, and honey. This was to be applied to the head. Three other formulas for pains in the head, the last for a pain on one side of the head (migraine), are given, and then there is a break in the manuscript, and afterwards some interesting instructions are given for the medicinal employment of the ricinus (degm) tree. The stems infused in water will make a lotion which will cure headache; the berries chewed with beer will relieve constipation; the berries crushed in oil will make a woman's hair grow; and pressed into a salve will cure abscesses if applied every morning for ten days. The paragraph ends (but on the next page), as many of them do, with the curious idiom, "As it shall be a thousand times." The translation is given in full (in German) in Dr. Joachim's *Papyros Ebers. Das älteste Buch über Heilkunde* (Berlin, Georg. Reimer. 1890).

To draw the blood from a wound:—Foment it four times with a mixture made from wax, fat, date wine, honey, and boiled horn; these ingredients boiled with a certain quantity of water.

To prevent the immoderate crying of children a mixture of the seeds of the plant Sheben with some fly-dirt is recommended. It is supposed that Sheben may have been the poppy. Incidentally it is remarked that if a new-born baby cries "ny" that is a good sign; but it is a bad sign if it cries "mbe."

To prevent the hair turning grey anoint it with the blood of a black calf which has been boiled in oil; or with the fat of a rattlesnake. When it falls out one remedy is to apply a mixture of six fats, namely those of the horse, the hippopotamus, the crocodile, the cat, the snake, and the ibex. To strengthen it anoint with the tooth of a donkey crushed in honey.

A few other prescriptions are appended.

As Purges:—Mix milk, one part, yeast and honey, two parts each. Boil and strain. A draught of this to be taken every morning for four days. Pills compounded of equal parts of honey, absinth powder, and onion. In another formula "kesebt" fruits are ordered with other ingredients. Ebers conjectures that kesebt may have been the castor oil tree.

For Headache:—Equal parts of frankincense, cummin, berries of u'an tree and goosegrease are to be boiled together; the head to be anointed with the mixture.

For Worms:—Resin of acanthus, peppermint flowers, lettuce, and "as" plant. Equal parts to make a plaster.

For too much urine (diabetes):—Twigs of kadet plant ¼, grapes ⅛, honey ¼, berries of u'an tree 1/32, sweet beer 1⅙.

As a Tonic:—Figs, sebestens, grapes, yeast, frankincense, cummin, berries of u'an tree, wine, goosegrease, and sweet beer are recommended.

An Application for Sore Eyes. Dried excrement of a child 1, honey 1, in fresh milk.

To make the hair grow:—Oil of the Nile horse 1, powder of mentha montana 1, myrrh 1, mespen corn 1, vitriol of lead 1. Anoint. Another formula prescribed for the same purpose was prepared for Schesch (a queen of the 3rd dynasty) and consisted of equal parts of the heel of the greyhound (from Abyssinia), of date blossoms, and of asses' hoofs boiled in oil.

A long formula for an ointment "which the god Ra made for himself" contains honey, wax, frankincense, onions, and a number of unidentified plants. The dust of alabaster and powdered statues are prescribed as applications for wounds.

To stop Diarrhœa:—Green bulbs (? onions) ⅛, freshly cooked groats ⅛, oil and honey ¼, wax 1/16, water ⅓ dena (a dena is about a pint). Take four days.

A plaster to remove pains from one side of the stomach:—Boil equal parts of lettuce and dates in oil, and apply.

Medicines against worms are numerous. Heftworms, believed to be thread worms, are treated with pomegranate bark, sea-salt, ricinus, absinth, and other unidentified drugs. For tape worms, mandrake fruits, castor oil, peppermint, a preparation of lead, and other drugs are prescribed.

Remedies which the God Su (god of the air), the God Seb (god of the earth), the Goddess Nut (goddess of the sky), and other divinities had devised are comprised in this collection. This is an application which Isis prescribed for Ra's headache:—Coriander, opium, absinth, juniper, (another fruit), and honey.

Remedies are also prescribed in this papyrus for diseases of the stomach, the abdomen, and the urinary bladder; for the cure of swellings of the glands in the groin; for the treatment of the eye, for ulcers of the head, for greyness of the hair, and for promoting its growth; to heal and strengthen the nerves; to cure diseases of the tongue, to strengthen the teeth, to remove lice and fleas; to banish pain; to sweeten the breath; and to strengthen the organs of hearing and of smell.

Quantities are indicated on the prescriptions by perpendicular lines thus: | one, || two, ||| three. Each of these lines represents a unit. Ebers calls the unit a drachm and supposes it to be equivalent to the Arabic dirhem, about forty-eight English grains. The Egyptian system of numeration was decimal. Up to nine lines were used; ⌒ was ten, and two, three or more of these figures followed each other up to ninety. Then came ꓛ a hundred, ⸕ a thousand, and so on. Fractions were shown by the figure ○, and this with three dots under it meant one-third, with four dots one-fourth, or with the 10 sign under it, ⵕ one-tenth. Half was represented by ⊏. The unit of liquid measure is believed to have been the tenat, equal to three-fifths of a litre, or rather more than an English pint.

In the British Museum "Guide" Dr. Budge quotes the following prescription "for driving away wrinkles of the face," and gives the same in hieroglyphics:—"Ball of incense, wax, fresh oil, and cypress berries, equal parts. Crush, and rub down, and put in new milk, and apply it to the face for six days. Take good heed." Generally medicines are directed to be taken or applied for four days; the ingredients are very often four; and in many cases incantations are to be four times repeated. The Pythagoreans swore by the number 4, and probably their master acquired his reverence for that figure from Egypt.

A sacred perfume called kyphi is prescribed to perfume the house and clothes for sanitary reasons. It was composed of myrrh, juniper berries, frankincense, cyprus wood, aloes wood, calamus of Asia, mastic, and styrax.

Among the Greek Papyri discovered in the last decade of the 19th century at Oxyrinchus one quoted by Messrs. Grenfell and Hunt in their work on these papyri (Vol. II., p. 134) gives about a dozen formulas for applications for the earache. These are believed to have been written in the 2nd or 3rd century A.D. One is:—Dilute some gum with balsam of lilies; add honey and rose-extract. Twist some wool with the oil in it round a probe, warm, and drop in. Onion juice, the gall of an ox, the sap of a fir tree, alum and myrrh, and frankincense in sweet wine, are among the other applications recommended.

III
PHARMACY IN THE BIBLE

> Pour bien entendre le Vieux Testament il est absolument nécessaire d'approfondir l'Histoire Naturelle, aussi bien que les mœurs des Orientaux. On y trouve à peu près trois cents noms de végétaux; je ne sais combien de noms tirés du règne animal, et un grand nombre qui désignent des pierres précieuses.—T. D. MICHAELIS, *Göttingen*, 1790.

To some extent the habits and practices of the Israelites were based on those of the Egyptians. But in the matter of medicines the differences are more notable than the resemblances. In Egypt the practice of medicine was entirely in the hands of the priesthood, and was largely associated with magical arts. It appears, too, that the Egyptian practitioners had acquired experience of a fairly wide range of internal medicines. Among the Israelites the priests did not practise medicine at all. Some of the prophets did, and they were expected to exercise healing powers. Elijah and Elisha were frequently called upon for help in this way, and the prescription of Isaiah of a lump of figs to be laid on Hezekiah's boil (2 Kings, xx, 7) will be recalled. But among the Israelites physicians formed a distinct profession, though it cannot be said that in all the history covered by the Scriptures they performed the same functions. The physicians of Joseph's household whom he commanded to embalm his father (Genesis 1, 2) were rather apothecaries. That, of course, was in Egypt. There is a curious allusion to physicians in 2 Chronicles, xvi, 12, where it is said that when Asa was exceedingly ill with a disease in his feet "he sought not to the Lord, but to the physicians." Possibly this means that he employed physicians who practised incantations. Some commentators think, however, that the passage has reference to himself, his name signifying a physician. In the apocryphal Book of Ecclesiasticus physicians are alluded to in language which suggests that at the time it was written there were doubts about the necessity of physicians. Until recently this work was attributed to Joshua or Jesus, the son of Sirach. It so appeared in the Greek manuscripts. But a Hebrew manuscript discovered in 1896 shows that the author was Simon, son of Jeshua, and critics agree that the date of its composition was rather less than 200 years before Christ.

This book, "Ecclesiasticus," is professedly a collection of the grave and short sentences of wise men. Those relating to medicine and physicians are brought together in the first part of the 38th chapter. They appear to be quoted from different authors, and several of the verses are merely parallels. Thus we have, "Honour a physician with the honour due unto him for the uses which ye may have of him; for the Lord hath created him." And again, "Then give place to the physician, for the Lord hath created him; let him not go from thee, for thou hast need of him." But the author of a verse inserted between these appears to regard the physician as less essential. He says, "My son, in thy sickness be not negligent; but pray unto the Lord, and He will make thee whole." The 15th verse is somewhat enigmatic, and may or may not be complimentary. It runs, "He that sinneth before his Maker, let him fall into the hand of the physician." In the recently discovered manuscript is the passage not previously known, "He that sinneth against God will behave arrogantly before his physician." Probably into this may be read the converse idea that he that behaves arrogantly towards his physician sinneth before God.

In the same chapter we are told that "the Lord hath created medicines out of the earth, and he that is wise will not abhor them." Possibly this was directed against the Jewish prejudice against bitter flavours. Then the writer asks, "Was not the water made sweet with wood?" and he says "of such" (the medicines) men to whom God hath given skill heal men and take away their pains; and "of such doth the apothecary make a confection."

The idea that physicians get their skill direct from God is prominent in these passages, and is perhaps truer than we are willing to admit in this age of curricula and examinations.

MEDICINES OF THE JEWS.

The Papyrus Ebers was supposed by its discoverer to have been compiled about the time when Moses was living in Egypt, a century before the Exodus. There is no evidence in the Bible that the Jews brought with them from the land of their captivity any of the medical lore which that and other papyri not much later reveal. It is not certain that in the whole of the Bible there is any distinct reference to a medicine for internal administration. It is assumed that Rachel wanted the mandrakes which Reuben found to make a remedy for sterility, but that is not definitely stated. Nor is it certain that the Hebrew word Dudaim, translated mandrakes, meant the shrub we know by that name. Violets, lilies, jasmin, truffles, mushrooms, citrons, melons, and other fruits have been proposed by various critics. There are three passages in Jeremiah where Balm of Gilead is mentioned in a way which may have meant that it was to be used as an internal remedy. These are c. viii. v. 12, c. xlvi. v. 11, and c. li. v. 8. In two of these the expression "take balm" is used, but it is quite possible to understand this as meaning employ balm, and in all the passages the sense is metaphorical.

The Mishnah, the book of Jewish legends, which forms part of the Talmud, mentions a treatise on medicines believed to have been compiled by Solomon. Hezekiah is said to have "hidden" this work for fear that the people should trust to that wisdom rather than to the Lord. The Talmud also cites a treatise on pharmacology called Megillat-Sammanin, but neither of these works has been preserved. In the Talmud an infusion of onions in wine is mentioned as a means of healing an issue of blood. It was necessary at the same time for someone to say to the patient, "Be healed of thine issue of blood." This remedy and the formula to be spoken are strongly reminiscent of Egypt.

The Talmud, though it was compiled in the early centuries of our era, undoubtedly reflects the Jewish life and thought of many previous ages, and consequently indicates fairly enough the condition of therapeutics among the ancient Hebrews. Among its miscellaneous items are cautions against the habit of taking medicine constantly also against having teeth extracted needlessly. It advises that patients should be permitted to eat anything they specially crave after. Among its aphorisms are salt after meals, water after wine, onions for worms, peppered wine for stomach disorders, injection of turpentine for stone in the bladder. People may eat more before 40, drink more after 40. Magic is plentifully supplied for the treatment of disease. To cure ague, for instance, you must wait by a cross-road until you see an ant carrying a load. Then you must pick up the ant and its load, place them in a brass tube which you must seal up, saying as you do this, "Oh ant, my load be upon thee, and thy load be upon me."

Towards the time of Christ the sect of the Essenes, ascetic in their habits and communistic in their principles, cultivated, according to Josephus, the art of medicine, "collecting roots and minerals" for this purpose. Their designation may have been derived from this occupation.

THE APOTHECARY

is, or was, familiar to readers of the Old Testament, but in the revised translation he has partially disappeared. The earliest allusion to him occurs in Exodus xxx., 25, where the holy anointing oil is prescribed to be made "after the art of the apothecary"; and in the same chapter, v. 29, incense is similarly ordered to be made into a confection "after the art of the apothecary, tempered together." The Revised Version gives in both cases "the art of the perfumer," and instead of the incense being "tempered together" (c. xxx, v, 35) the instruction is now rendered "seasoned with salt." A further mention of the art of the apothecary, or in the Revised Version, the perfumer, is found again in connection with the same compounds in Exodus xxxvii., 29. In 2 Chronicles xvi., 14, the apothecaries' art in the preparation of sweet odours and divers kinds of spices for the burial of King Asa is again alluded to, and this time without any apparent reason the Revised Version retains the old term. The next quotation (Nehemiah, iii, 8) is particularly interesting. The Authorised Version says "Hananiah, the son of one of the apothecaries," worked on the repair of the walls of Jerusalem by the side of Haraiah of the goldsmiths. In the Revised Version Hananiah is described as "one of the apothecaries." Hebrew scholars tell us that the idiom employed shows that these men belonged to guilds of apothecaries and goldsmiths respectively; a pretty little insight into ancient Jewish trade history.

In Ecclesiastes, x, 1, we come to the oft quoted parallel, "Dead flies cause the ointment of the apothecary to send forth a stinking savour," this being likened to a little folly spoiling a reputation for wisdom. The revisers have substituted perfumer for apothecary in this text. They certainly ought to have changed ointment for pomade in the same text to explain their view of the meaning of the passage.

In the passage already quoted from the apocryphal book of Ecclesiasticus, xxxviii, 8, "Of such doth the apothecary make a confection," and in xlix, 1, "The remembrance of Josias is like the composition of the perfume made by the art of the apothecary," the revisers have not seen fit to alter the trade designation.

The words translated apothecary, compound, ointment, and confection in the passages cited, and in many others in the Hebrew scriptures, are all inflexions of the root verb, Rakach (in which the final ch is a strong aspirate or guttural). Gesenius says of this root, "The primary idea appears to be in making the spices small which are mixed with the oil." The apothecary, therefore, may be regarded as a crusher, or pounder.

PHARMACY, DISGRACEFUL.

The Greek word, pharmakeia, the original of our "pharmacy," had a rather mixed history in its native language. It does not seem to have exactly deteriorated, as words in all languages have a habit of doing, for from the earliest times it was used concurrently to describe the preparation of medicines, and also through its association with drugs and poisons and the production of philtres, as equivalent to sorcery and witchcraft. It is in this latter sense that it is employed exclusively in the New Testament. St. Paul, for instance (in Galatians, v, 20), enumerating the works of the flesh names it after idolatry. The word appears as witchcraft in the Authorised, and as sorcery in the Revised Version. Pharmakeia or one of its derivatives also occurs several times in the Book of Revelations (ix, 21; xviii, 23; xxi, 8, and xxii, 15), and is uniformly rendered sorcery or sorcerers in both versions, and is associated with crime. Hippocrates uses the verb Pharmakeuein with the meaning of to purge, but he elsewhere employs the same word with the meaning of to drug a person, to give a stupefying draught. In Homer the word "Pharmaka" appears in the senses of both noxious and healing drugs, and also to represent enchanted potions or philtres. The word "pharmakoi" in later times came to be used for the criminals who were sacrificed for the benefit of the communities, and thus it acquired its lowest stage of signification. It is remarkable and unusual for a word which has once fallen as this one did to recover its respectable position again.

DRUGS NAMED IN THE BIBLE.

BALM OF GILEAD

is now usually identified with the exudation from the Balsamum Gileadense, known as Opobalsamum, a delicately odorous resinous substance of a dark red colour, turning yellow as it solidifies. It is not now used in modern pharmacy, except in the East. The London Pharmacopœia of 1746 authorised the substitution of expressed oil of nutmeg for it in the formula for Theriaca. Some Biblical commentators have preferred to regard mastic as the original Balm of Gilead, and others have thought that styrax has fulfilled the description. At this day the monks of Jericho sell to tourists an oily gum extracted from the Takkum, or Balanites Egyptiaca, as Balm of Gilead. It is put up in tin cases, and is said to be useful in the treatment of sores and wounds; but it cannot be the true Balm of the Bible.

The references to Balm of Gilead in the Old Testament show that it was exported from Arabia to Egypt from very early times. The Ishmaelites "from Gilead" who bought Joseph, were carrying it down to Egypt with other Eastern gums and spices (Genesis, xxxvii, 25). "A little balm" was among the gifts which Jacob told his sons to take to the lord of Egypt (Genesis, xliii, 11). This was the same substance: tsora in Hebrew. The translation "balm" in the Authorised Version is said in the Encyclopedia Biblica to be "an unfortunate inheritance from Coverdale's Bible." Why it is unfortunate is not clear, unless it is that the English word suggests the idea of a medicine. In the Genesis references to the substance there is no indication that the tsora was employed as a remedy, but in the Book of Jeremiah it is mentioned three times (viii, 22; xlvi, 11; li, 8), and in all these allusions its healing virtues are emphasised. Wyclif translates tsora in Genesis "sweete gum," and, in Jeremiah, "resyn." Coverdale adopts "triacle" in Jeremiah. The Septuagint rendered the Hebrew tsora into the Greek retiné, resin.

The text of the prophetic book leaves it open to doubt whether the balm was for internal or external administration. Probably it was made into an ointment.

Gilead was the country on the East of the Jordan, not very defined in extent, a geographical expression for the mountainous region which the Israelites took from the Amorites. But it is not necessary to suppose that the balsam was produced in that district. Josephus states that the Balsamum Gileadense, the Opobalsamum tree, was grown in the neighbourhood of Jericho; but he also reports the tradition that it was brought to Judea by the Queen of Sheba when she visited Solomon. This is not incompatible with the much earlier record of the Ishmaelites carrying it "from Gilead" to Egypt. For the Sabaeans who inhabited the southern part of Arabia were from very early times the great traders of the East, and they would have supplied the balm to these Ishmaelites in the regular course of commerce. The Sabaeans are believed to have colonised Abyssinia, and the Queen of Sheba may have come from that country. But whether the tree was originally grown in Africa or Arabia, there is no doubt about the esteem in which it was held by many nations. Strabo (B.C. 230) says: "In that most happy land of the Sabaeans grow frankincense, myrrh, and cinnamon; and on the coast that is about Saba, the balsam also." Many later writers allude to its costliness and to its medicinal virtues; Pliny tells us that it was preferred to all other odours. He also states that the tree was only grown in Judea, and there only in two gardens, both belonging to the King.

INCENSE.

The formula for the holy incense given in Exodus, xxx, 35, is sufficiently definite. Taking it as it is translated in the Revised Version, the prescription orders stacte, onycha, galbanum and frankincense, equal parts; seasoned with salt; powdered.

The word translated incense in that passage, and also in Deuteronomy, xxxiii, 10, and in Jeremiah, xliv, 21, is Ketorah, which originally meant a perfumed or savoury smoke. In the Septuagint the word used for Ketorah is Thymiana. In other passages (Isaiah, xliii, 33, lx, 6, lxvi, 3; Jeremiah, vi, 20; xvii, 26, and xli, 5), the word used in Hebrew was Lebonah. This in our Authorised Version appears each time as incense, but in the Revised Version the name frankincense is uniformly adopted. Lebonah meant whiteness, probably milkiness being understood in this connection, and travellers state that when the gum exudes from the tree it is milky-white. The Greek equivalent, libanos, occurs severed times in the New Testament (Matt., ii, 11; Revelations, xviii, 3). The Arabic term was luban, and apparently olibanum is a modification of this Arabic name with the article prefixed, Al-luban. The common trade term "thus" is the Greek word for incense, and is derived from the verb thuein, to sacrifice. Thurible was the Greek equivalent of the censer. The same word has been modified into fume in English. There is, besides, a common gum thus, obtained from the pines which yield American turpentine.

Olibanum, or frankincense, derived from various species of the Boswellia, was greatly prized among many of the ancient nations, especially by the Egyptians, the Assyrians, and the Phœnicians. The finest qualities were grown in Somaliland, but the stocks of these were always bought up by the Arabs, who monopolised the commerce in olibanum. It was believed for centuries that the shrub from which it was obtained was a native of South

Arabia, and an old Eastern legend alluded to in the Apocalypse of Moses declares that Adam was allowed to bring this tree with him when he was expelled from the Garden of Eden. Bruce, the African traveller, first ascertained its African origin. The historical notes on Olibanum in "Pharmacographia" are extremely interesting and complete.

Stacte, in Hebrew Nataph, is frequently identified with opobalsamum, and this interpretation is given in the margin of the Revised Version. But there are reasons for regarding it as a particularly fine kind of myrrh in drops or tears. Nataph meant something dropped or distilled.

Galbanum, it is not disputed, was the galbanum known to us by the same name. Its Hebrew name was Helbanah or Chelbanah. It has been an article of commerce from very early times, but the exact plant from which it is obtained is very uncertain. Hanbury states that the Irvingite chapels in London still use galbanum as an ingredient in their incense in imitation of the ancient Jewish custom.

Onycha has been the subject of much discussion. The balance of learned opinion favours the view that it is the operculum of a species of sea-snail found on the shores of the Red Sea. It is known as Unguis odoratus, blatta Byzantina, and devil's claw. Nubian women to this day use it with myrrh, cloves, frankincense, and cinnamon, to perfume themselves.

The incense made from the formula just quoted was reserved specially for the service of the tabernacle, and it was forbidden, under the penalty of being cut off from his people, for any private person to imitate it. It does not appear, however, that the Israelites continued to use the same formula for their Temple services. Josephus states that the incense of his day consisted of thirteen ingredients. These were, as we learn from Talmudic instructions, in addition to the four gums named in the Exodus formula, the salt with which it had to be seasoned, myrrh, cassia, spikenard, saffron, costus, mace, cinnamon, and a certain herb which had the property of making the smoke of the incense ascend straight, and in the form of a date palm. This herb was only known to the family of Abtinas, to whom was entrusted the sole right of preparing the incense for the Temple. Rooms were provided for them in the precincts, and they supplied 368 minas (about 368 lbs.) to the Temple for a year's consumption; that was 1 lb. per day and an extra 3 lbs. for the Day of Atonement. In the first century (A.D.) this family were dismissed because they refused to divulge their secret. The Temple authorities sent to Alexandria for some apothecaries to succeed them, but these Egyptian experts could not make the smoke ascend properly, so the Abtinas had to be re-engaged at a considerably increased salary. They gave as a reason for their secrecy their fear that the Temple would soon be destroyed and their incense would be used for idolatrous sacrifices.

The incense now used in Catholic churches is not made according to the Biblical formula. The following is a typical recipe in actual use:—Olibanum, 450; benzoin, 250; storax, 120; sugar, 100; cascarilla, 60; nitre, 150.

Olive Oil.

Among all the ancient Eastern nations olive oil was one of the most precious of products. It was used lavishly by the Egyptians for the hair and the skin, as well as in all sorts of ceremonies. The Israelites held it in the highest esteem before they went to Egypt, the earliest allusion to it in the Scriptures being in Genesis, xxviii, 18, where we read that Jacob poured oil on the stone which he set up at Bethel, evidently with the idea of consecrating it. The Apocalypse of Moses has a legend of Adam's experience of its medicinal virtues in the Garden of Eden. When he was in his 930th year he was seized with great pain in his stomach and sickness. Then he told Eve to take Seth and go as near as they could get to the Garden, and pray to God to permit an angel to bring them some oil from the tree of mercy so that he might anoint himself therewith and be free of his pain. Eve and Seth were, however, met by the Archangel Michael, who told them to return to Adam, for in three days the measure of his life would be fulfilled.

To the Israelites in the Desert the anticipation of the "corn and wine and oil" of Canaan was always present, and throughout their history there are abundant evidences of how they prized it.

The prescription for the "holy anointing oil" given in Exodus, xxx, 23, is very remarkable. It was to be compounded of the following ingredients:—

Flowing myrrh	500	shekels.
Sweet cinnamon	250	"
Sweet calamus	250	"
Cassia (or costus)	500	"
Olive oil	One	hin.

It is the Revised Version which gives "flowing myrrh," apparently the gum which exudes spontaneously. The Authorised Version reads "pure myrrh." The Revised Version also suggests costus in the margin as an alternative to cassia. This oil was to be kept very sacred. Any one who should compound any oil like it was to be cut off from his people.

A hin was a measure equivalent to about 5½ of our quarts. The shekel was nearly 15 lbs., and some of the Rabbis insist that the "shekel of the sanctuary" was twice the weight of the ordinary shekel. At the lowest reckoning, less than 6 quarts of oil were to take up the extract from nearly 90 lbs. of solid substance. It will be seen on reference that the shekel weights are not definitely stated, but the verses can hardly be otherwise read. Some critics have suggested that so many shekels' worth is intended, but this reading under the circumstances is almost inadmissible. Maimonides, a great Jewish authority, says the method was to boil the spices and gum in water until their odours were extracted as fully as possible, and then to boil the water and the oil together until the former was entirely evaporated. Doubtless the expression "after the art of the apothecary" (or "perfumer," R.V.) was a sufficient explanation to those Israelites who had practised that art in Egypt. The consistence of the oil could not have been thick, for when used it trickled down on Aaron's beard.

Rabbinical legends say that the quantity of the holy oil prepared at the time when it was first prescribed was such as would miraculously suffice to anoint the Jewish priests and kings all through their history. In the reign of Josiah the vessel containing the holy oil was mysteriously hidden away with the ark, and will not be discovered until the Messiah comes. Messiah, it need hardly be said, means simply anointed; and Christ is the Greek equivalent of the Hebrew word.

Manna.

The manna of the wilderness provided for the children of Israel on their journey towards Canaan has no claim to be regarded as a drug, except that a drug has in modern times usurped its name. When the Israelites first saw the small round particles "like hoar frost on the ground" (Exodus, xvi, 14) they said, according to the Authorised Version, "It is manna; for they wist not what it was." The Revised Version makes the sentence read more intelligibly by translating the Hebrew word Man-hu interrogatively thus:—"What is it? For they wist not what it was." This Hebrew interrogation has been widely adopted as the origin of the name, but it is more probable that the Hebrew word man, a gift, is the true derivation. Ebers suggested the Egyptian word "manhu," food, as a probable explanation. The Arabic word for the manna of Sinai is still "man." This is the substance which scientific investigators have agreed is the manna described in Exodus. It is an exudation from the Tamarisk mannifera, a shrub which grows in the valleys of the Sinai peninsula, the manna being yielded from the young branches after the punctures of certain insects. Another Eastern manna, a Persian product from a leguminous plant, Alhagi Maurorum, and a manna yielded by an evergreen oak in Kurdistan, are still sold and used in some Eastern countries for food and medicine. But in Europe, and to some extent in the East also, Sicilian manna, the product of an ash tree, Fraxinus ornus, has displaced the old sorts since the fifteenth century. The commerce in this article and its history were investigated by Mr. Daniel Hanbury and described by him in Science Papers and in Pharmacographia.

The rabbinical legends concerning the manna of the wilderness are many and strange. One is to the effect that when it lay on the ground all the kings of the East and of the West could see it from their palace windows. According to Zabdi ben Levi it was provided in such abundance that it covered every morning an area of 2,000 cubits square and was 60 cubits in depth. Each day's fall was sufficient to nourish the camp for 2,000 years. The Book of Wisdom (xvi, 20, 21) tells us that the manna so accommodated itself to every taste that it proved palatable and pleasing to all. "Able to content every man's delight, and agreeing to every taste." The rabbinical legends enlarge this statement and assure us that to those Israelites who did not murmur the manna became fish, flesh, fowl at will. This is in a degree based on the words in Ps. lxxviii, 24, 25, in which it is described as "corn of heaven, bread of the mighty, and meat to the full." But the traditions say it could not acquire the flavours of cucumbers, melons, garlic, or onions, all of which were Egyptian relishes which were keenly regretted by the tribes. It is also on record among the legends that the manna was pure nourishment. All of it was assimilated; so that the grossest office of the body was not exercised. It was provided expressly for the children of Israel. If any stranger tried to collect any it slipped from his grasp.

BDELLIUM.

Bdellium (Heb. Bedoloch) is mentioned in Genesis, ii, 12, as being found along with gold and onyx in the land of Havilah, near the Garden of Eden. The association with gold and onyx suggests that bdellium was a precious stone. The Septuagint translates the word in Genesis, anthrax, carbuncle; but renders the same Hebrew word in Numbers, xi, 7, where the manna is likened to bdellium, by Krystallos, crystals. The Greek bdellion described by Dioscorides and Pliny was the fragrant gum from a species of Balsamodendron, and this word was almost certainly derived from an Eastern source, and might easily have been originally a generic term for pearls. Pearls would better than anything else fit the reference in Numbers ("like coriander seed, and the appearance thereof as the appearance of bdellium"), and this is the meaning attached to the word in the rabbinical traditions. Some authorities have conjectured that the "ד" (d) of bedolach may have been substituted for "ר" (r) berolach, so that the beryl stone may have been intended.

ALOES WOOD.

References to aloes are frequent in the Scriptures. The first allusion is found in Numbers, xxiv, 6, when in his poetic prophecy Balaam describes Israel flourishing "as lign-aloes which the Lord hath planted." The other allusions occur in Psalm xlv, 8, Proverbs, vii, 17, Canticles, iv, 14, and John, xix, 39. In the four last-named passages aloes is associated with myrrh as a perfume. Of course it is understood that the lign or lignum aloes, the perfumed wood of the aquilaria agallocha, the eagle wood of India, is meant, but as that tree is believed not to have been known except in the Malayan peninsula in the days of Balaam, critics have remarked on the extraordinary circumstance that it should be used as a simile by an orator in Palestine who would naturally select objects for comparison familiar to his hearers. It has been suggested, and with much force, that the original word in Balaam's prophecy may have been the Hebrew word for the palm or date tree. The Septuagint translates the word "tents."

Myrrh.

It has been stated that the stacte ordered in the formula for incense was probably a very fine kind of liquid myrrh (the flowing myrrh of the holy oil formula). But myrrh (Heb. mur) is several times directly mentioned. Esther purified herself for six months with oil of myrrh (ii, 12); myrrh, aloes, and cassia are grouped as sweet odours in Ps. xlv, 8; with cinnamon in the place of cassia in Prov., vii, 17, and in numerous verses of the Song of Songs. In the New Testament it is named among the gifts which the wise men brought to the Saviour. Nicodemus brought myrrh and aloes to embalm the body of Jesus. On the cross St. Matthew (xxvii, 34) names vinegar mixed with gall as a drink given to Christ by the soldiers; in an apparently parallel passage in St. Mark's Gospel (xv, 23) wine with myrrh is the mixture described. It is possible that Matthew writing in Syriac may have used the word mur (myrrh) and that his translator into Greek read from his manuscript Mar (gall). In Genesis, xxxvii, 25, and xliii, 11, the word translated myrrh is Loth (not mur) in the Hebrew. The best opinion is that this meant ladanum, the gum from the cistus labdaniferus which Dioscorides states was scraped from the beards of goats which had fed on the leaves of this shrub and had taken up some of the exuding gum.

Wormwood.

The Israelites had great objection to bitter flavours, and the coupling of "gall and wormwood" expresses something extremely unpleasant. The Hebrew word is La'anah, and the Septuagint twice renders this hemlock (Hos., x, 4 and Amos, vi, 12) but in other places wormwood. The star which fell from heaven and made the rivers bitter (Rev., viii, 11) was called by the Greek name for wormwood, Apsinthos.

Hyssop.

Hyssop is a word which has occasioned much difference of opinion among interpreters. The Hebrew word hezob was translated in the Septuagint by hyssopos, and this word is used twice in the New Testament. From references used in the Pentateuch it is clear that "a bunch of hyssop" was employed in the Israelitish ritual for sprinkling purposes (Exodus, xii, 22; Leviticus, xiv, 4 and 6; Numbers, xix, 6 and 18). From 1 Kings, iv, 33, it appears that it was a shrub that grew in crevices of walls; from Psalm li, 7, "Purge me with hyssop and I shall be clean," it has been assumed to have possessed purgative properties, though it is more likely that the allusion was to the ceremonial purification of the law; according to St. John its stem was used to hand up the sponge of vinegar to the Saviour on the cross, but St. Matthew and St. Mark use the term calamus, or a reed. It may have been that a bunch of hyssop was fixed to the reed and the sponge of vinegar placed on the hyssop. Some learned commentators have conjectured that the word hyssopos in St. John's account was originally hysso, a well-known Greek word for the Roman pilum or javelin. The other allusion in the New Testament occurs in Hebrews, ix, 19, and is merely a quotation from the Pentateuch.

It has been found impossible to apply the descriptions quoted to any one plant. That which we now call hyssop (Hyssopus officinalis) does not grow in Palestine. It is generally agreed that it was not that shrub. The caper has been suggested and strongly supported, but the best modern opinion is that the word was applied generically to several kinds of origanum which were common in Syria.

JUNIPER.

The Hebrew word rothem, translated juniper in our Authorised Version, has given much trouble to translators. The Septuagint merely converted the Hebrew word into a Greek one, and the Vulgate followed the Septuagint. The allusions to the tree are in 1 Kings, xix, 4 and 5, where Elijah slept under a juniper tree; Job, xxx, 4, speaks of certain men so poor that they cut up mallows by the bushes, and juniper roots for their meat; and Psalm cxx, 4, "Sharp arrows of the mighty with coals of juniper." The tree alluded to was almost certainly the Broom, and it is so rendered in the Revised Version either in the text or in the margin in all the instances. The Arabic name for the broom is ratam, evidently a descendant of rothem. The Genista roetam is said to be the largest and most conspicuous shrub in the deserts of Palestine, and would be readily chosen for its shade by a weary traveller. The mallows in the Book of Job are translated salt wort in the Revised Version. Renan gives "They gather their salads from the bushes." Salads were regarded as indispensable by the poorest Jews. The coals of juniper (or broom) are supposed to have reference to the lasting fire which this wood furnishes, but other translations suggest as the proper reading of the verse "The arrows of a warrior are the tongues of the people of the tents of Misram."

Jonah's Gourd.

The Gourd, of which we read in Jonah, iv, 6–10, is Kikaion in Hebrew, and there has been some doubt what the plant could have been which grew so rapidly and was so quickly destroyed. It is stated that the Lord made this grow over the booth which the prophet had erected in a single night, and provide a shade of which Jonah was "exceedingly glad." The next morning, however, a worm attacked it, and it withered.

The author of "Harris's Natural History of the Bible," Dr. Thaddeus M. Harris, of Dorchester, Massachusetts (1824), quotes from an earlier work, "Scripture Illustrated," a curious account of a violent dispute between St. Jerome and St. Augustine in reference to the identification of this plant. According to this author "those pious fathers ... not only differed in words, but from words they proceeded to blows; and Jerome was accused of heresy at Rome by Augustine. Jerome thought the plant was an ivy, and pleaded the authority of Aquila, Symmachus, Theodotion, and others; Augustine thought it was a gourd, and he was supported by the Seventy, the Syriac, the Arabic, &c. Had either of them ever seen the plant? Neither. Let the errors of these pious men teach us to think more mildly, if not more meekly, respecting our own opinions; and not to exclaim Heresy, or to enforce the exclamation, when the subject is of so little importance as—gourd *versus* ivy."

While endorsing the practical lesson which the author just cited extracts from his rather unpleasant story, I think I ought to append to this narrative another which is given in Gerard's Herbal (1597) which seems to be incompatible with the previously quoted account of the quarrel. This is what Gerard writes:—

"Ricinus, whereof mention is made in the fourth chapter and sixt verse of the prophecie of Jonas, was called of the Talmudists kik, for in the Talmud we reade Velo beschemen kik, that is in English, And not with the oile of kik; which oile is called in the Arabian toong Alkerua, as Rabbi Samuel the sonne of Hofni testifieth. Moreover a certain Rabbine mooveth a question saying What is kik? Hereunto Resch Lachisch maketh answer in Ghemara, saying Kik is nothing else but Jonas his kikaijon. And that this is true it appeareth by that name kiki which the ancient Greeke phisicions and the Aegyptians used, which Greeke word cometh of the Hebrew kik. Hereby it appeereth that the olde writers long ago, though unwittingly, called this plant by his true name. But the olde Latine writers knew it by the name Cucurbita which evidently is manifested by an Historie which St. Augustine recordeth in his Epistle to St. Jerome where in effect he writeth thus:—That name kikaijon is of small moment yet so small a matter caused a great tumult in Africa. For on a time a certaine Bishop having occasion to intreat of this which is mentioned in the fourth chapter of Jonas his prophecie (in a collation or sermon which he made in his cathedral church or place of assemblie), said that this plant was called Cucurbita, a Gourde, because it increased to so great a quantitie in so short a space, or else (saith he) it is called Hedera. Upon the novelty and untruth of this doctrine the people were greatly offended, and there arose a tumult and hurly burly, so that the bishop was inforced to go to the Jews to aske their judgement as touching the name of this plant. And when he had received of them the true name which was kikaijon, he made his open recantation and confessed his error, and was justly accused of being a falsifier of Holy Scripture."

I quote the letter as Gerard gives it without quite understanding it, and I have not been able to trace its origin. But it is clear that if St. Augustine thought it was such a small matter he would hardly have quarrelled so violently with St. Jerome about it. Probably, however, the story of the quarrel is founded on this letter. Moreover the conclusion seems to be that the gourd was not a cucurbita but the Palma Christi.

The importance of Jerome's translation of the word representing the plant to be Ivy (Hedera) is that he incorporated it into his Latin version of the Bible known as the Vulgate. The much older Septuagint (Greek) translation gives "kolokyntha," the bottle gourd, as the rendering of the Hebrew kikaion. The Swedish botanist and theologian Celsius strongly supported the view that Jonah's gourd was the Palma Christi in his "Hierobotanicon; sive de Plantis Sacrae Scripturae," 1746. But though this tree is of very rapid growth, and is planted before houses in the East for its shade, and though philological arguments are in its favour, Dr. Hastings ("Encyclopædia Biblica") rejects the suggestion and prefers the Septuagint version because he thinks the passage clearly indicates that a vine is intended. He considers there is no support, either botanical or etymological, for the selection of ivy to represent the gourd.

THE WILD GOURDS

mentioned in 2 Kings, iv, 39, are generally supposed to have been colocynth fruit, though the squirting cucumber (Ecbalium purgans) has also been suggested. The plant on which this grows, however, would hardly be called a wild vine, for it has no tendrils. The Jews were in the habit of shredding various kinds of gourds in their pottage, and as narrated, someone had brought a lapful of these gourds, the fruit of a wild vine, and shredded them into the pottage which was being prepared for the sons of the prophets. The mistake could hardly have been made with the squirting cucumber, which is very common throughout Palestine, but the colocynth only grew on barren sands like those near Gilgal, and might easily be mistaken for the globe cucumber. The mistake was discovered as soon as the pottage was tasted, and the alarm of "death in the pot" was raised. Elisha, however, casting some meal in the pot destroyed the bitter taste, and apparently rendered the pottage quite harmless.

THE HORSE LEECH

mentioned in Proverbs, xxx, 15, "The horse-leech hath two daughters, crying Give, Give," is a translation of Hebrew Aluka, the meaning of which is not without doubt. The Hebrew word is interpreted by corresponding terms in Arabic, but of these there are two, one meaning the leech, and the other fate or destiny. The latter word is supposed to have been derived from the former from the idea that every person's fate clings to him. Another similar Arabic word is Aluk, a female ghul or vampire, who, it was believed, sucked the blood of those whom she attacked.

NITRE

is mentioned twice in the Old Testament, first in Proverbs, xxv, 20, "As vinegar upon nitre, so is he that singeth songs to a heavy heart." In the Revised Version soda is given instead of nitre in the margin. The other reference is in Jeremiah, ii, 22, "Though thou wash thee with nitre, and take thee much sope." In this passage the Revised Version changes nitre to lye. The Hebrew word is Nether, the natrum of the East, an impure carbonate of sodium which was condensed from certain salt lakes, or obtained from marine plants. Vinegar would cause effervescence with this substance, but not with nitrate of potash. The soap in the same passage in Jeremiah, in Hebrew Borith, was either the soap wort or a salt obtained from the ashes of herbs by lixiviation.

MUSTARD SEEDS

are mentioned twice by the Saviour as illustrations of something very small: first as the small seed which grows into a tree, and second as the measure of even a minute degree of faith. The weed did in fact grow in Palestine to some ten or twelve feet in height.

VINEGAR.

Homez in Hebrew, Oxus in Greek, is mentioned five times in the Old Testament, and five times in the New Testament. It was used as a relish by the Jews, the food being dipped into it before eating. The passages where vinegar is mentioned in the accounts of the Crucifixion in the several Gospels are not fully explained by Biblical scholars. The first administration of vinegar to the Saviour was, according to St. Matthew, vinegar mixed with gall; according to St. Mark, vinegar mixed with myrrh. There are linguistic reasons for assuming that the additional ingredient may have been opium, given with a merciful intention. But both evangelists state that Jesus refused it. The second time vinegar was given to him on a sponge, and St. Luke seems to suggest that this was given in mockery. It is supposed that the vinegar was the posca, a sour wine which was largely drunk by the Roman soldiers.

ANETHON.

All translators agree that dill and not anise was the "anethon" named with mint and cummin in the passage, Matthew, xxiii, 23. Anise was never grown in Palestine. The other herbs were common in gardens, and the allusion to paying tithe on them, and to rue in a similar connection in Luke, xi, 42, appears to refer to the scrupulous observance of the letter of the law by the Pharisees, even down to such an insignificant matter as the tithe on these almost valueless herbs. The law did not, in fact, require tithe to be paid except on productions which yielded income. It was therefore rather to satisfy their own self-righteousness that the Pharisees insisted on paying the contribution on mint and anise and cummin.

SAFFRON

is only mentioned in the Song of Solomon, iv, 14, as one of the many valuable products of an Eastern garden. There is not much doubt that this was the crocus sativa known to medicine from the earliest times. The Hebrew word, karkum, was kurkum in ancient Arabic, and this is given in Arab dictionaries as equivalent to the more modern za-faran from which our word is derived.

POMEGRANATES

are always referred to in the Scriptures as luxuries. The spies sent by Moses to see the land of Canaan brought back pomegranates with figs and grapes (Numbers, xiii, 23); the same fruits are promised in Deut. (viii, 8); the withering of the pomegranate tree is, with that of the vine and fig tree, noted by the prophet Joel (i, 12) as a sign of desolation. It is still highly prized as a fruit in the East.

THE POULTICE OF FIGS

applied to Hezekiah's boil (2 Kings, xx, 7) is an interesting reminiscence of Israelitish home medicine. The fig tree often appears in the Bible. Some very learned Biblical commentators (Celsius, Gesenius, Knobel, among them) have believed that the fig leaves with which Adam and Eve made aprons were in fact the very long leaves of the banana tree. This, however, is scarcely possible, as the banana is a native of the Malay Archipelago, and there is no evidence that it was known to the Jews at the time when the Pentateuch was written.

SPIKENARD

is mentioned three times in the Song of Songs (i, 12, iv, 13, iv, 14), and in the New Testament on two occasions (Mark xiv, 3, and John xii, 3), a box of spikenard ointment, "very costly" and "very precious" is, in the instance recorded by St. Mark, poured on the Saviour's head, and in the narrative of St. John, is used to anoint His feet. On both occasions we are told that the value of this box or vase was three hundred pence. It is explained in the Revised Version that the coin named was equivalent to about 8½d. The price of the ointment used was therefore over ten pounds.

In the Greek text the word used is nardos pitike. It has been variously conjectured that the adjective may have meant liquid, genuine or powdered; the word lends itself to either of those meanings. Or it may have been a local term, or possibly it may have been altered from a word which would have meant what we understand by "spike" in botany. The most likely meaning is "genuine," for we know that this product was at that period a perfume in high esteem, and that there were several qualities, the best, and by far the costliest, being brought from India. The ointment employed was really an otto, and it was imported into Rome and other cities of the Empire in alabaster vessels. Dioscorides and Galen refer to it as nardostachys. The Arab name for it was Sumbul Hindi, but this must not be confounded with the sumbul which we know. The word sumbul simply means spike. The botanical origin of the Scripture spikenard, the nardostachys of Dioscorides, was cleared up, it is generally agreed, by Sir William Jones in 1790. He traced it to a Himalayan plant of the valerian order which was afterwards exactly identified by Royle. A Brahman gave some of the fibrous roots to Sir William Jones, and told him it was employed in their religious sacrifices.

Pliny mentions an ointment of spikenard composed of the Indian nard, with myrrh, balm, custos, amomum, and other ingredients, but the "genuine" nard alluded to in the Gospels was probably the simple otto. Pliny also states that the Indian nard was worth, in his time, in Rome, one hundred denarii per pound.

Horace mentions an onyx box of nard which was considered of equal value with a large vessel of wine:

> Nardo vinum merebere
>
> Nardi parvus onyx eliciet cadum.

EASTERN IMAGERY

In Ecclesiastes, xii, 5, the familiar words "and desire shall fail," have been changed in the Revised Version to "the caper-berry shall fail." This alteration does not strike the ordinary reader as an improvement, but it appears that the Revised Version translation is a reversion to that of the Septuagint, and is probably exactly correct. It is supposed to mean the same thing. The caper has always been recognised as a relish to meat, as we use it; and there is evidence that it was given as a stimulating medicine among the Arabs in the Middle Ages, and perhaps from very ancient times. The idea would be therefore that even the caper-berry will not now have any effect. The Revisers also suggest in the margin "burst" for "fail." It is only a question of points in Hebrew which word is intended, and some think that the berry when fully ripe and bursting may have been an emblem of death.

The other clauses in the same verse have given rise to much difference of opinion. "The almond tree shall flourish" is generally supposed to indicate the white locks of the old man. But against this it is objected that the almond blossom is not white, but pink; and by a slight alteration of the original it is possible to read "the almond (the fruit) shall be refused" or rejected; it is no longer a tempting morsel.

The almond and the almond tree (the same word may mean either) are mentioned several times in the Bible. Jacob's gifts to Joseph from Canaan to Egypt included almonds. They were grown in Canaan and were a luxury in Egypt. In Jeremiah, i, 11, the almond branch is used as symbolical of hastening or awakening, which is the primary meaning of the word, derived from the early appearance of the blossoms on the almond tree.

The third clause, "the grasshopper shall be a burden," similarly presents difficulties, but these hardly concern us here. Probably all the metaphors conveyed distinct ideas to Eastern readers at that time, but have lost their point to us.

The interpretation of the beautiful Hebrew poetry of the twelfth chapter of Ecclesiastes, as given in Leclerc's "History of Medicine," may be of interest. Leclerc says the chapter is an enigmatic description of old age and its inconveniences, followed by death. The sun, the light, the moon, and the stars are respectively the mind, the judgment, the memory, and the other faculties of the soul, which are gradually fading. The clouds and the rain are the catarrhs and the fluxions incident to age. The guards of the house and the strong man are the senses, the muscles, and the tendons. The grinders are the teeth; those who look out through the windows is an allusion to the sight. The doors shall be shut in the streets, and the sound of the grinding is low, means that the mouth will scarcely open for speaking, and that eating must be slow and quiet. The old man must rise at the voice of the bird, for he cannot sleep. There is no more singing, and reading and study are no longer pleasures. The fear of climbing, even of walking, are next expressed;

the white hair is signalised by the almond blossom, and the flesh falling away by the grasshopper, though the word burden may indicate the occasional unhealthy fattening of old persons. The caper failing indicates the loss of the various appetites. The silver cord represents the spinal marrow, the golden bowl the brain or the heart; the pitcher, the skull; and the wheel, the lung. The long home is the tomb.

IV
THE PHARMACY OF HIPPOCRATES.

> When we search into the history of medicine and the commencement of science, the first body of doctrine that we meet with is the collection of writings attributed to Hippocrates. Science ascends directly to that origin and there stops. Everything that had been learned before the physician of Cos has perished; and, curiously, there exists a great gap after him as well as before him.... So that the writings of Hippocrates remain isolated amongst the ruins of ancient medical literature.—LITTRÉ. Introduction to the *Translation of the Works of Hippocrates*.

About eight hundred years separated the periods of Æsculapius and Hippocrates. During that long time the study of medicine in all its branches was proceeding in intimate association with the various philosophies for which Greece has always been famous. Intercourse between Greece and Egypt, Persia, India, and other countries brought into use a number of medicines, and probably these were introduced and made popular by the shopkeepers and the travelling doctors, market quacks as we should call them.

Leclerc has collected a list of nearly four hundred simples which he finds alluded to as remedies in the writings of Hippocrates. But these include various milks, wines, fruits, vegetables, flits, and other substances which we should hardly call drugs now. Omitting these and certain other substances which cannot be identified I take from the author named the following list of medicines employed or mentioned in that far distant age;—

- Abrotanum.
- Absinthe.
- Adiantum (maidenhair).
- Agnus castus.
- Algae (various).
- Almonds.
- Althaea.
- Alum.
- Amber.
- Ammoniac.

- Amomum.
- Anagallis (a veronica).
- Anagyris.
- Anchusa.
- Anemone.
- Anethum.
- Anise.
- Anthemis.
- Aparine (goose grease).
- Aristolochia.
- Armenian stone.
- Asphalt.
- Asphodel.
- Atriplex.
- Baccharis.
- Balm.
- Basil.
- Bistort.
- Blite.
- Brass (flowers, filings, ashes).
- Briar.
- Bryony.
- Burdock.
- Cabbage.
- Cachrys.
- Calamus aromaticus.
- Cantharides.
- Capers.

- Cardamom.
- Carduus benedictus.
- Carrot.
- Castoreum.
- Centaury.
- Centipedes.
- Chalcitis (red ochre).
- Chenopodium.
- Cinnamon.
- Cinquefoil.
- Clove.
- Colocynth.
- Coriander.
- Crayfish.
- Cress.
- Cucumber (wild).
- Cummin.
- Cyclamen.
- Cytisus.
- Dictamnus.
- Dog.
- Dracontium.
- Earths (various).
- Elaterium.
- Elder.
- Erica.
- Euphorbia.
- Excrement of ass, goat, mule, goose, fox.

- Fennel.
- Fig tree (leaves, wood, fruit).
- Foenugreek.
- Frankincense.
- Frogs.
- Galbanum.
- Galls.
- Garlic.
- Germander.
- Goat (various parts).
- Hawthorn.
- Heather.
- Hellebore (white and black).
- Hemlock.
- Henbane.
- Honey.
- Horehound.
- Horns of ox, goat, stag.
- Hyssop.
- Isatis.
- Ivy.
- Juniper.
- Laserpitium.
- Laurel.
- Lettuce.
- Licorice.
- Linseed.
- Loadstone.

- Lotus.
- Lupins.
- Magnesian stone.
- Mallow.
- Mandragora.
- Mecon (?).
- Melilot.
- Mercurialis.
- Minium.
- Mints (various).
- Mugwort.
- Myrabolans.
- Myrrh.
- Myrtle.
- Narcissus.
- Nard.
- Nitre.
- Oak.
- Oenanthe.
- Oesypus.
- Olive.
- Onions.
- Origanum.
- Orpiment.
- Ostrich.
- Ox-gall.
- Ox (liver, gall, urine).
- Panax.

- Parthenium.
- Pennyroyal.
- Peony.
- Pepper.
- Persea (sebestens).
- Persil.
- Peucedanum.
- Phaseolus.
- Philistium.
- Pine.
- Pitch.
- Pomegranate.
- Poppy.
- Quicklime.
- Quince.
- Ranunculus.
- Red spider.
- Resin.
- Rhamnus.
- Rhus.
- Ricinus.
- Rock rose.
- Rose.
- Rosemary.
- Ruby.
- Rue.
- Saffron.
- Sagapenum.

- Sage.
- Salt.
- Samphire.
- Sandarach.
- Scammony.
- Sea water.
- Secundines of a woman.
- Sepia.
- Serpent.
- Sesame.
- Seseli.
- Silver.
- Sisymbrium.
- Solanum.
- Spurge.
- Squill.
- Stag (horns, &c.).
- Stavesacre.
- Styrax.
- Succinum.
- Sulphur.
- Sweat.
- Tarragon.
- Tetragonon.
- Thaspia.
- Thistles (various).
- Thlapsi.
- Thuja.

- Thyme.
- Torpedo (fish).
- Trigonum.
- Tribulus.
- Turpentine.
- Turtle.
- Umbilicus veneris.
- Verbascum.
- Verbena.
- Verdigris.
- Verjuice.
- Violet.
- Wax.
- Willow.
- Woad.
- Worms.
- Worm seed.

This list may be taken to have comprised pretty fairly the materia medica of the Greeks as it was known to them when Hippocrates practised, and as it is not claimed that he introduced any new medicines it may be assumed that these formed the basis of the remedies used in the temples of Æsculapius, though perhaps some of them were only popular medicines.

The temples of Æsculapius were in all those ages the repositories of such medical and pharmaceutical knowledge as was acquired. The priests of these temples were called Asclepiades, and they professed to be the descendants of the god. Probably the employment of internal medicines was a comparatively late development. Plato remarks on the necessarily limited medical knowledge of Æsculapius. Wounds, bites of serpents, and occasional epidemics, he observes, were the principal troubles which the earliest physicians had to treat. Catarrhs, gout, dysentery, and lung diseases only came with luxury. Plutarch and Pindar say much the same. The latter specially mentions that Æsculapius had recourse to prayers, hymns, and incantations in mystic words and in verses called epaioide, or carmina, from which came the idea and name of charm.

In later times these temples were beautiful places, generally situated in the most healthy localities, and amid lovely scenery. They were either in forests or surrounded by gardens. A stream of pure water ran through the grounds, and the neighbourhood of a medicinal spring was chosen if possible. The patients who resorted to them were required to purify themselves rigorously, to fast for some time before presenting themselves in the temple, to abstain from wine for a still longer preliminary period, and thus to appreciate the solemnity of the intercession which was to be made for them. On entering the temple they found much to impress them. They were shown the records of cures, especially of diseases similar to their own; their fasts had brought them into a mental condition ready to accept a miracle, the ceremonies which they witnessed were imposing, and at last they were left to sleep before the altar. That dreams should come under those circumstances was not wonderful; nor was it surprising that in the morning the priests should be prepared to interpret these dreams. Not unfrequently the patients saw some mysterious shapes in their dreams which suggested to the priests the medicines which ought to be administered. For no doubt they did administer medicines, though for many centuries they observed the strictest secrecy in reference to all their knowledge and practices.

It need hardly be added that offerings were made to the god, to the service of the temple, and to the priests personally by grateful patients who had obtained benefit. At one of the temples it is said it was the custom to throw pieces of gold or silver into a well for the god. At others pieces of carving representing the part which had been the seat of disease were sold to those who had been cured, and these were again presented to the temple, and, it may be surmised, sold again. That cures were effected is likely enough. The excitement, the anticipation, the deep impressions made by the novel surroundings had great influence on many minds, and through the minds on the bodies. Records of these cures were engraved on tablets and fixed on the walls of the temples.

Sprengel gives a translation of four of these inscriptions found at the Temple of Æsculapius which had been built on the Isle of the Tiber, near Rome. The first relates that a certain Gaius, a blind man, was told by the oracle to pray in the temple, then cross the floor from right to left, lay the five fingers of his right hand on the altar, and afterwards carry his hand to his eyes. He did so, and recovered his sight in the presence of a large crowd. The next record is also a cure of blindness. A soldier named Valerius Aper was told to mix the blood of a white cock with honey and apply the mixture to his eyes for three successive days. He, too, was cured, and thanked the god before all the people. Julian was cured of spitting of blood. His case had been considered hopeless. The treatment prescribed was mixing seeds of the fir apple with honey, and eating the compound for three days. The fourth cure was of a son of Lucius who was desperately ill with pleurisy. The god told him in a dream to take ashes from the altar, mix them with wine, and apply to his side.

The legend of the foundation of this Roman temple is curious. In the days of the republic on the occasion of an epidemic in the city the sibylline books were consulted, with the result that an embassy was sent to Epidaurus to ask for the help of Æsculapius. Quintus Ogulnius was appointed for this mission. On arriving at Epidaurus the Romans were astonished to see a large serpent depart from the temple, make its way to the shore, and leap on the vessel, where it proceeded at once to the cabin of Ogulnius. Some of the priests followed the serpent and accompanied the Romans on the return journey. The vessel stopped at Antium, and the serpent left the ship and proceeded to the Temple of Æsculapius in that city. After three days he returned, and the voyage was continued. Casting anchor at the mouth of the Tiber the serpent again left the vessel and settled itself on a small island. There it rolled itself up, thus indicating its intention of settling on that spot. The god, it was understood, had selected that island as the site for his temple, and there it was erected.

As might be expected, some of the less reverent of the Greek writers found subjects for satire in the worship of Æsculapius. Aristophanes in one of his comedies makes a servant relate how his master, Plautus, who was blind, was restored to sight at the Æsculapian temple. Having placed their offerings on the altar and performed other ceremonies, this servant says that Plautus and he laid down on beds of straw. When the lights were extinguished the priest came round and enjoined them to sleep and to keep silence if they should hear any noise. Later the god himself came and wiped the eyes of Plautus with a piece of white linen. Panacea followed him and covered the face of Plautus with a purple veil. Then on a signal from the deity two serpents glided under the veil, and having licked his eyes Plautus recovered his sight.

It cannot be doubted that in the course of the centuries a large amount of empiric knowledge was accumulated at these temples, and probably the pretence of supernatural aid was far more rare than we suppose. In an exhaustive study of the subject recently published by Dr. Aravintinos, of Athens, that authority expresses the opinion that the temples served as hospitals for all kinds of sufferers, and that arrangements were provided in them for prolonged treatment. He thinks that in special cases the treatment was carried out during the mysterious sleep, when it was desired to keep from the patient an exact knowledge of what was being done; but generally he supposes a course of normal medication or hygiene was followed. Forty-two inscriptions have been discovered, but on analysing these Dr. Aravintinos comes to the conclusion that they record in most cases only cures effected by rational means, and not by miracles. He finds massage, purgatives, emetics, diaphoresis, bleeding, baths, poulticing, and such like methods indicated, and though the sleeps, possibly hypnotic, are often mentioned, this is not by any means the case invariably.

About a century before Hippocrates wrote and practised, the Asclepiads began to reveal their secrets. The revolt against the mysteries and trickeries of the temples was incited by the infidelity to their oaths of certain of the Italian disciples of Pythagoras. The school of philosophy and medicine founded by that mystic aimed also to keep his doctrines secret, but when the colony he had established at Crotona, in South Italy, was dispersed by the attacks of the mob, a number of the initiates travelled about under the title of Periodeutes practising medicine often in close proximity to an Æsculapian temple. The first of the Asclepiads to yield to this competition were those of Cnidos, but the school of Cos was not long after them. The direct ancestors of Hippocrates were among the teachers of the temple who became eager to make known the accumulated science in their possession, and thus by the time when the famous teacher was born (460 B.C.) the world was ripe for his intellect to have free play.

HIPPOCRATES.

Hippocrates was born in Cos, as far as can be ascertained, about the year 460 B.C., and is alleged to have lived to be 99, or, as some say, 109 years of age. It is claimed that his father, Heraclides, was a direct descendant of Æsculapius, and that his mother, Phenarita, was of the family of Hercules. His father and his paternal ancestors in a long line were all priests of the Æsculapian temples, and his sons and their sons after them also practised medicine in the same surroundings. The family, traceable for nearly 300 years, among whom were seven of the name of Hippocrates, were all, it would appear, singularly free from the charlatanism which the Greek dramatists attributed to the Æsculapian practitioners, from the superstition which overlaid the medical science of so many older and later centuries, and especially from the fantastic pharmacy which was to develop to such an absurd extent in the following five hundred years.

It is not possible to distinguish with any confidence the genuine from the spurious writings attributed to Hippocrates which have come down to us. But the note which even his imitators sought to copy was one of directness, lucidity, and candour. He tells of his failures as simply as of his successes. He does not seek to deduce a system from his experience, and though he is reputed to be the originator of the theory of the humours, he does not allow the doctrine to influence his treatment, which is based on experience.

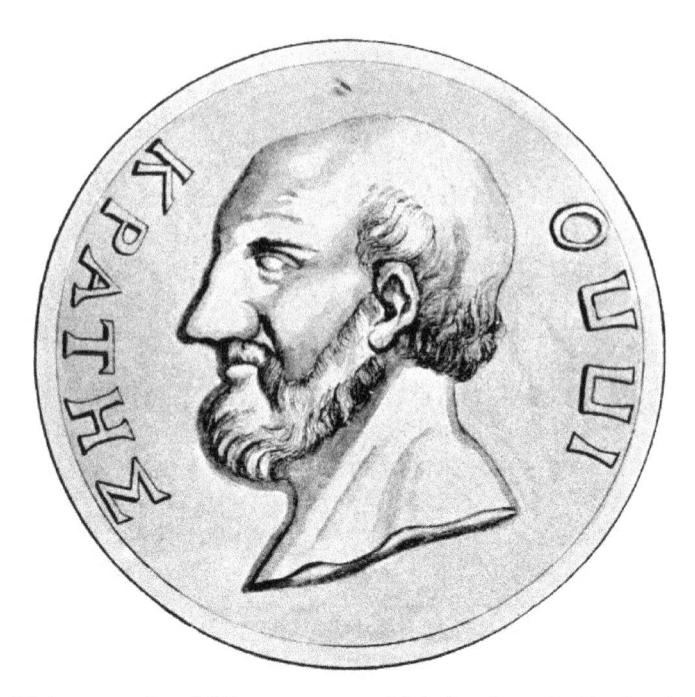

This portrait of Hippocrates, which is given in Leclerc's "History of Medicine," is stated to be copied from a medal in the collection of Fulvius Ursinus, a celebrated Italian connoisseur. It is believed that the medal was struck by the people of Cos at some long distant time in honour of their famous compatriot. A bust in the British Museum, found near Albano, among some ruins conjectured to have been the villa of Marcus Varro, is presumed to represent Hippocrates on the evidence of the likeness it bears to the head on this medal.

The medical views of Hippocrates do not concern us here except as they affect his pharmaceutical practice; but a very long chapter might be written on his pharmacy, that is to say, on the use he made of drugs in the treatment of disease. Galen believed that he made his preparations with his own hand, or at least superintended their preparation. Leclerc's list of the medicaments mentioned as such in the works attributed to Hippocrates have been already quoted, and it will be found that after deducting the fruits and vegetables, the milks of cows, goats, asses, mules, sheep, and bitches, as well as other things which perhaps we should hardly reckon as medicaments, there remain between one hundred and two hundred drugs which are still found in our drug shops. There are a great many animal products, some copper and lead derivatives, alum, and the earths so much esteemed; but evidently the bulk of his materia medica was drawn from the vegetable kingdom.

Hippocrates was considerably interested in pharmacy. Galen makes him say, "We know the nature of medicaments and simples, and make many different preparations with them; some in one way, some in another. Some simples must be gathered early, some late; some we dry, some we crush, some we cook," &c. He made fomentations, poultices, gargles, pessaries, katapotia (things to swallow, large pills), ointments, oils, cerates, collyria, looches, tablets, and inhalations, which he called perfumes. For quinsy, for example, he burned sulphur and asphalte with hyssop. He gave narcotics, including, it is supposed, the juice of the poppy and henbane seeds, and mandragora; purgatives, sudorifics, emetics, and enemas. His purgative drugs were generally drastic ones: the hellebores, elaterium, colocynth, scammony, thapsia, and a species of rhamnus.

Hippocrates describes methods for what he calls purging the head and the lungs, that is, by means of sneezing and coughing. He explains how he diminishes the acridity of spurge juice by dropping a little of it on a dried fig, whereby he gets a good remedy for dropsy. He has a medicine which he calls Tetragonon, or four-cornered. Galen conjectures that this was a tablet of crude antimony. Leclerc more reasonably suggests that it was a term for certain special kinds of lozenges, and points out that not long after Hippocrates physicians used a trochiscus trigonus, or three-cornered lozenge for another purpose.

Although he used many drugs, Hippocrates is especially insistent on Diet as the most important aid to health. He claims to have been the first physician who had written on this subject, and this assertion is confirmed by Plato, who, however, somewhat grimly commends the ancient doctors for neglecting this branch of treatment, for, he says, the modern ones have converted life into a tedious death. Barley water is repeatedly recommended by the physician of Cos, with various additions to suit the particular case under consideration. Oxymel is the usual associate, but dill, leeks, oil, salt, vinegar, and goats' fat also figure.

Particular instructions are also given about the wine to be drunk, the kind, and the quantity of water with which it is to be diluted in spring, summer, autumn, and winter. In one place, at the end of the 3rd Book on Diet, a word is used which apparently means that persons fatigued with long labour should "drink unto gaiety" occasionally; but there is some doubt about the correct translation of that word.

V
FROM HIPPOCRATES TO GALEN.

> Medicine is a science which hath been more professed than laboured, and yet more laboured than advanced; the labour having been, in my judgment, rather in circle than in progression. For I find much iteration, but small addition.—BACON, "Advancement of Learning."—Book 2.

The fame of Hippocrates caused naturally a great multiplication of works attributed to him. The Ptolemies when founding the Library of Alexandria, which they were determined should be more important than that of Pergamos, commissioned captains of ships and other travellers to buy manuscripts of the Greek physician at almost any price; an excellent method of encouraging forgeries. The works attributed to Hippocrates have been subject to the keenest scrutiny by scholars, but even now the verdict of Galen in regard to their genuine or spurious character is the consideration which carries the greatest weight. Even the imitations go to prove how free the physician of Cos was from superstitious practices or prejudiced theories.

Between him and Galen an interval of some six hundred years elapsed and, especially in the latter half of that period, pharmacy developed into enormous importance. Not that it necessarily advanced. But the faith in drugs, and especially in the art of compounding them, and the wild polypharmacy which grew up in Alexandria and Rome in the first two centuries of our era, of which Galen shows so much approval, add inestimably to the chronicles of pharmacy. It was during the interval between Hippocrates and Galen that the many sects of ancient medicine, the Dogmatics, the Stoics, the Empirics, the Methodics, and the Eclectics were born and flourished. Some of these encouraged the administration of special remedies. But probably a far greater influence was exercised on the pharmacy of the ancient world by the new commerce with Africa and the East which the Ptolemies did so much to foster, and by the travelling quacks and the prescribing druggists who exploited the drugs of foreign origin which now came into the market.

Serapion of Alexandria, one of the most famous of the Empirics, who is supposed to have lived in the second century, was largely responsible for the introduction of the animal remedies which were to figure so prominently in the pharmacy of the succeeding seventeen centuries. Among his specifics were the brain of a camel, the excrements of the crocodile, the heart of the hare, the blood of the tortoise, and the testicles of the wild boar.

The Empirics were the boldest users of drugs, and so far as can be judged, were the practitioners who brought opium into general medicinal esteem.

One of the most famous doctors of this sect, Heraclides, made several narcotic compounds which are commended by Galen. One of these formulæ prescribed for cholera was 2 drms. of henbane seeds, 1 drm. of anise, and ½ drm. of opium, made into 30 pills, one for a dose. Another which was recommended for coughs was composed of 4 drms. each of juice of hemlock, juice of henbane, castorum, white pepper, and costus; and 1 drm. each of myrrh and opium.

Musa, a freed slave of Augustus, and apparently a sort of medical charlatan, but a great favourite with the Emperor, is alleged to have introduced the flesh of vipers into medical use especially for the cure of ulcers.

Celsus, Dioscorides, and Pliny, whose works are recognized as the storehouses of the science of Imperial Rome, belonged to the period under review. Celsus wrote either a little before or a little after the commencement of our era. He was the first eminent author who wrote on medicine in Latin. Pliny died A.D. 79, suffocated by the gases from Vesuvius, which in his eagerness to observe he had approached too near during an eruption. Dioscorides is supposed to have lived a little before Pliny, who apparently quotes him, but curiously never mentions his name, though usually most scrupulous in regard to his authorities.

Themison, who lived at Rome in the reign of Augustus Cæsar, and who is said to have been the first physician to have distinguished rheumatism from gout, is noted in pharmacy as the author of the formulæ for Diagredium and Diacodium. He praised the plantain as a universal remedy, and is also the earliest medical writer to mention the use of leeches in the treatment of illness.

Several of the writers on medical subjects of this period adopted the method of prescribing their formulas and the instructions for compounding them in verse. The most famous instance is that of Andromachus, physician to Nero, whose elegiac verses describing the composition of his Theriakon are quoted by Galen. The idea was that the formula thus presented was less likely to be tampered with. Theriakon as invented contained 61 ingredients. Its principal improvement on the more ancient Mithridatum was the addition of dried vipers. Andromachus appears to have acquired a large and lucrative practice in Rome at the time when wealth was most lavishly squandered.

Among other medical verse writers were Servilius Damocrates, who lived in the reign of the Emperor Tiberius, and who invented a famous tooth powder, a number of malagmata, (emollient poultices), acopa (liniments for pains), electuaries, and plasters; and Herennius Philon, a physician of Tarsus (about A.D. 50), whose fame rests on his philonium, a compound designed to relieve colic pains, which appear to have been specially frequent at that period. This philonium was composed of opium, saffron, pyrethrum, euphorbium, pepper, henbane, spikenard, and honey.

Menecrates, physician to Tiberius, and said to have written 155 works, was the inventor of diachylon plaster, but his diachylon was a compound of many juices (as the name implies) along with lead plaster.

The Romans were curiously badly off for regular doctors until Julius Cæsar specially tempted some to come from Greece and Egypt by offers of citizenship. Augustus, too, warmly encouraged the settlement in the city of trained medical men.

Pharmacy in the Roman Empire.

The separation of the practices of medicine, pharmacy, and surgery, which became general though never universal, was of course a gradual process. Galen expresses the opinion that Hippocrates prepared the medicines he prescribed with his own hands, or at least superintended the production of them. According to Celsus, it was in Alexandria and about the year 300 B.C. that the division of the practice of medicine into distinct branches was first noticeable. The sections he names were Dietetics, Surgery and Pharmaceutics.

The physicians who practised dietetics were like our consultants, only more so. They were above all things philosophers, the recognised successors of the Greek thinkers and theorists, and but too often their imitators. Although they owed their designation to their general authority on régime, they prescribed and invented medicines. The pharmaceutical section came to be called in Latin medicamentarii, and their history corresponds closely with that of our English apothecaries. At first they prepared and administered the medicines which the physicians ordered. But in Alexandria and Rome they gradually assumed the position of general practitioners. To another class, designated by Pliny Vulnerarii, was left the treatment of wounds, and probably of tumours and ulcers. The necessity of a lower grade of medical practitioners in Rome is manifest from a remark of Galen's to the effect that no physician, meaning a person in his own rank, would attend to diseases of minor importance.

It is worthy of note that the Latin designation medicamentarius, which was nearly equivalent to the Greek pharmacopolis, was similarly used to mean a poisoner, while pharmakon in Greek and medicamentus in Latin might mean either a medicine or a poison.

It is noted elsewhere (page 52) that the word pharmakeia when it occurs in the New Testament is universally translated in our versions by the term sorcery or some similar word. At the time when the Apostles wrote this was evidently the prevalent meaning attached to the term. But in earlier Greek literature the reputable and the disgraceful ideas associated with the word seem to have run side by side for centuries. Homer uses pharmakon in both senses; Plato makes pharmakeuein mean to administer a remedy, while Herodotus adopts it to signify the practice of sorcery. Apparently this word came from an earlier, pharmassein, which was derived from a root implying to mix, and the gradual sense development was that of producing an effect by means of drugs. They might produce purging, they might produce a colour, or they might produce love.

The multiplication of names for the various classes connected with medicine and pharmacy in the Roman world is rather confusing. As the language of medicine up to and including Galen was largely Greek, many of the designations employed were those which had been drawn from that tongue. The name Pharmacopeus, used in Greek to denote certain handlers of drugs, had always a sinister signification. It suggested a purveyor of noxious drugs, a compounder of philtres, a vendor of poisons. The men who kept shops for the sale of drugs generally were called pharmacopoloi. This term was not free from reproach, because it was a common appellation, not only of the shopkeepers strictly so-called, but was also applied to the periodeutes, or agyrtoi, travelling quacks or assembly gatherers, or as they came to be named in Latin, circulatores or circumforanei.

These itinerant drug sellers are occasionally referred to by the classic authors. Lucian speaks of one hawking a cough mixture about the streets; and Cicero, in his Oratia pro Cluentio, suggests that the travelling pharmacopolists who attended the markets of country towns were not unwilling to sell poisons as well as medicines when they were wanted. One of these is specifically named, Lucius Clodius, and the orator suggests that he was bribed to supply medicines to a certain lady which were to have a fatal effect.

The designation Periodeutes meant originally, and always in strict legal terminology, physicians who visited their patients. The term was also used among the Christians to describe the ministers charged to visit the sick and poor in their dioceses.

The tramp doctor in time gets tired of his vagabond life, and, it may be, a little weary of hearing his own voice. If he has saved a little money, therefore, the attractions of a shop in the city, where he can exercise his healing on people who seek him, appeal strongly to him. So in Greece and in the Roman Empire the charlatans settled in little shops and were called iatroi epidiphrioi or sellularii medici, meaning sedentary doctors. But all these were pharmacopoloi.

Peculiarly interesting is the suggestion made by Epicurus and intended as a sneer, that Aristotle was one of these pharmacopoloi in his younger days. According to Epicurus the philosopher having first wasted his patrimony in riotous living and then served as a soldier, afterwards sold antidotes in the markets up to the time when he joined Plato's classes.

Seplasia was the ordinary name in Rome for a druggist's shop, and those who kept them were designated Seplasiarii or Pigmentarii. These names appear to have been used without much recognition of their original meanings. Strictly the Seplasiarii were ointment makers, and though the Pigmentarii were no doubt at first sellers of dyes and colours, they evidently came to include medicines in their stocks of pigments, and Coelius Aurelianus, in writing on stomach complaints, alludes to aloes as a pigment. Greek designations corresponding to those just quoted were Pantopoloi and Kadolikoi (the latter used by Galen in referring to the trader who supplied the drugs for the theriacum prepared in the palace of the Emperor Antoninus). Kopopoloi, and Migmatopoloi, both of which words meant dealers in all sorts of small wares, were like the mercers in this country when shopkeeping first began. The shops of perfumers were myropolia or myrophecia, the perfumers themselves were myrepsi. A general term in Latin for any sort of shop where medicines were sold or surgical operations performed was Medicina. This was in the days before the Empire, when there was no usual distinction between the branches of the healing art.

Pharmacotribae, strictly drug-grinders, may have been compounders, and it has also been conjectured that they were the assistants employed by the Seplasiarii or Roman druggists.

Herbalists were of very ancient Greek lineage, under the names of Botanologoi, who were collectors of simples, and who, to enhance the price of their wares, pretended to have to gather them with many superstitious observances; and Rhizotomoi, or root-cutters. The name Apothek, which came to be appropriated to the warehouse where medicinal herbs were kept, and which is to-day the German equivalent of our pharmacy, or chemist's shop, meant originally any warehouse, and from it has been derived the French boutique and the Spanish bodega.

The earlier Greek and Roman physicians were in the habit of themselves preparing the medicines they prescribed for their patients. But naturally they did not gather their own herbs, and as many of those used for medicine were exotics, it is obvious that they could not have done so if they had wished. The herbalists who undertook this duty (botanologoi in Greek) developed into the seplasiarii, pharmacopoloi, medicamentarii, and pigmentarii already mentioned. Beckmann says they competed with the regular physicians, having acquired a knowledge of the healing virtues of the commodities they sold, and the methods of compounding them. This could not help happening, but it ought to be remembered that the physicians of all countries had themselves developed from herbalists, that is, if we abandon the theories of miraculous instruction which are found among the legends of Egypt, Assyria, India, and Greece.

How similar the relations of the doctors and druggists of ancient Rome were with those still prevailing in this country may be gathered from a reproach levelled by Pliny against physicians contemporary with him (Bk. xxxiv, 11) to the effect that they purchased their medicines from the seplasiarii without knowing of what they were composed.

VI
ARAB PHARMACY.

> In the science of medicine the Arabians have been deservedly applauded. The names of Mesua and Geber, of Razis and Avicenna, are ranked with the Grecian masters; in the city of Bagdad 860 physicians were licensed to exercise their lucrative profession; in Spain the lives of the Catholic princes were entrusted to the skill of the Saracens; and the School of Salerno, their legitimate offspring, revived in Italy and Europe the precepts of the healing art.—GIBBON: "Decline and Fall of the Roman Empire," Chap. LII.

No period of European history is more astonishing than the records of the triumphant progress of the Arab power under the influence of the faith of Islam. From the earliest times this grand Semitic race was distinguished for learning of a certain character, for gravity, piety, superstition, a poetic imagination, and eloquence. Centuries of independence, jealously guarded, and innumerable local feuds made the material of perfect soldiers, and when Mohammed had grafted on the native religious character his own faith and missionary zeal the Arab army, the Saracens, as they came to be called, filled with fanatic fervour, and utterly indifferent to death, or, rather, eager for it as the introduction to the Paradise which their prophet had seen and told them of, formed such an irresistible force as on a small scale has only been reproduced by Cromwell in our nation.

But the rapidity of the conquests of Mohammedanism was perhaps less remarkable than the extraordinary assimilation of ancient learning and the development of new science among these hitherto unlettered Arabs. Mohammed was born in the year 569 of our era. The Koran was the first substantial piece of Arabic literature. Alexandria was taken and Egypt conquered by the Moslems under Amrou in A.D. 640, Persia and Syria having been previously subdued. Amrou was himself disposed to yield to the solicitations of some Greek grammarians, who implored him to spare the great Library of the city, the depository of the learning of the ancient world. But he considered it necessary to refer the request to the Caliph Omar. The reply of the Commander of the Faithful is one of the most familiar of the stories in Gibbon's fascinating history. "If the writings support the Koran they are superfluous; if they oppose it they are pernicious; burn them." It is declared that the papers and manuscripts served as fuel for the baths of the city for six months.

The destruction of the Alexandrian Library is often alluded to as a signal triumph of barbarism over civilisation. Gibbon cynically remarks that "if the ponderous mass of Arian and Monophysite controversy were indeed consumed in the public baths a philosopher may allow with a smile that it was ultimately devoted to the benefit of mankind." But at least the spirit which animated Omar in 640 may be noted for comparison with the encouragement of learning which was soon to characterise the Arab rulers.

Only a lifetime later, in A.D. 711, the sons of the Alexandrian conquerors invaded Spain, and within the same century made their western capital, Cordova, the greatest centre of learning, civilisation, and luxury in Europe. The following quotation from Dr. Draper's "History of the Intellectual Development of Europe" will give an idea of this achievement:

> Scarcely had the Arabs become firmly settled in Spain than they commenced a brilliant career. Adopting what had become the established policy of the Commanders of the Faithful in Asia, the Emirs of Cordova distinguished themselves as patrons of learning, and set an example of refinement strongly contrasting with the condition of the native European Princes. Cordova under their administration, at the highest point of their prosperity, boasted of more than two hundred thousand houses, and more than a million inhabitants. After sunset a man might walk through it in a straight line for ten miles by the light of the public lamps. Seven hundred years after this time there was not so much as one public lamp in London. Its streets were solidly paved. In Paris, centuries subsequently, whoever stepped over his threshold on a rainy day stepped up to his ankles in mud. Other cities, as Granada, Seville, Toledo, considered themselves rivals of Cordova. The palaces of the Khalifs were magnificently decorated. Those sovereigns might well look down with supercilious contempt on the dwellings of the rulers of Germany, France, and England, which were scarcely better than stables—chimneyless, windowless, with a hole in the roof for the smoke to escape, like the wigwams of certain Indians.

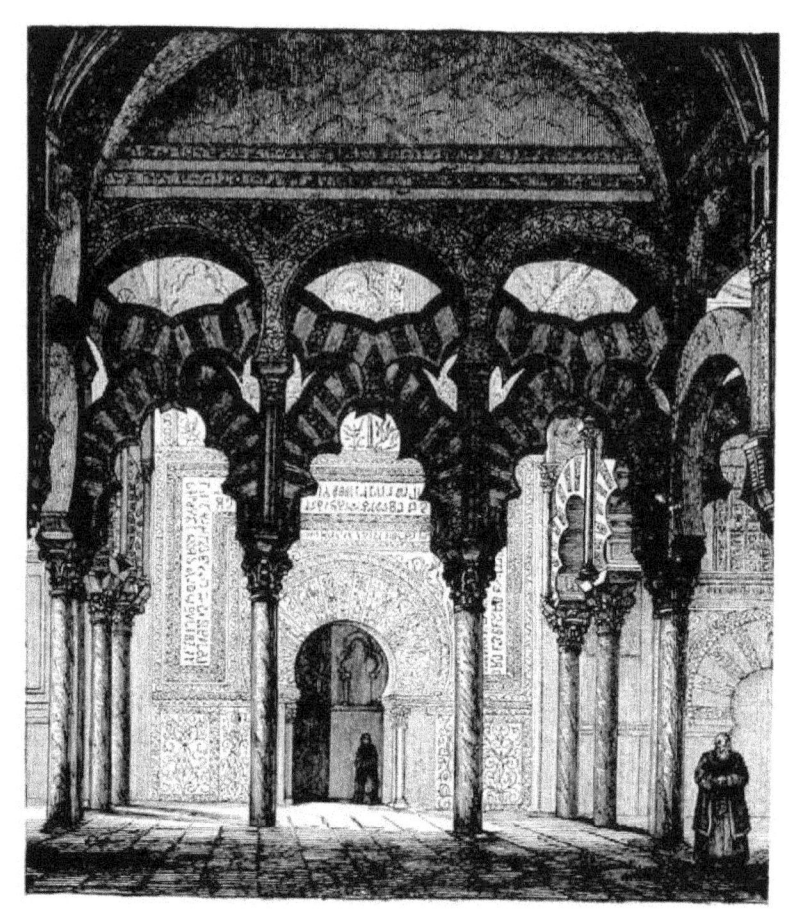

Interior of Mosque, Cordova.

About the same time the passion for learning was growing in the East. Bagdad was founded A.D. 762, and about the year 800 Haroun Al-Raschid founded the famous university of that city. Libraries and schools were established throughout the two sections of the Saracenic dominions. Greek and Latin works of philosophy and science were translated, but the licentious and blasphemous mythology of the classical poets was abhorred by this serious nation, and no Arabic versions of Olympian fables were ever made. Astronomy, mathematics, metaphysics, and the arts of agriculture, of horticulture, of architecture, of war, and of commerce, were advanced to an extent which this century does not realise, while amid all this progress the study of chemistry, medicine, and pharmacy was pursued with particular eagerness.

Curiously the Arabs owed their instruction in these branches of knowledge to those whom we are accustomed to regard as their traditional foes. The dispersion of the Nestorians after the condemnation of their doctrines by the Council of Ephesus in A.D. 431 resulted in the foundation of a Chaldean Church and the establishment of famous colleges in Syria and Persia. In these the science of the Greeks, the philosophy of Aristotle, and the medical teaching of Hippocrates were kept alive when they had been banished by the Church from Constantinople. The Jews had also acquired special fame for medical skill throughout the East, and they and the Nestorians appear to have associated in some of the schools. It was to these teachers the Arabs turned when, having assured their military success, they demanded intellectual advancement. The Caliphs not only tolerated, they welcomed the assistance of the "unbelievers," and, in fact, depended on them for the equipment of their own schools, and for the private tuition of their children. To John Mesuë, a Nestorian, and a famous writer on medicine and pharmacy, Haroun Al-Raschid entrusted the superintendence of the public schools of Bagdad.

The first Nestorian college is believed to have been established in the city of Dschondisabour in Chuzistan (Nishapoor), before the revelation of Mohammed. Theology and Medicine were particularly studied at this seat of learning, and a hospital was established to which the medical students were admitted, but they had first to be examined in the Psalms, the New Testament, and in certain books of prayers.

It was the Caliph Almansor and his immediate successor, Haroun Al-Raschid, who between them made Bagdad a centre of study. Students and professors came thither from all parts of the then civilised world, and the Caliphs welcomed, and indeed invited, both Christians and Jews to teach there. Hospitals were established in the city, and the first public pharmacies or dispensaries were provided in Bagdad by Haroun Al-Raschid. It is on record that in A.D. 807 envoys from that monarch came to the court of Charlemagne bringing gifts of balsams, nard, ointments, drugs, and medicines.

Arabic medicine was based on the works of Hippocrates and Galen, which were for the most part translated first into Syriac, and then into Arabic. It does not come within the scope of this work to narrate or estimate the advance in medicine which may be accredited to the Arabian writers and practitioners. Medical historians do not allow that they contributed much original service to either anatomy, physiology, pathology, or surgery; but it is admitted by every student that their maintenance of scholarship through the half dozen centuries during which Europe was sunk in the most abject ignorance and superstition entitles them to the gratitude of all who have lived since. The medicine of Avicenna was perhaps much the same as that of Galen. Both were accepted by the physicians of England, France, and Germany with the slavish deference which the long burial of the critical faculties had made inevitable, and which needed the vigorous abuse of Paracelsus to quicken into activity.

Whatever may have been the case with medicine it cannot be denied that the Arabs contributed largely to the development of its ministering arts, chemistry and pharmacy. The achievements attributed to Geber in the eighth century were probably not due to any single adept. Tradition assigned the glory to him and, likely enough, if such a chemist really lived and acquired fame, other investigators who followed him for a century or two adopted the pious fraud so frequently met with in other branches of study in the early centuries of our era of attributing theories or discoveries to some venerated teacher in order to assure for them immediate acceptance. However this may be, it is not the less established that the chemistry of Geber, or of Geber and others, was in fact the fruit of Arab industry and genius.

Our language indicates to some extent what Pharmacy owes to the Arabs. Alcohol, julep, syrup, sugar, alkermes, are Arabic names; the general employment in medicine of rhubarb, senna, camphor, manna, musk, nutmegs, cloves, bezoar stones, cassia, tamarinds, reached us through them. They first distilled rose water. They first established pharmacies, and from the time of Haroun Al-Raschid there is evidence that the Government controlled the quality and prices of the medicine sold in them. Sabor-Ebn-Sahel, president of the school of Dschondisabour, was the author of the earliest pharmacopœia, which was entitled "Krabadin"; and Hassan-Ali-Ebno-Talmid of Bagdad in the tenth century, and Avicenna (Al-Hussein-Ben-Abdallah-Ebn-Sina) in the eleventh century prepared collections of formulas which were used as pharmacopœias.

It was the Arabs who raised pharmacy to its proper dignity. We do not read of any noted pharmacists among them who were not physicians, but the latter were all keen students of the materia medica, and occupied themselves largely with pharmaceutical studies. But it is evident that there was a distinct profession of pharmacy. We read of Avicenna, for example, taking refuge with an apothecary at Hamdan, and there composing some of his famous works. Elsewhere a quotation from Rhazes gives some indication of the irregular practice of medicine which has prevailed in every country and among all nations; and Sprengel quotes some translated items from various Arabic authors which show that as early as the ninth century the Government sanctioned the book of pharmaceutical formulas, compiled by Sabor-Ebn-Sahel, director of the School of Dschondisabour, already mentioned. His work was frequently imitated in later times. The first London Pharmacopœia was professedly based largely on the Formulary of Mesuë.

There is also evidence that both in civil life and in the army the pharmacists were closely supervised. Their medicines were inspected, and the prices at which they were sold to the public were controlled by law.

The development and progress of medicine and its associated sciences among the Arabs may be very concisely sketched. The flight of Mohammed from Mecca to Medina, the Hejira as it is called, from which the Mohommedan era is dated, corresponds in our chronology with A.D. 622. The prophet died in 632. Contemporary with him lived a priest at Alexandria named Ahrun or Aaron, who compiled from Greek writers thirty books which he called the Pandects of Physic. These were translated into Syriac and Arabic about 683 by a Jew of Bassora named Maserdschawaih-Ebn-Dschaldschal. It is not in existence, and is only known by references to it made by Rhazes. The first allusion to small-pox known to history was contained in these Pandects. Serapion quotes a number of formulas which he says were invented by Ahrun. In 772 Almansor, the Caliph who founded the city of Bagdad, brought thither from Nishabur (Dschondisabour) in Persia, a famous Christian physician named George Baktischwah, who stayed for some time, and at the request of Almansor translated into Arabic certain books on Physic. He then returned to his own land, but his son was afterwards a physician in great favour with the two succeeding Caliphs, Almohdi and Haroun Al-Raschid. Freind states that when the elder Baktischwah returned to Persia Almansor presented him with 10,000 pieces of gold, and that Al-Raschid paid the younger Baktischwah an annual salary of 10,000 drachmas. The last-named ruler also brought to Bagdad the Nestorian Christian, Jahiah-Ebn-Masawaih, who, under the name of Mesuë the Elder, retained a reputation for his formulas even up to the publication of the London Pharmacopœia.

Mesuë is noted for his opposition to the violent purgative medicines which the Greek and Roman physicians had made common, and he had much to do with the popularisation, if not with the introduction of, senna, cassia, tamarinds, sebestens, myrabolans, and jujube. He modified the effects of certain remedies by judicious combinations, as, for example, by giving violet root and lemon juice with scammony. He gave pine bark and decoction of hyssop as emetics, and recommended the pancreas of the hare as a styptic in diarrhœa.

A disciple of Mesuë's, Ebn-Izak, added greatly to the medical resources of the Arabs by translations of the works of Hippocrates, Galen, Pliny, Paul of Egineta, and other Greek authors.

Abu-Moussah-Dschafar-Al-Soli, commonly called Geber, the equivalent of his middle name, is supposed to have lived in the eighth century. It has already been remarked that the chemical discoveries attributed to this philosopher were probably the achievements of many workers, and were afterwards collected and passed on to posterity as his alone. From him are dated the introduction into science, to be adopted later in medicine, of corrosive sublimate, of red precipitate, of nitric and nitro-muriatic acids, and of nitrate of silver.

These chemical discoveries must have been made within the hundred years from 750 to 850, because Rhazes, who wrote in the latter half of the ninth century, mentions them. Geber has been supposed to have claimed to have discovered the philosopher's stone, and to have made the universal medicine. But it is not at all certain that he contemplated medicine at all. His language is highly figurative, and probably when he says his gold had cured six lepers he meant only that he had, or thought he had, extracted gold from six baser metals.

Rhazes, whose Europeanised name is the modification of Arrasi, which was the final member of a long series of Eastern patronymics, was of Persian birth, and commenced his studies in that country with music and astronomy. When he was thirty he removed to Bagdad, and it was not until then that he took up the sciences of chemistry and medicine. Subsequently he was made director of the hospital of Bagdad, and his lectures on the medical art were attended by students from many countries. His principal work was entitled Hhawi, which has been translated Continent, apparently because it was supposed to contain all there was to know about medicine. The style of this treatise is that of notes without method, and it is certain that it could not have been written entirely by Rhazes, as authorities are named who did not live until after he had died. The theory is that Rhazes left a quantity of notes of his lectures and cases, and that some of his disciples afterwards published them with additions, but without much editing.

Among the methods of treatment for which Rhazes is responsible may be mentioned that of phthisis, with milk and sugar; of high fever, with cold water; of weakness of the stomach and of the digestive organs, with cold water and buttermilk; and he advises sufferers from melancholia to play chess. He states that fever is not itself a disease, but an effort of nature to cast out a disease. He was particularly careful in the use of purgatives, which he said were apt to occasion irritation of the intestinal canal, and in dysentery he relied usually on fruits, rice, and farinaceous food, though in severe cases he ordered quicklime, arsenic, and opium. In Freind's History of Medicine (1727) a translation of some comments of Rhazes on the impostors of his day shows better than the citations already given how just and, it may be said, modern were the ideas of this practitioner of more than a thousand years ago. It may be added that Freind is not very complimentary to Rhazes generally. I append an abbreviation of this interesting notice of the quackery of the ninth century.

There are so many little arts used by mountebanks and pretenders to physic that an entire treatise, had I mind to write one, would not contain them. Their impudence is equal to their guilt in tormenting persons in their last hours. Some of them profess to cure the falling sickness (epilepsy) by making an issue at the back of the head in form of a cross, and pretending to take something out of the opening which they held all the time in their hands. Others give out that they will draw snakes out of their patients' noses; this they seem to do by putting an iron probe up the nostril until the blood comes. Then they draw out an artificial worm, made of liver. Other tricks are to remove white specks from the eye, to draw water from the ear, worms from the teeth, stones from the bladder, or phlegm from various parts of the body, always having concealed the substance in their hands which they pretend to extract. Another performance is to collect the evil humours of the body into one place by rubbing that part with winter cherries until they cause an inflammation. Then they apply some oil to heal the place. Some assure their patients they have swallowed glass. To prove this they tickle the throat with a feather to induce vomiting, when some particles of glass are ejected which were put there by the feather. No wise man ought to trust his life in their hands, nor take any of their medicines which have proved fatal to many.

Rhazes writes of aqua vitæ, but it is now accepted that he only means a kind of wine. The distillation of wine was not practised till a century after him. Mercury in the form of ointment and corrosive sublimate were applied by him externally, the latter for itch; yellow and red arsenic and sulphates of iron and copper were also among his external remedies. Borax (which he called tenker), saltpetre, red coral, various precious stones, and oil of ants, are included among the internal remedies which he advises.

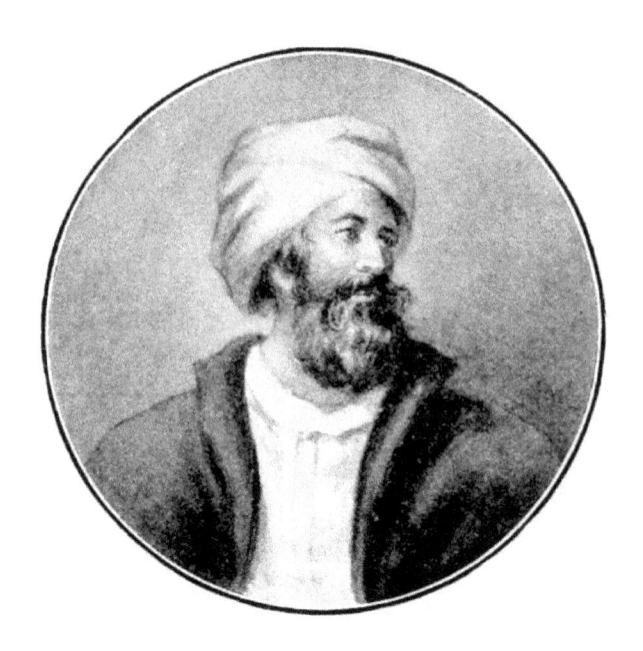

Avicenna.

As represented on the diploma of the Pharmaceutical Society.

The Arab author who acquired by far the greatest fame in Western lands, and who, indeed, shared with Galen the unquestioning obedience of myriads of medical practitioners throughout Europe until Paracelsus shook his authority five hundred years after his death, was Al-Hussein-Abou-Ali-Ben-Abdallah-Ebn-Sina, which picturesque name loses its Eastern atmosphere in the transmutation of its two concluding phrases into Avicenna. This famous man was born at Bokhara in 980; at twelve years of age he knew the Koran by heart; at sixteen he was a skilful physician; at eighteen he operated on the Caliph Nuhh with such brilliant success that his fame was established. In the course of a varied life he was at one time a Vizier, and soon afterwards in prison for being concerned in some sedition. He escaped from prison and lived for a long time concealed in the house of a friendly apothecary, where he wrote a large part of his voluminous "Canon." He spent the later years of his life at Ispahan, where he was in great favour with the Caliph Ola-Oddaula, and he died at Hamdan in 1038 in the fifty-eighth year of his age. He had led an irregular life, and it was said of him that all his philosophy failed to make him moral, and all his knowledge of medicine left him unable to take care of his own health.

Competent critics who have studied the medical teaching of Avicenna have not been able to discover wherein its merits have justified the high esteem to which it attained. The explanation appears to be that what Avicenna lacked in originality he made up in method. The main body of his "Canon" is a judicious selection from the Greek and Latin physicians, and from Rhazes and other of his Arabic predecessors. He wrote a great deal on drugs and remedies, but it has been found impossible to identify many of the substances of his Materia Medica, as in many cases the names he gives evidently do not apply to those given by Serapion, Rhazes, and other writers. He often prescribed camphor, and alluded to several different kinds; a solution of manna was a favourite medicine with him; he regarded corrosive sublimate as the most deadly of all poisons, but used it externally; iron he had three names for, probably different compounds; he had great faith in gold, silver, and precious stones; it was probably he who introduced the silvering and gilding of pills, but his object was not to make them more pleasant to take, but to add to their medicinal effect.

Serapion the younger, and Mesuë the younger, who both lived soon after the time of Avicenna, were principally writers on Materia Medica, from whose works later authors borrowed freely.

The subsequent Arab authorities of particular note came from among the Western Saracens. Albucasis of Cordova, Avenzoar of Seville, and Averrhoes of Cordova, who are all believed to have flourished in the twelfth century, were the most celebrated. Albucasis was a great surgeon and describes the operations of his period with wonderful clearness and intelligence. Avenzoar was a physician who interested himself largely in pharmacy. He was reputed to have lived to the age of 135 and to have accumulated experience from his 20th year to the day of his death. Averrhoes knew Avenzoar personally, but was younger. He was a philosopher and somewhat of a freethinker who interested himself in medical matters. We are naturally more concerned with Avenzoar than with the others.

It is evident from the books left by Avenzoar, whose full name was Abdel-Malek-Abou-Merwan-Ebn-Zohr, that in his time the practices of medicine, surgery, and pharmacy were quite distinct in Spain, and he apologises to the higher branch of the profession for his interest in those practices which were usually left to their servants. But he states that from his youth he took delight in studying how to make syrups and electuaries, and a strong desire to know the operation of medicines and how to combine them and to extract their virtues. He writes about poisons and antidotes; has a chapter on the oil alquimesci, which Freind renders oil of eggs, and Sprengel calls oil of dates. Avenzoar says his father brought it from the East, and that it was a marvellous lithontryptic. He tells how mastic corrects scammony, and sweet almonds colocynth. He is the earliest writer to refer to the medicinal virtues of the bezoar stones. He gives a different account of the origin of these stones from that of other authors. The best, he says, comes from the East and is got from the eyes of stags. The stags eat serpents to make them strong, and at once to prevent any injury their instinct impels them to run into streams and stand in the water up to their necks. They do not drink any water. If they did they would die immediately; but standing in the stream gradually reduces the force of the poison, and then a liquor exudes by the eyelids which coagulates and forms a stone which may grow to the size of a chestnut, which ultimately falls off. According to another Arab author, Abdalanarack, the bezoar stone acquired such a celebrity in Spain that a palace in Cordova was given in exchange for one.

Moses Maimonides, the most famous Jewish scholar and theologian of the middle ages, must be mentioned among the exponents of Arab pharmacy. He was born at Cordova in 1139, and studied medicine under Averrhoes, but when he was twenty-five the then Mohammedan ruler of Spain required him to be converted or quit the kingdom. Maimonides therefore went to Cairo, and became physician to Saladin, the well-known hero of Crusade wars, who was then Sultan of Egypt. Among his duties he had to superintend the preparation of theriaca and mithridatium for the Court. The drugs for these compounds, Maimonides says, had to be brought from the East and the West at great expenditure of time and money. Consequently, "the illustrious Kadi Fakhil," (who was apparently one of Saladin's ministers), "whose days may God prolong, ordered the most humble of his servants in 595 (A.D. 1198) to compose a treatise, small, and showing what ought to be done immediately for a person bitten by a venomous animal." The treatise which Maimonides composed, in obedience to this order, he called "Fakhiliteh." This small popular manual reflects in general the pharmacy of Spain and is of no particular interest. The author considers that for all kinds of poisons and venoms the most efficacious antidote is an emerald, laid on the stomach or held in the mouth; and he notes the virtues of theriaca, mithridatium, and of bezoar. But the Kadi was thinking of poor people, and therefore more ordinary remedies were also named. A pigeon killed and cut in two pieces might be applied to painful wounds, but if this was not available warm vinegar with flour and olive oil might be substituted. Vomiting must be excited, and to destroy the virus a mixture of asafœtida, sulphur, salt, onions, mint, orange-pips, and the excrement of pigeons, ducks, or goats, compounded with honey and taken in wine, was recommended. The wisdom of Rhazes, of Avenzoar, and of other great authorities was also drawn from.

VII
FROM THE ARABS TO THE EUROPEANS

> "Mediciners, like the medicines which they employ, are often useful, though the one were by birth and manners the vilest of humanity, as the others are in many cases extracted from the basest materials. Men may use the assistance of pagans and infidels in their need, and there is reason to think that one cause of their being permitted to remain on earth is that they might minister to the convenience of true Christians."—The Archbishop of Tyre in Sir Walter Scott's *Talisman*.

It would require a very long chapter and would be outside the scope of this work to attempt to trace in any detail the manner in which the ancient wisdom and science of the Greek and Latin authors, which was so marvellously preserved by the iconoclastic Arabs, was transferred, when their passion for study and research began to fail, to European nations. It has been alleged that the Crusades served to bring the attainments of the Eastern Saracens to the knowledge of the West through learning picked up by the physicians and others who accompanied the Christian armies against the Mohammedans.

But there is no evidence and not much probability that Europeans acquired any Eastern science of value through the Crusades. Indirectly medicine ultimately profited greatly by the commerce which these marvellous wars opened up between the East and the West, and the diseases which were spread as the consequence of the intimate association of the unwholesome hordes from all the nations concerned, resulted in the establishment of thousands of hospitals all over Europe. The provision of homes for the sick was far more common among the Mohammedans than among the Christians of that period. Activity of thought was stimulated, and medical science must have shared in the effects of spirit of inquiry. Some historians have supposed that the infusion of astrological superstitions into the teaching and practice of medicine was largely traceable to the communion with the East in these Holy Wars: but this idea is not supported by anything that we know of the Arab doctors. "I have not found the union of astrology with medicine taught by any writer of that nation," says Sprengel; and his authority is very great. On the other hand the philosophers and theologians of that age were only too eager to seize upon anything mystic, and plenty of materials for their speculations were found in the Greek and Latin manuscripts handed down to them. Superstitions entered into the mental furniture of the age much more directly from Rome and Alexandria than from Bagdad.

That the Arabs of the East could have taught their Christian foes much useful knowledge cannot be doubted. The letter from the Patriarch of Jerusalem to Alfred the Great (see page 131), for example, is proof of the pharmaceutical superiority of the Syrians over the Saxons at that time.

M. Berthelot has shown by abundant evidence in his "History of Alchemy" that the Latin works dealing with chemistry of the thirteenth, fourteenth, and fifteenth centuries which were very numerous in Christendom, were almost exclusively drawn from Arabic sources. Such chemical learning as the Arabs had collected from Greek writers, as well as that which they had added from their own investigations, in this way found its way back to the heirs of the original owners as they may be called.

We read likewise of Constantine the African, who, about the year 1050, came to Salerno after a long residence in the East, and gave to the medical school of that city the translations he had made from Arab authors. But, notwithstanding these evidences of Eastern culture, it is certain that the actual introduction of pharmacy into the Northern European countries is much more largely due to the Spanish Mohammedans. In the Middle Ages poor Arabs and Jews who had studied medicine in the schools of Cordova and Seville tramped through France and Germany, selling their remedies, and teaching many things to the monks and priests who, in spite of repeated papal edicts forbidding them to sell medicines, did in fact cultivate all branches of the art of healing, including many superstitions. The edicts themselves are evidence that they sold their services to those who could afford to pay for them.

The Medical School of Salerno, already mentioned, was the principal link between the later Greek physicians and the teaching institutions which remain with us to this day, as, for instance, the universities of Paris, Naples, Oxford, Padua, Vienna, and others of later fame. The origin of the school of Salerno is unknown, but it was certainly in existence in the ninth century. It was long supposed to have developed from a monastic institution, but it is now generally believed to have been always a secular school. Its historian, Mazza of Naples, 1681, quotes an ancient chronicle which names Rabbi Elinus (a Jew), Pontus (a Greek), Adala (a Saracen), and Salernus (a Roman) as its founders, but there is no evidence of the epoch to which this refers. Although other subjects were taught at Salerno, it became specially noted for its medical school, and in the ninth century it had assumed the title of Civitas Hippocratica. William of Normandy resorted to Salerno prior to his conquest of England, and a dietetic treatise in verse exists dedicated to his son Robert. It has been claimed that the works of Hippocrates and Galen were studied at Salerno from its earliest days, but so far as this was the case it was by the intermediary of Jewish doctors, who themselves derived their knowledge from Arab sources, that these were available. The original texts of the Greek and Latin authors were not in the hands of European scholars till Aldus of Venice began to reproduce them early in the sixteenth century.

The pharmaceutical knowledge to which the famous school attained may be judged by the reputation which attended the Antidotary of Nicolas Prepositus, who was director of the school in the first half of the twelfth century. In this Antidotary are found the absurd formulas pretending to have been invented or used by the Apostle Paul and others. "Sal Sacerdotale quo utebantur sacerdotales tempore Heliae prophetae" is among these. In the course of the next century or two medical students from England, Germany, Italy, and France went to Cordova, Toledo, and Seville, and there wrote translations of the medical works used in those schools. These translations by the end of the thirteenth century were so universally accepted as to eclipse Salerno, which from then began to decline in fame, Bologna, Montpellier, Padua, and Leyden gradually partitioning among themselves its old reputation. But the medical school of Salerno actually existed until 1811, when it was dissolved by a decree of Napoleon I.

As evidence of the monopoly of Avicenna in the medical schools of Europe at the beginning of the sixteenth century, and doubtless for a long period previously, the following from the preface to a Latin translation of the works of Paulus Egineta is quoted by Leclerc:—

> Avicenna, who is regarded as the Prince and most excellent of all physicians, is read and expounded in all the schools; and the ninth book of Rhazes, physician to the Caliph Almansor, is similarly read and commented on. These are believed to teach the whole art of healing. A few later writers, such as Betruchius, Gatinaria, Guaynerius, and Valescus, are occasionally cited, and now and then Hippocrates, Galen, and Dioscorides are quoted, but all the other Greek writers are unknown. The Latin translations of a few of the books of Galen and Hippocrates which are in use are very corrupt and barbarous, and are only admitted at the pleasure of the Arabian Princes, and this favour is but rarely conceded.

The most notable event in the history of pharmacy after the earlier Crusades was an edict regulating the practice of both medicine and pharmacy issued by Frederick II, the Holy Roman Emperor and King of Sicily. This monarch, probably the ablest ruler in the Middle Ages, who died in 1250, had great esteem for Arab learning. Mohammedans and Jews were encouraged to come to Naples during his reign, and he facilitated by all means in his power the introduction of such innovations as had been acquired from Cordova and Bagdad.

The edict referred to mentions "apotheca," meaning thereby only the warehouses where prepared medicines were stored. Those who compounded the medicines were termed "confectionarii," the places or shops where they were sold were called "stationes," and the persons who supplied them, "stationarii." It is not quite clear whether the confectionarii and the stationarii were the same persons. Probably they were sometimes, but not necessarily always. Apparently the stationarii were generally the drug importers and dealers, and the confectionarii were the compounders. Both had to be licensed by the Medical School of Salerno; and among the duties imposed upon the physician, one was to inform the authorities if he came to discover that any "confectionarius" had falsified medicines. Longfellow alludes to this provision in the "Golden Legend"—

> To report if any confectionarius
> Mingles his drugs with matters various.

The physician was strictly forbidden to enter into any arrangement with a druggist whereby he would derive any profit by the sale of medicaments, and he was not permitted himself to conduct a pharmacy. The "confectioners" were required to take an oath to prepare all medicines according to the Antidotary of the Salernian School. Their profits were limited and graduated, less being allowed on those of frequent consumption than on those which they had to keep for more than a year. Pharmacies were only allowed in the principal cities, and in each such city two notable master-apothecaries were appointed to supervise them. The "confectioners" had to make their syrups and electuaries and other compounds in the presence of these two inspectors, and if they were detected in any attempt at fraud their property was subject to confiscation. If one of the inspectors was found to have been a party to the fraud his punishment was death.

> "It is well known," says Beckmann in "Ancient Inventions," "that almost all political institutions on this side the Alps, and particularly everything that concerned education, were copied from Italian models. These were the only patterns then to be found; and the monks despatched from the papal court saw they could lay no better foundation for the Pontiff's power and their own aggrandizement than by inducing other States to follow the examples set them in Italy. Medical establishments were formed, therefore, everywhere at first according to the plan of that at Salerno. Particular places for vending medicines were more necessary in other countries than in Italy. The physicians of that period used no other drugs than those recommended

by the ancients; and as these had to be procured from the Levant, Greece, Arabia, and India, it was necessary to send thither for them. Besides, herbs, to be confided in, could only be gathered when the sun and planets were in certain constellations, and certificates of their being so were necessary to give them reputation. All this was impossible without a distinct employment, and it was found convenient to suffer dealers in drugs gradually to acquire monopolies. The preparation of medicines was becoming more difficult and expensive. The invention of distillation, sublimation, and other chemical processes necessitated laboratories, furnaces, and costly apparatus; so that it was thought proper that those who devoted themselves to pharmacy should be indemnified by an exclusive trade; and monopolists could be kept under closer inspection so that the danger of their selling improper drugs or poisons was lessened or entirely removed. They were also allowed to deal in sweetmeats and confectionery, which were then great luxuries; and in some places they were required to give presents of these delicacies to the magistrates on certain festivals."

This extract shows how the German provision of protected pharmacy originated. In many of the chief cities the apothecaries' shops were established by, and belonged to, the King or Queen, or the municipality. Sometimes, as at Stuttgart, there was a contract between the ruler and the apothecary, the former agreeing to provide a certain quantity of wine, barley, and rye; while the apothecary in return was to supply the Court with its necessary confectionery.

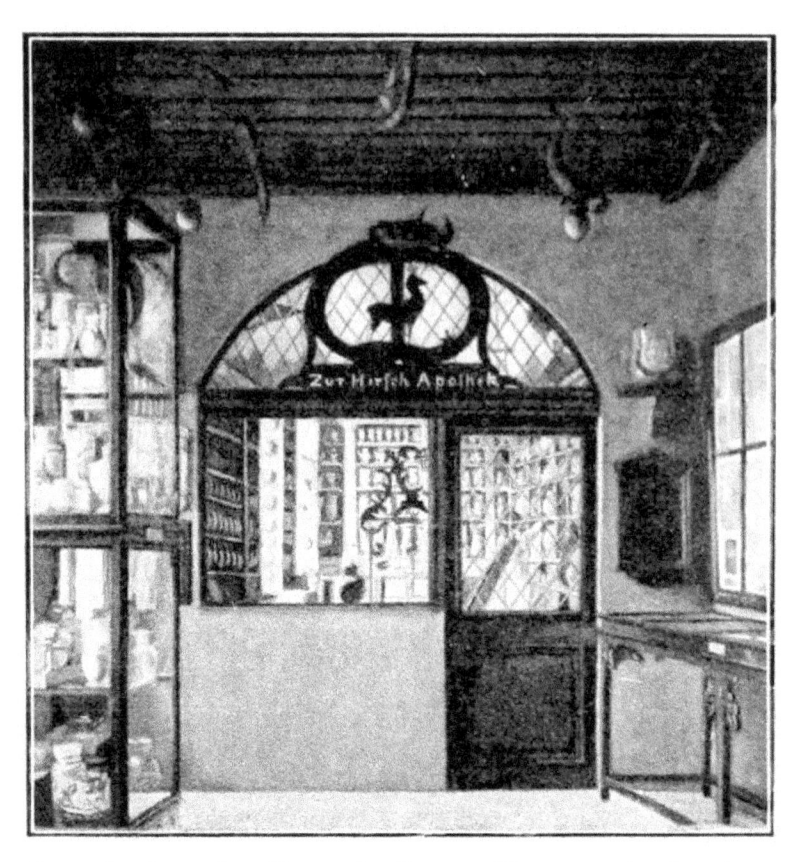

The Reproduction of a Sixteenth Century Pharmacy in the Germanic Museum at Nuremberg.

Beckmann gives much minute information concerning the establishment of apothecaries' shops in the chief cities of Germany.[1] He mentions a conjecture that there was a pharmacy at Augsburg in the thirteenth and fourteenth centuries, but exact dates begin with the fifteenth century. There was a female apothecary established at Augsburg in 1445, and the city paid her a salary. At Stuttgart, in 1458, Count Ulric authorised one Glatz to open a pharmacy. There was one existing at Frankfort in 1472. The police regulations of Basle in 1440 mention the public physician and his duty, adding that "what costly things people may wish to have from the apothecary's shop they must pay for." The magistrates of Berlin, in 1488, granted to one Hans Zebender a free house, a certain provision of rye, no taxes, and the assurance that no other apothecary should reside in the city. But the Elector Joachim granted a new patent to another apothecary in 1499. At Halle there was only one apothecary. In that year the Archbishop, with the confirmation of the Chapter, granted to his physician, von Wyke, the privilege of opening another, but gave at the same time the assurance that no more should be permitted in the city "to eternity."

In France apothecaries were in business as such certainly before 1250. A charter of the church of Cahors, dated 1178, describes the retail shopkeepers of the town as "apothecarii," the term being used evidently as "boutiquiers" is now, and signifying nothing more than shopkeepers. The meaning, however, soon became restricted to dealers in drugs and spices. In the middle of the next century John of Garlande alludes to "appotecarii," who sold confections and electuaries, roots and herbs, ginger, pepper, cumin, and other spices, wax, sugar, and licorice. Officially, however, these tradesmen were classed at that time among the "espiciers." The two guilds, indeed, continued in formal association until 1777, but royal ordinances of 1484 and 1514 clearly established the distinction between them. Even in 1271 the Faculty of Medicine of Paris forbade "herborists and apothecaries" to practise medicine. Special responsibilities, duties, and privileges were expressly provided for the apothecaries, and in the ordinance of 1514 it is specifically declared that though the apothecary is always a grocer, the grocer is not necessarily an apothecary. ("Qui est espicier n'est pas apothicaire, et qui est apothicaire est espicier.")

In the fourteenth century the apothecaries of Paris were required to subscribe to a formal oath before they were permitted to practise. They swore to live and die in the Christian faith, to speak no evil of their teachers or masters, to do all in their power for the honour, glory, ornament, and majesty of medicine, to give no remedy or purge without the authority of a physician, to supply no drugs to procure abortion, to prepare exactly physicians' prescriptions, neither adding, subtracting, nor substituting anything without the express permission of the physician, to avoid the practices of charlatans as they would the plague, and to keep no bad or old drug in their stocks. An ordinance of 1359 provides that no one shall be granted the title of master-apothecary unless he can show that he can read recipes.

The edict of 1484, issued during the minority of Charles VIII, sets forth that, "We, of our certain science, especial grace, full power, and royal authority, do say, declare, statuate, and ordain" the curriculum to be observed by those who desire to learn the trade of an apothecary. A four years' apprenticeship was essential, and the aspirant had to dispense prescriptions, recognise drugs, and prepare "chefs d'œuvres" in wax and confectionery in the presence of appointed master-apothecaries. Latin was added to the examination in 1536, and ten years' experience after the apprenticeship was also insisted upon ultimately before the candidate could be admitted as a master-apothecary. One of the ordinances of the sixteenth century gave to the apothecaries the monopoly in the manufacture and sale of gingerbread.

These edicts all related particularly to the apothecaries of Paris. There were similar ones in the provinces, with some peculiarities. At Dijon, for example, it was provided that no apothecary could receive a legacy from one of his clients. *En revanche* he had the first claim on the estate of a deceased debtor for the payment of his account.

In 1629 the Hotel de Ville of Paris granted to the apothecaries of that city a banner and blazon, the latter, which I do not venture to translate, being thus described:—"Couppé d'azur et d'or, et sur l'or deux nefs de gueulle flottantes aux bannieres de France, accompagnés de deux estoiles a cinq poincts de gueulle avec la devise 'Lances et pondera servant,' et telles qu'elles sont cy-dessous empreinctes."

In 1682, under Louis XV, after the Brinvilliers panic, the poison register was introduced, and regulations were framed forbidding apothecaries to sell any arsenic, sublimate, or drug reputed to be a poison except to persons known to them, and who signed the register stating what use they intended to make of their purchase. Earlier in the same reign the practice of pharmacy was strictly forbidden to persons professing the reformed religion.

The last of the royal edicts applying to pharmacy was issued in 1777 by Louis XVI, and, as already stated, this was the authority which finally separated the apothecaries from the grocers. Then came the Revolution, and in 1791 all restrictions on trades or professions, including pharmacy, were abolished. Some accidents having occurred, the Assembly passed an ordinance on April 14, 1791, declaring that the old laws, statutes, and regulations governing the teaching and practice of pharmacy should remain in force until a new code should be framed. This did not appear until April, 1803, under Napoleon's Consulate, and the law, which is still in force, is to this day cited in legal proceedings as the law of Germinal, year XI.

VIII
PHARMACY IN GREAT BRITAIN.

> For none but a clever dialectician
>
> Can hope to become a great physician:
>
> That has been settled long ago.
>
> Logic makes an important part
>
> Of the mystery of the healing art;
>
> For without it how could you hope to show
>
> That nobody knows so much as you know.
>
> —LONGFELLOW: "Golden Legend."

BRITISH PHARMACY IN SAXON ENGLAND.

The condition of medicine and pharmacy in Saxon times has been carefully portrayed in three volumes published, in 1864, under the authority of the Master of the Rolls at the expense of the Treasury. These were edited by the Rev. Oswald Cockayne, M.A., and appeared under the title of "Leechdoms, Wortcunning, and Starcraft." Many old documents were translated and explained, and from these the ideas of medicine in these islands a thousand years ago were made manifest.

Mr. Cockayne gave at length a Saxon Herbarium, written, he supposed, about the year 1000, and professing to be a translation from Apuleius, a Roman physician of the second century, with additions from Dioscorides, and some from native science. A few specimens will suffice to show the character of the herb treatment in England before the Conquest.

CRESS, WATERCRESS (Nasturtium officinale).

1. This wort is not sown, but it is produced of itself in wylls (springs), and in brooks, also it is written that in some lands it will grow against walls.

2. In the case that a man's hair fall off take juice of the wort which one nameth nasturtium, and by another name cress; put it on the nose; the hair shall wax (grow).

3. For sore of head, that is for scurf and for itch, take seed of this same wort and goose grease. Pound together. It draws from the head the whiteness of the scurf.

4. For soreness of the body (the Latin word is ad cruditatem, indigestion) take this same wort nasturtium, and pennyroyal; seethe them in water, give to drink; then amendest thou the soreness of the body, and the evil departs.

5. Against swellings, take this same wort, and pound it with oil; lay over the swellings; then take leaves of the same wort, and lay them thereto.

6. Against warts, take this same wort and yeast, pound together, lay thereto, they be soon taken away.

MAYTHE (Anthemis nobilis).

For sore of eyes, let a man take ere the upgoing of the sun, the wort which is called Chamaimelon, and by another name Maythe, and when a man taketh it let him say that he will take it against white specks, and against soreness of the eyes; let him next take the ooze, and smear the eyes therewith.

POPPY (Papaver somniferum).

1. For sore of eyes, that is what we denominate blearedness, take the ooze of this wort, which the Greeks name Makona and the Romans Papaver album, and the Engles call white poppy, or the stalk with the fruit; lay it to the eyes.

2. For sore of temples or of the head, take ooze of this same wort, pound with vinegar, and lay upon the sore; it alleviates the sore.

3. For sleeplessness, take ooze of this same wort, smear the man with it, and soon thou sendest the sleep on him.

Many of the herbs named in the Herbarium were employed for other purposes than those for which they were used in later practice. Comfrey is recommended for one "bursten within." It was to be roasted in hot ashes and mixed with honey; then to be taken fasting. But nothing is said of its bone-setting property. Mullein, subsequently famous as a pectoral medicine, is recommended in the Herbarium as an external application in gout, and to carry about to prevent the attacks of wild beasts. Dill is prescribed as a remedy against local itching; fennel in cough and sore bladder; and madder for broken legs, which it would cure in three days.

To prevent sea-sickness the traveller had to smear himself with a mixture of pennyroyal and wormwood in oil and vinegar. Peony laid over a lunatic would soon cause him to upheave himself whole; and vervain or verbena if carried on the person would ensure a man from being barked at by dogs.

A Professed Translation.

The next document presented is the Medicina de Quadrupedibus of Sextus Placitus, an unknown personage, who adds to the interest of his narrative by pretending that "a king of the Egyptians, Idpartus he was highten," sent this treatise to the Emperor Octavius Cæsar, "for," he said, "I wist thee worthy of this." Probably this manuscript was not a translation at all; if it was, the pretended authors were almost certainly fictitious. Most of the instructions here given relate to the medicinal uses of animals. The idea that foxes' lungs will strengthen ours is hardly dead yet. Here it is in this old Saxon document:—

"For oppressive hard drawn breathing, a fox's lung sodden and put into sweetened wine, and administered, is wonderfully healthy."

The fox had many other uses. Foxes' grease would heal many kinds of sores. His sinews soaked in honey would cure a sore throat; his "naturam" wrapped round the head would banish headache; his "coillon" rubbed on warts would break them up and remove them; and dimness of sight could be relieved by his gall mingled with honey. The worst recipe is:

For disease of joints. Take a living fox and seethe him till the bones alone are left. Let the man go down therein frequently, and into another bath. Let him do so very oft. Wonderfully it healeth.

There are scores of cures from parts of animals, some of them very disgusting. A few more specimens of decent ones must suffice.

For oversleeping, a hare's brain in wine is given for a drink. Wonderfully it amendeth.

To get sleep a goat's horn laid under the head turneth waking into sleep.

For sleep lay a wolf's head under the pillow; the unhealthy shall sleep.

Let those who suffer apparitions eat lion's flesh; they will not after that suffer any apparition.

For any fracture, take a hound's brain laid upon wool and bind upon the broken place for fourteen days; then will it be firmly amended, and there shall be a need for a firmer binding up.

If thou frequently smearest and touchest children's gums with bitches' milk, the teeth wax without sore.

Various Leechdoms.

Some "Fly-Leaf Leechdoms" of unknown authorship follow. In these information concerning the four humours is given, hot and cold, moist and dry remedies are distinguished, and we are told of the forty-five dies caniculares "in which no leech can properly give aid to any sick man." It is carefully noted that the same disorder may occur from different causes, and quite scientifically the practitioner is advised to vary his treatment accordingly. Thus, for example, dealing with "host" (cough) we are told that "it hath a manifold access, as the spittles are various. Whilom it cometh of immoderate heat, whilom of immoderate cold, whilom of immoderate dryness." The remedies must depend on the causes of the complaint. The "tokens" of "a diseased maw" of "a half head's ache" (megrims) and of other distempers are set forth with graphic simplicity, and often sensible advice as to diet and medicine is given. But not infrequently the remedy may not be an easily procurable one. For instance "If one drink a creeping thing in water, let him cut open a sheep instantly and drink the sheep's blood hot"; and "if a man will eat rind which cometh out of Paradise no venom will damage him." The writer considerately adds that such rind is "hard gotten."

The following is apparently adapted from Alexander of Tralles, or some other of the later classical authors.

"Against gout and against the wristdrop; take the wort hermodactylus, by another name titulosa, that is in our own language the great crow leek; take this leek's heads and dry them thoroughly, and take thereof by weight of two and a half pennies, and pyrethrum and Roman rinds, and cummin, and a fourth part of laurel berries, and of the other worts, of by weight of a halfpenny, and six pepper corns, unweighed, and grind all to dust, and add wine two egg-shells full; this is a true leechcraft. Give it to the man to drink till that he be hole."

A few other recipes in the Leechbooks may be quoted:—

For headache take a vessel full of leaves of green rue, and a spoonful of mustard seed, rub together, add the white of an egg, a spoonful, that the salve may be thick. Smear with a feather on the side which is not sore.

For ache of half the head (megrim) take the red nettle of one stalk, bruise it, mingle with vinegar and the white of an egg, put all together, anoint therewith.

For mistiness of the eyes take juice of fennel and of rose and of rue, and of dumbledores' honey; (the dumbledore is apis bombinatrix); and kid's gall, mixed together. Smear the eyes with this. Again, take live periwinkles burnt to ashes; and let him mix the ashes with dumbledores' honey.

For sore and ache of ears take juice of henbane, make it lukewarm, and then drip it on the ear; then the sore stilleth. Or, take garlic and onion and goose fat, melt them together, squeeze them on the ear. Or, take emmets' eggs, crush them, squeeze them on the ear.

For the upper tooth ache:—Take leaves of withewind (convolvulus), wring them on the nose. For the nether tooth ache, slit with the tenaculum till they bleed.

For coughs, mugwort, marrubium, yarrow, red nettle, and other herbs are recommended generally boiled in ale, sometimes in milk.

Pock disease (small-pox) is dealt with, but not very seriously. It is of interest because the classical writers do not mention it. The Arab Rhazes wrote a treatise on it about A.D. 923. A few herb drinks are prescribed in the Leechbooks, and to prevent the pitting "one must delve away each pock with a thorn, then drip wine or alder drink within them, then they will not be seen."

Against lice:—One pennyweight of quicksilver and two of old butter.

Against itch:—Take ship tar, and ivy tar, and oil, rub together, add a third part of salt; smear with that.

In case a man should overdrink himself, let him drink betony in water before his other drink.

For mickle travelling over land, lest he tire, let him take mugwort to him in hand or put it in his shoe, lest he should weary, and when he will pluck it, before the upgoing of the sun, let him say these words, "I will take thee, artemisia, lest I be weary on the way." Sign it with the sign of the cross when thou pullest it up.

HELIAS TO ALFRED.

In one of the Leechbooks translated by Mr. Cockayne is found a letter on medicines from Helias, Patriarch of Jerusalem, to King Alfred the Great. Mr. Cockayne believes it to be authentic. There was a patriarch of that name at Jerusalem contemporary with Alfred, and the medicines he recommends are such as were obtainable in the Syrian drug shops at that date. It is to be presumed that the information was given in reply to a request for some recipes from the king. Helias recommends scammony, ammoniacum, gum dragon, aloes, galbanum, balsam, petroleum, triacle, and alabaster. Of petroleum he writes:—

"It is good to drink simple for inward tenderness, and to smear on outwardly on a winter's day, since it hath very much heat; hence one shall drink it in winter; and it is good if for anyone his speech faileth, then let him take it; and make the mark of Christ under his tongue, and swallow a little of it. Also if a man become out of his wits, then let him take part of it, and make Christ's mark on every limb, except the cross on the forehead, that shall be of balsam, and the other on the top of his head."

The patriarch had strong faith in Theriaca, and the directions he gives for its administration are minute, and would be explicit if he had only explained how much he meant by "a little bit."

"Theriaca," he says, "is a good drink for all inward tenderness, and the man who so behaves himself as is here said, he may much help himself. On the day on which he will drink Triacle he shall fast until midday, and not let wind blow on him that day; then let him go to the bath, let him sit there till he sweat; then let him take a cup, put a little warm water in it, then let him take a little bit of the triacle, and mingle with the water, and drain through some thin raiment, then drink it, and let him then go to his bed and wrap himself up warm, and so lie till he sweat well; then let him arise and sit up and clothe himself, and then take his meat at noon (three hours after midday), and protect himself earnestly against the wind that day; then I believe to God it will help the man much."

Early English Medical Practice.

In the thirteenth century Roger Bacon, the great man of science, wrote on medicine, alchemy, magic, and astrology, as well as most other sciences. He believed that a universal remedy was attainable, and urged Pope Clement IV to give his powerful aid to its discovery. Nothing particular remains of his medical studies.

Gilbert Anglicanus, who was a contemporary of Bacon, and wrote a Compendium of Medicine, a tedious collection of the most fantastic theories of disease, was more advanced in pharmacy than in the treatment of disease. He describes at considerable length the manner of extinguishing mercury to make an ointment, recommending particularly the addition of some mustard seed to facilitate the process. He gives particulars of the preparation of the oil of tartar per deliquium, and proposes a solution of acetate of ammonia in anticipation of Mindererus four hundred years later. Gilbert's formula is thus expressed:—

"Conteratur sal armoniacum minutim, et superinfundatur frequenter et paullatim acetum, et cooperiatur et moveatur, ut evanescet sal."

Ant's eggs, oil of scorpions, and lion's flesh is his prescription for apoplexy, but he does not explain how the last ingredient was to be obtained in England. Several of his formulas are quoted in the first London Pharmacopœia. For the expulsion of calculi he prescribes the blood of a young goat which has been fed on diuretic herbs such as persil and saxifrage.

Chaucer, whose writings belong to the latter half of the fourteenth century, has left on record a graphic picture of the "Doctour of Phisike" of his day, and the old poet is as gently sarcastic about his pilgrim's "science" as a writer of five hundred years later might have been. "He was grounded in astronomy," we are told, and—

> Well could he fortune the ascendant
>
> Of his images for his patient
>
> He knew the cause of every malady
>
> Were it of cold, or hot, or moist, or dry,
>
> And where engendered and of what humour.
>
> He was a very perfect practisour.

His library was a wonderful one considering the rarity of books at that time.

> Well knew he the olde Esculapius
>
> And Dioscorides, and eek Rufus
>
> Old Ypocras, Haly, and Galien,
>
> Serapyon, Razis, and Avicen,
>
> Averrois, Damascien, and Constantyn,
>
> Bernard, and Gatesden, and Gilbertyn.

The doctor was careful about his food, "his study was but little on the Bible," he dressed well, but was inclined to save in his expenses.

> He kept that he won in the pestilence.
>
> For gold in phisike is a cordialle
>
> There fore he loved gold in special.

The original of Chaucer's "Doctour of Phisike" has been sometimes supposed to have been the well-known John of Gaddesden, physician to Edward II, Professor of Medicine at Merton College, Oxford, a Prebendary of the Church, and the author of "Rosa Anglicana." This work, although full of absurdities and crude ideas of medicine and pharmacy, became the popular medical treatise in England, was translated into several European languages, and reprinted many times in this country during the two hundred years which followed its first appearance. The author named it the Rose, he says, because, as the rose has five sepals, his book is divided into five parts; and as the rose excels all other flowers, so his book is superior to all other treatises on medicine. It was probably published between 1310 and 1320.

John of Gaddesden's work well illustrates the pharmacy of the period, for he was great on drugs. He taught that aqua vitæ (brandy) was a polychrest, or complete remedy; that swines' excrement was a sovereign cure for hæmorrhage; that a sponge steeped in a mixture of vinegar, roses, wormwood, and rain-water, and laid on the stomach, would check vomiting and purging; that toothache and other pains might be cured by saying a Paternoster and an Ave for the souls of the father and mother of St. Phillip; a boar's bladder, taken when full of urine and dried in an oven, is recommended as a cure for epilepsy; a wine of fennel and parsley for blindness; and a mixture of whatever herbs came into his mind—for example, "apium, petroselinum, endive, scolopendron, chicory, liver-wort, scariola, lettuce, maidenhair, plantain, ivory shavings, sandal wood, violets, and vinegar"—is ordered as a digestive drink. Add to such senseless recipes as these a number of equally unintelligent charms, and a fair idea of the condition of medical science in England in the fourteenth century is obtained. It does not compare at all favourably with the condition to which the Arabs in Spain had elevated the art two and three hundred years before.

Bernard of Gordon, who wrote from Montpellier, but is believed to have been a Scotchman, was the author of the "Lilium Medicinæ," published about 1307 or 1309. The work was known to John of Gaddesden, for he quotes from it. Perhaps he had it in his mind when he observed that the rose excels all other flowers. Mainly it was a compilation from Arabic writers with the addition of many scholastic subtleties and astrological reveries. It is noticeable in this author and in John of Gaddesden how careful both are to distinguish between the treatment of the rich and the poor. The latter, for example, states that dropsy can be cured by spikenard, but he advises practitioners never to give this costly medicine without first receiving pay for it. Gordon recommends for a poor person's cough that he should be ordered to hold his breath frequently during the day for as long as possible, and if that does not cure he is to breathe fire.

John Mirfield also wrote his "Breviarium Bartholomei" in the latter part of the fourteenth century. Dr. Norman Moore in his "History of the Study of Medicine" has freely quoted from this old work, and gives several facsimile pages from some of the earliest manuscript copies of it. Dr. Moore regards the Breviarium with special interest as it is the first book on medicine in any way connected with his hospital, the oldest in London. Mirfield, relating some of the cures performed by his master, mentions that a woman came to him having lost her speech. The master rubbed her palate with some "theodoricon emperisticon" and with a little "diacostorium." She soon recovered. An apothecary brought a youth to the hospital with a carbuncle on his face, and his throat and neck swollen beyond belief. The master said the youth must go home to die. "Is there then no remedy?" asked the apothecary. The physician replied, "I believe most truly that if thou wert to give tyriacum in a large dose, there would be a chance that he might live." The apothecary gave two doses of ʒij. each, which caused a profuse perspiration, and in due course the youth recovered. He advises smelling and swallowing musk, aloes wood, storax, calamita, and amber to prevent infection in cold weather, and in warm weather sandal wood, roses, camphor, acetositas citri, sour milk, and vinegar, taking syrup of vinegar in the morning and syrup of violets at midday. For gout he prescribes an ointment the principal constituent of which is goose grease. The preparation of this remedy is explained metrically. The verses begin thus:—

> Anser sumatur, Veteranus qui videatur,
>
> Post deplumetur, Intralibus evacuetur.

Rheumatism was to be treated with olive oil, and the pharmacist is directed to warm it while he repeats the Psalm "Quare fremerunt gentes" as far as "Postula a me et dabo tibi gentes hereditatem tuam," then the Gloria and two prayers. This recitation was to be repeated seven times. There were no clocks available at that time, and this therefore was the method of prescribing the length of an operation. Dr. Moore says he finds this direction would cover about a quarter of an hour.

Medical treatises in verse were frequent and popular in England in the fourteenth and fifteenth centuries. There are several in the British Museum. A curious specimen is preserved in the Royal Library at Stockholm, and it is reproduced in readable English in "Archeologia," Vol. XXX, with notes by the translator, Mr. George Stephens, and by Dr. Pettigrew. They both believe it was written in the fourteenth century. It consists of 1485 lines. Of these it will suffice to give the first four, and one specimen of its sections. It begins thus:—

> In foure parties of amā
>
> Be gynneth ye sekenesse yt yie han
>
> In heed, in wombe, or i ye splene
>
> Or i bleddyr, yese iiij I mene.

The following is entitled in the margin "Hed werk."

    Amedicyn I hawe i Myde
    For hedwerk to telle as I fynde
    To taken eysyl pulyole ryale
    And camamyle to sethe wt all;
    And wt ye jous anoyte yi nosthryll well
    A make aplaister of ye toyerdel;
    And do it in a good grete clowte
    And wynde yi heed yer wt abowte;
    As soon as it be leyde yeron
    All yi hedwerk xal away gon.

Two other specimens of these early poetical recipes from other authors may be quoted:—

    ffor defhed of ye hed.

        For defhed of hed & for dullerynge
        I fynde wrete dyuers thynge
        Take oporcyon (a portion) of boiys vryne
        And mege it wt honey good & fyne
        And i ye ere late it caste
        Ye herynge schal amede in haste.

    ffor to slepe well

        Qwo so may not slepe wel
        Take egrimonye afayre del
        And ley it vnder his heed on nyth
        And it schall hym do slepe aryth
        For of his slepe schal he not wakyn
        Tyll it be fro vnder his heed takyn.

THE EARLY ENGLISH DRUG TRADE.

The development of pharmacy as a separate organisation was later in England than on the Continent, and was very gradual. In the Norman period the retail trade in drugs and spices and most other commodities was in the hands of the mercers. These were, in fact, general shopkeepers, deriving their designation from merx, merchandise. They attended fairs and markets, and in the few large towns had permanent booths. Under the Plantagenets a part of the south side of "Chepe" roughly extending from where is now Bow Church to Friday Street was occupied by their stores, and was known as the Mercery. Behind these booths were the meadows of Crownsild, sloping down to what it may be hoped was then the silvery Thames. Probably sheep and cattle fed on the pastures which Cannon Street and Upper Thames Street have since usurped.

But English traders were beginning to feel their feet, and other guilds were pushing forward. The Easterlings (East Germans from the Baltic coasts and the Hanse towns) brought goods from the East and placed them on the English market, and the Pepperers and Spicers distributed them to the public. The Easterlings, it may be mentioned, have left us the word sterling to commemorate their sojourn among us. The Mercers meanwhile were getting above the shop. They were becoming merchant adventurers, and had no desire to contest the trade in small things with the Pepperers of Sopers' Lane, or the Spicers of Chepe. Their other small wares fell into the hands of the Haberdashers.

There is evidence of a guild of Pepperers in London as early as 1180. As a company they appear to have been ruined by the demands of Edward III for subsidies for his French and Scottish campaigns. From their ashes, including those of the Spicerers, arose the Grocers, the sellers "en gros." They are heard of in the fourteenth century, and were apparently incorporated by letters patent from Edward III in 1345, but their first known charter was granted by Henry VI in 1429, while in 1453 that King conferred on them the charge of the King's beam, by which all imported merchandise was weighed, a charge of 1d. per 20 lbs. being authorised for the service. In 1457 they were given the exclusive power of garbling (cleansing and separating) drugs, spices, and other imported merchandise, and they also had the duty of examining the drugs and medicinal wares sold by the apothecaries. The law requiring certain drugs to be officially "garbled" before they could be sold was repealed by an Act passed in the sixth year of Queen Anne's reign.

The earliest record of the exercise of their authority over apothecaries is found in 1456, when the minutes of the Company show that they imposed a fine on John Ashfield "for making untrue powder of ginger, cinnamon, and saunders." Other similar items appear from time to time. In 1612 Mr.

Lownes, apothecary to Prince Charles, complained to the Company that Michael Easen, a grocer-apothecary, "had supplied him with divers defective apothecaries' wares," and the offender was committed to the Poultry Comptoir.

BUCKLERSBURY.

Bucklersbury was the centre and headquarters of the London drug trade, at least from the Tudor to the Hanoverian periods. Shakespeare in "The Merry Wives of Windsor" makes Falstaff refer to "the lisping hawthorn buds that come like women in men's apparel, and smell like Bucklersbury in sample time." Stow (1598) says of this thoroughfare that "This whole street on both sides throughout is possessed of grocers and apothecaries." Ben Jonson calls it "Apothecarie Street." This dramatist in "Westward Ho!" makes Mrs. Tenderhook say "Go into Bucklersbury and fetch me two ounces of preserved melons; look there be no tobacco taken in the shop when he weighs it." Later in a self-asserting poem to his bookseller, Ben Jonson says of one of his books, objecting to vulgar advertising methods,

> If without these vile arts it will not sell,
>
> Send it to Bucklersbury, there 'twill well.

In Charles II's reign Mouffet speaks of Bucklersbury being replete with physic, drugs, and spicery, and says it was so perfumed at the time of the plague with the pounding of spices, melting of gums, and making of perfumes, that it escaped that great plague. A quotation from Pennant in Cassell's "Old and New London" shows that in the reign of William III Bucklersbury was the resort of ladies of fashion to purchase teas, furs, and other Indian goods; and the king is said to have been angry with the queen for visiting these shops, which appear from some lines of Prior to have been sometimes perverted to places of intrigue.

The street acquired its name from a family called the Bokerells or Buckerells, who lived there in the thirteenth century. Stow gives a different account. He states that there was a tower in the street named Carnet's Tower, and that a grocery named Buckle who had acquired it was assisting in pulling it down, intending to erect a goodly frame of timber in its place, when a part fell on him, which so sore bruised him that it shortened his life.

A CHEMIST'S ADVERTISEMENT IN THE SEVENTEENTH CENTURY.

A London chemist's advertisement (about 1680–1690) runs thus:—

"Ambrose Godfrey Hanckwitz, chemist in London, Southampton Street, Covent Garden, continues faithfully to prepare all sorts of remedies, chemical and galenical. He hopes that his friends will continue their favours.

Good cordials can be procured at his establishment, as well as Royal English drops, and other articles such as Powders of Kent, Zell, and Contrajerva, Cordial red powder, Gaskoins powder, with and without bezoar, English smelling salts, true Glauber's salt, Epsom salt, and volatile salt of ammonia, stronger than the former. Human skull and hartshorn, essence of Ambergris, volatile essence of lavender, musk and citron, essence of viper, essence for the hair, vulnerary balsam, commendeur, balsam for apoplexy, red spirit of purgative cochliaria, spirit of white cochliaria, and others. Honey water, lavender water of two kinds, Queen of Hungary water, orange flower water, arquebusade.

"For the information of the curious, he is the only one in London who makes inflammable phosphorus, which can be preserved in water. Phosphorus of Bolognian stone, flowers of phosphorus, black phosphorus, and that made with acid oil, and other varieties. All unadulterated. Every description of good drugs he sells, wholesale and retail.

"Solid phosphorus, wholesale, 50s. an ounce, and retail, £3 sterling, the ounce."

THE ENGLISH APOTHECARIES.

Although the Grocers were the recognised drug dealers of this country, apothecaries who were associated in their Guild were also recognised. Some authorities name Richard Fitznigel as apothecary to Henry II before he was made Bishop of London. But this evidence cannot be trusted. The first definite allusion to an apothecary in England occurs in 1345, when Edward III granted a pension of sixpence a day for life to Coursus de Gangeland, an apothecary of London, in recognition of his services in attending on the king during his illness in Scotland. The record of this grant is found in Rymer's "Foedera," which was not published until 1704, but Rymer was historiographer royal, appointed by William III, and his work was a compilation from official archives. An earlier mention of an apothecary is found in the Scottish Exchequer Rolls wherein it appears that on the death of Robert the Bruce, in 1329, payments were made to John the Apothecary, presumably for materials for embalming the king's body. Dr. J. Mason Good, who wrote a "History of Medicine, so far as it relates to the Profession of the Apothecary," in 1795, mentions, on the authority of Regner, that J. de Falcand de Luca publicly vended medicines in London in 1357, while Freind ("History of Medicine," 1725) states that Pierre de Montpellier was appointed Apothecary to Edward III in 1360.

It is clear, therefore, that the apothecary was a familiar professional personage in England five hundred years ago. Conclusive evidence of his practice is given by Chaucer, who, in the Prologue to the "Canterbury Tales" (written in the last quarter of the fourteenth century), describing a "Doctour of Phisike" says—

> Ful reddy hadde he his apothecaries
>
> To send him dragges and his lettuaries
>
> For eche of hem made other for to Winne.

The satirical suggestion of the mutual obligations of physicians and apothecaries has been familiar for all these centuries.

It seems certain that in Henry VIII's reign the apothecaries were doing a considerable amount of medical practice, besides selling drugs. The Act of 1511 incorporating the College of Physicians and giving them the exclusive right to practise physic in London and for seven miles round, was largely used, if not intended, against apothecaries. In 1542, however, an Act was passed which rather modified the severe restrictions of the original statute, and under the new law apothecaries became more aggressive. In Mary's reign the Physicians again got the legislative advantage, and there is a record in the archives of the College of Physicians (preserved by Dr. Goodall, who wrote "A History of the Proceedings of the College against Empiricks," in 1684) stating that in Queen Elizabeth's reign the President and Censors of the College summoned the Wardens of the Grocers' Company and all the apothecaries of London and the suburbs to appear before them, "and enjoyned them that when they made a dispensation of medicine they should expose their several ingredients (of which they were composed) to open view in their shops for six or eight days that so the physicians passing by might judge of the goodness of them, and prevent their buying or selling any corrupt or decayed medicines." The grocers and apothecaries do not appear to have raised any objection to this decree. Whether they obeyed it or not is not stated.

INCORPORATION OF THE APOTHECARIES.

The first Charter of Incorporation was granted to the apothecaries by James I in 1606, but this did not separate them from their old foes, the grocers. They continued their efforts, however, and with the aid of friends at Court they obtained a new Charter in 1617, which gave them an entirely independent existence as a City Guild under the title of the Society of the Apothecaries. This is the only London guild which has from its incorporation to the present time admitted only actual apothecaries to its fraternity.

Another peculiarity claimed by one of the Company's historians (Dr. J. Corfe: "The Apothecary") is that the Guild of Apothecaries is the only City Company which is called a Society. He believes that this may be attributed to the supposed fact that the corporation was modelled on a similar association founded at Naples in 1540 under the name of Societa Scientifica.

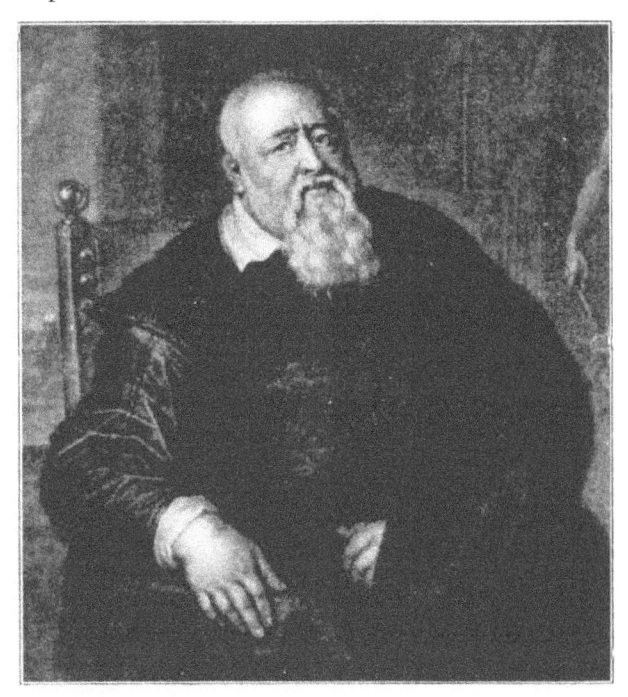

Sir Theodore Mayerne.

> The original painting by Rubens, of which the above is a copy, was in the collection of Dr. Mead, and was sold in 1754 for £115. It passed into the possession of the Earl of Bessborough and the Marquis of Lansdowne, and then through the hands of some dealers, and in 1848 was bought by the Royal College of Physicians for £33 12*s*.

Sir Theodore de Mayerne, the King's first physician, and Gideon de Laune, pharmacien or apothecary to the Queen, Anne of Denmark, were the supporters of the apothecaries in rescuing them from the control of the grocers. Both of these men deserve honourable mention in the chronicles of British pharmacy. It happens that both were of foreign origin and of the Protestant faith, two of that eminent crowd of immigrants of high principle and distinguished ability who served England so well in the seventeenth century when they found themselves "not wanted" in France.

Mayerne was a Swiss by birth, but a Frenchman by education and adoption, and had been physician to Henri IV. But he incurred the bitter animosity of the Paris Faculty, led by the fanatic Gui Patin, partly on account of his religious heresy, and partly because he prescribed chemical medicines. By a unanimous vote the Paris College of Physicians resolved in 1603 that he must not be met by any of its members in consultation. He continued, however, to practise in Paris until an English peer whom he had treated took him to London and introduced him to James I, who made him physician to the Queen. Mayerne, however, soon returned to Paris, but in 1611 he settled in London on the invitation of the King, who made him his first physician. He had a great deal to do with the compilation of the first London Pharmacopœia, and is reputed to have introduced calomel and black wash into medical practice. Subsequently he was appointed physician to Charles I and Queen Henriette, but after the execution of the King he retired into private life, and though nominally physician to Charles II he never practised at that Court. He died at Chelsea in 1665.

Gideon de Laune was also a man of considerable influence. Dr. Corfe regards him as almost the founder of the Society of Apothecaries, but Mr. Barrett, who recently wrote a history of that Society, suggests that he could not have been so much thought of by his contemporaries, as he was only elected to the Mastership some years after the Charter had been granted, and then only after a contest. At any rate the apothecaries must have largely owed the Charter to his influence. He lived in Blackfriars and called himself a "Pharmacopœius," but we also read of him as an importer of drugs, and it is probable that he traded as a merchant. That he was a man of position is evident from the fact that on one occasion he fetched the Queen, Anne of Denmark, from Norway.

Gideon de Laune was born at Rheims in 1565, and was brought to England as a boy by his father, who was a Protestant pastor. A Nonconformist writer of the same surname who got into trouble in the reigns of Charles II and James II, and was befriended by De Foe, referring to Gideon as a relative, says of him that when he died at the age of 97 he had near as many thousands of pounds as he had years; that he had thirty-seven children by one wife; and that his funeral was attended by sixty grandchildren. It has been ascertained, however, that his children only numbered seventeen, and that he died at the age of 94; so that the later De Laune who wrote in 1681 cannot be implicitly relied upon when figures are concerned. Another thing he tells us of Gideon is that "his famous pill is in great request to this day notwithstanding the swarms of pretenders to pill-making."

The Grocers' Company warmly resented the secession of the apothecaries who had been their subordinate partners so long, but their formal petition of complaint called forth a cruel snub from the King. Grocers were but merchants, said James, the business of the apothecaries was a mystery; "Wherefore I think it fitting they should be a corporation of themselves." The grocers, however, got some of their own back a few years later when

James demanded a subsidy from the city for the relief of the Palatinate. The grocers and the apothecaries were assessed at £500 between them. Towards this the apothecaries, pleading poverty, offered £20. The grocers ridiculed this offer, and having paid £300 as their share, left their old associates to find the other £200, which they had to do somehow.

About the same time the new corporation vigorously opposed an application for a Charter made by the distillers of London. The grocers supported the distillers, and the apothecaries failed in their opposition. Sir Theodore Mayerne told them that their monopoly of distillation was only intended to extend to the distillation of medicinal spirits and waters. Mr. Barrett quotes from the old records another curious instance of the contest for monopolies which was characteristic of the period. In 1620, one John Woolf Rumbler having obtained from the King a concession of the sole right of making "mercuric sublimate," applied to the Court of Apothecaries that he might enjoy the same without their contradiction. This "upon advised consideration," the Court refused to grant. It is not stated whether the will of the King or that of the apothecaries prevailed in the end.

The story of the jealousies which arose between the physicians and the apothecaries is a long and tedious one; innumerable pamphlets were written on both sides of the controversy, and the dispute figures in English literature of the seventeenth and eighteenth centuries. Pope very neatly expressed the views of the physicians in the familiar verse in the "Essay on Criticism" in which, comparing the old critics of Greece who "fanned the poet's fire, And taught the world with reason to admire," with those of his own day who

> Against the poets their own arms they turned
> Sure to hate most the men from whom they learn'd,

illustrated the position by introducing the

> Modern pothecaries, taught the art
> By doctors' bills to play the doctors' part,
> Bold in the practice of mistaken rules,
> Prescribe, apply, and call their masters fools.

This was written in 1709.

The apothecaries strengthened their position as medical practitioners in the public esteem by remaining at their posts during the Great Plague in London in 1665 when most of the physicians fled from the stricken city. Between this date and the end of the seventeenth century the quarrel between the two sections of the profession constantly grew in bitterness. Some of the allegations of extortion made against the apothecaries are almost incredible. In Dr. Goodall's "Historical Account of the Proceedings of the Royal College of Physicians against Empiricks and Unlicensed Practisers" (1684), it is reported that George Buller who gave the college some trouble in 1633 had charged 30s. each for 25 pills; £37 10s. for the boxful. Three were given to a Mrs. Style for a sore leg, and she died the same night. A Dr. Tenant prosecuted by the college in James I's reign "was so impudent and unconscionable in the rating of his medicines that he charged £6 for one pill and the same for an apozeme."

Dr. R. Pitt, F.R.S., in "Crafts and Frauds of Physic Exposed," 1703 (a book written expressly to defend the establishment of dispensaries by the Physicians), states that apothecaries had been known to make £150 out of a single case, and that in a recent instance (which had apparently come before the law courts) the apothecary had made £320. In every bill of £100 Dr. Pitt says the charges were £90 more than the shop prices for the medicine.

In Jacob Bell's "Historical Sketch of the Progress of Pharmacy in Great Britain" an apothecary's bill for medicines for one day, supplied to a Mr. Dalby of Ludgate Hill, is quoted from a pamphlet called "The Wisdom of the Nation is Foolishness." It is as follows:

> An Emulsion, 4s. 6d. A Mucilage, 3s. 4d. Gelly of Hartshorn, 4s. Plaster to dress Blister, 1s. An Emollient Glister, 2s. 6d. An ivory pipe, armed 1s. A Cordial Bolus, 2s. 6d. The same again, 2s. 6d. A cordial draught, 2s. 4d. The same again, 2s. 4d. Another bolus, 2s. 6d. Another draught, 2s. 4d. A glass of cordial spirits, 3s. 6d. Blistering plaster to the arm, 5s. The same to the wrists, 5s. Two boluses again, 5s. Two draughts again, 4s. 8d. Another emulsion, 4s. 6d. Another pearl julep, 4s. 6d.

Mr. Dalby's bill for five days came to £17 2s. 10d., and this was declared to be not an isolated case but illustrative of the practice of apothecaries when attending patients of the higher classes.

Contest between the Physicians and Apothecaries.

In 1687 the College of Physicians adopted a resolution binding all Fellows, Candidates, and Licentiates of the College to give advice gratis to their neighbouring sick poor when desired within the city of London or seven miles round. But in view of the gross extortions of the apothecaries it was asked, What was the use of the physicians' charity if the cost of compounding the medicines was to be prohibitory? The apothecaries, of course, denied that the examples of their charges which were quoted were at all general, and probably they were not. It was not to the interest of the apothecaries to destroy free prescribing. Indeed a proposal was made to the physicians on behalf of a numerous body of London apothecaries to accept a tariff for medicines dispensed for the poor to be fixed by the physicians themselves.

The relations of the two bodies had become, however, so strained that arrangement was no longer possible. The apothecaries had in fact obtained the upper hand. They treated many cases themselves, and calling in the physician was largely within their discretion. At this time (about 1700) the ordinary fee paid to a physician was 10*s*. University graduates expected more, but they too, in the majority of cases, were only too glad to take the half sovereign, and it was alleged that they would sometimes pay the apothecary who called them a percentage off this.

Such was the condition of affairs when in 1696 an influential section of the physicians, fifty-three of them, associated themselves in the establishment of Dispensaries, where medicines should be compounded and supplied to the poor at cost price. The fifty-three subscribed ten pounds each, and Dispensaries were opened at the College premises in Warwick Lane, in St. Martin's Lane, and St. Peter's Alley, Cornhill.

Needless to say, the war now waxed fiercer than ever. The physicians were divided among themselves, and the anti-dispensarians refused to meet the dispensarians in consultation. The apothecaries naturally recommended the anti-dispensarians to their patients, and consequently it was only the independent ones who could afford to maintain the struggle. Scurrilous pamphlets were written on both sides, and one long poem, Garth's Dispensary, which was less venomous than most of the literature on the subject, but which as a poem had no merits which could justify the reputation it attained, complicated the struggle from the physicians' point of view. Johnson says that in addition to its intrinsic merit it "co-operated with passions and prejudices then prevalent." His sympathies are indicated by his remark that "it was on the side of charity against the intrigues of interest, and of regular learning against licentious usurpation of medical authority." One line in the book (the last in the passage quoted below) has attained currency in the English language. Expressing satirically the complaints of the apothecaries, Garth says:

> Our manufactures now the doctors sell,
>
> And their intrinsic value meanly tell;
>
> Nay, they discover too (their spite is such)
>
> That health, than crowns more valued, costs not much;

Whilst we must shape our conduct by these rules,

To cheat as tradesmen or to fail as fools.

The Apothecaries Win.

Notwithstanding the sympathy of Dr. Johnson, Pope, and many other famous contemporaries, the quarrel ended in the comparative triumph of the apothecaries.

The physicians, though reluctant to enforce what they believed to be their statutory powers, were goaded into law, and at last brought an action against a London apothecary named William Rose, who they alleged had infringed the Act passed in the reign of Henry VIII. Rose had attended a butcher in St. Martin's-in-the-Fields named Seale, and had administered "proper medicines" to him. He had no licence from the Faculty, and in his treatment of Seale had not acted under the direction of any physician. He had neither taken nor demanded any fee for his advice.

Those were the facts found by the jury who first heard the case. The College claimed a penalty of five pounds per month for the period during which Rose had thus practised. The Charter granted to the physicians in the tenth year of Henry VIII, and confirmed by an Act of Parliament passed in the fourteenth and fifteenth year of that reign, contained a clause forbidding any person not admitted by the College to practise the faculty of medicine in London or within seven miles thereof under a penalty of one hundred solidi for every month during which he should thus infringe the law.

The jury having found the facts already quoted, referred to the Court of Queen's Bench the legal question whether the acts performed constituted the practice of medicine within the meaning of the Act. The case was argued three times in the Court of Queen's Bench—(so it is stated in the report of the proceedings in the House of Lords),—and ultimately the judges decided unanimously in favour of the contention of the College. Thereupon, on behalf of Rose a writ of error was moved for in the House of Lords demanding a reversal of the judgment. The counsel who argued the appeal were S. Dodd for Rose, and F. Brown for the College. The case was heard on the 15th of March, 1703.

In support of the appeal it was argued that if the judgment were allowed to stand it would ruin not only Rose but all other apothecaries. That the Act was a very old one, and that the constant usage and practice ought to be taken into account. That if this judgment were right the apothecary would not dare to sell a few lozenges or a little electuary to any person asking for a remedy for a cold, or in other common cases where a medicine had a known and certain effect. That to give a monopoly in the treatment of disease to physicians would have most mischievous consequences; both rich and poor would be seriously taxed, and in the case of sudden accidents or illnesses in the night when apothecaries were so frequently sent for, the danger of not permitting them to supply the necessary medicine might often be most serious.

To these contentions the counsel for the College replied that by several orders physicians had bound themselves to attend the poor free, either at their own offices, or, if sent for, at the patient's house. That out of consideration for the poor they had gone further by establishing Dispensaries where the medicines they prescribed could be obtained at not more than one-third of the price which the apothecaries had been in the habit of charging. That in sudden emergencies an apothecary or anyone else was justified in doing his best to relieve his neighbours, but that in London, at least, a skilled physician was as available as an apothecary, and that this emergency argument ought not to be used to permit apothecaries to undertake all sorts of serious diseases at their leisure. That there was nothing to prevent apothecaries selling whatever medicines they were asked for, but that to permit them to treat cases however slight involved both danger and expense, because a mistake made at the beginning of a distemper might lead to a long illness, and in any case the apothecary would charge for much more medicine than was necessary.

After hearing the arguments "it was ordered and adjudged that the judgment given in the Court of Queen's Bench be reversed."

THE APOTHECARIES AND THE CHEMISTS AND DRUGGISTS.

From this period the apothecaries became recognised medical practitioners, the Society granted medical diplomas, and a hundred years later (1815) they obtained an Act which gave them powers against other persons similar to those which the physicians thought they possessed against them. Persons not qualified by them were forbidden to "act or practise as apothecaries" under a penalty of £20; and the courts have held that to practise as an apothecary is to judge of internal disease by symptoms, and to supply medicine to cure that disease. The chemists and druggists who had largely succeeded to the old business of the apothecaries opposed this provision, and the apothecaries, to buy off their opposition, offered to insert a clause in their Act which would allow all persons who should at that time or thereafter carry on that business to do so "as fully and amply to all intents and purposes as they might have done in case this Act had not been made." The chemists were not content with this provision, and drafted another which defined their business as consisting in the "buying, preparing, compounding, dispensing and vending drugs, and medicinal compounds, wholesale and retail." The apothecaries accepted this alteration, and subsequently obtained penalties from chemists who had prescribed remedies for customers. Such prescribing would have been legal if the druggists had accepted the provision proposed by the apothecaries; but they had limited themselves out of it. In the actions which the Society of Apothecaries have brought against chemists the apothecaries have often reproduced with scrupulous fidelity the arguments used against themselves by the physicians in Rose's case.

The Dispensaries established by the physicians were not long maintained, but apparently they provided the material of the modern chemist and druggist. "We have reason to believe," writes Jacob Bell in his Historical Sketch of the Progress of Pharmacy in Great Britain, "that the Assistants employed and instructed by the Physicians at these institutions became dispensing chemists on their own account; and that some of the apothecaries who found their craft in danger followed the example, from which source we may date the origin of the chemists and druggists."

In the course of the eighteenth century chemists and druggists had to a large extent replaced apothecaries as keepers of shops where medicines were sold and dispensed, and even when the businesses were owned by apothecaries, they usually styled themselves chemists and druggists. In the year 1841 an attempt was made to get a Bill through Parliament which would have made it penal to recommend any medicine for the sake of gain. The Bill was introduced by a Mr. Hawes, and the chemists and druggists of London opposed it with such vigour that it was ultimately withdrawn. In order to be prepared against future attacks the victorious chemists and druggists then formed the Pharmaceutical Society of Great Britain, which was incorporated by Royal Charter in 1842. An Act protecting the title of pharmaceutical chemist was passed in 1852, and in 1868 another Act, requiring all future chemists and druggists to pass examinations and be registered, and restricting to them the sale of poisons, became law.

IX
MAGIC AND MEDICINE

"Amulets and things to be borne about I find prescribed, taxed by some, approved by others. Look for them in Mizaldus, Porta, Albertus, etc. A ring made with the hoof of an ass's right forefoot, carried about, etc. I say, with Renodeus, they are not altogether to be rejected. Piony doth help epilepsies. Pretious stones most diseases. A wolf's dung carried about helps the cholick. A spider an ague, etc. Such medicines are to be exploded that consist of words, characters, spells, and charms, which can do no good at all, but out of a strong conceit, as Pomponatious proves, or the devil's policy, that is the first founder and teacher of them."

BURTON: "Anatomy of Melancholy."

Charms, enchantments, amulets, incantations, talismans, phylacteries, and all the armoury of witchcraft and magic have been intimately mixed up with pharmacy and medicine in all countries and in all ages. The degradation of the Greek term pharmakeia from its original meaning of the art of preparing medicine to sorcery and poisoning is evidence of the prevalence of debasing superstitions in the practice of medicine among the cultivated Greeks. Hermes the Egyptian, Zoroaster the Persian, and Solomon the Hebrew were famous among the early practitioners and teachers of magic. These names served to conjure with. Those who bore them were probably wise men above the average who were above such tricks as were attributed to them. But it suited the purpose or the business of those who made their living out of the superstitions of the people to pretend to trace their practices to universally revered heroes of a dim past.

Not that the whole of the magical rites associated with the art of healing were based on conscious fraud. The beliefs of savage or untutored races in demons which cause diseases is natural, it may almost be said reasonable. What more natural when they see one of their tribe seized with an epileptic fit than to assume the presence of an invisible foe? Or if a contagious plague or small-pox or fever attacks their village, is it not an inevitable conclusion that angry spirits have attacked the tribe, perhaps for some unknown offence? From such a basis the idea of sacrifice to the avenging fiend follows obviously. In some parts of China if a person accidentally kicks a stone and soon afterwards falls ill the relatives go to that stone and offer fruit, wine, or other treasures, and it may be that the patient recovers. In that case the efficacy of the treatment is demonstrated, and only those who do not desire to believe will question it; if the patient should die the proof is not less conclusive of the demon's malignity.

In some primitive peoples, among the New Zealand natives, for example, it is believed that a separate demon exists for each distinct disease; one for ague, one for epilepsy, one for toothache, and so forth. This too, seems reasonable. Each of those demons has something which will please or frighten him. So amulets, talismans, charms come into use. The North American Indians, however, generally attribute all disease to one evil spirit only. Consequently, their treatment of all complaints is the same.

Egyptian, Jewish, and Arabic Magic.

The Egyptians, according to Celsus, believed that there were thirty-six demons or divinities in the air, to each of whom was attributed a separate part or organ of the human body. In the event of disease affecting one of these parts the priest-physician invoked the demon, calling him by his name, and requiring him in a special form of words to cure the afflicted part.

Solomon was credited among many Eastern people with having discovered many of the secrets of controlling diseases by magical processes. According to Josephus he composed and bequeathed to posterity a book of these magical secrets. Hezekiah is said to have suppressed this work because it was leading the people to pray to other powers than Jehovah. But some of the secrets of Solomon were handed down in certain families by tradition. Josephus relates that a certain Jew named Eleazor drew a demon from the nose of a possessed person in the presence of the Emperor Vespasian and a number of Roman officers, by the aid of a magic ring and a form of invocation. In order to prove that the demon thus expelled had a real separate existence, he ordered it to upset a vessel of water which stood on the floor. This was done. Books professing to give Solomon's secrets were not uncommon among Christians as well as Jews. Goethe alluded to such a treatise in "Faust" in the line

> Für solche halbe Höllenbrut, Ist Salomoni's Schlüssel gut.

Throughout their history the Jewish people have studied and practised magic as a means of healing. According to the Book of Enoch the daughters of men were instructed in "incantations, exorcisms, and the cutting of roots" by the sons of God who came to earth and associated with them. The Greeks and Romans always held Jewish sorcery in the highest esteem, and the Arabs accepted their teaching with implicit confidence. The Talmud is full of magical formulas, and the Kaballah, a mystic theosophy which combined Israelitish traditions with Alexandrian philosophy, and began to be known about the tenth century, was unquestionably the foundation of the sophistry of Paracelsus and his followers.

In the Middle Ages, and in some communities until quite recent times, belief in the occult powers of Jews, which they had themselves inculcated, was firm and universal, and became the reason, or at least the excuse, for much of the persecution they had to suffer. For the punishment of sorcery and witchcraft was not based on a belief that fraud had been practised, but resulted from a conviction of the terrible truth of the claims which had been put forward.

The Jews of Western Europe have lost or abandoned many of the traditional practices which have been associated with their popular medicines from time immemorial. But in the East, especially in Turkey and Syria, quaint prayers and antiquated materia medica are still associated as they were in the days of the Babylonian captivity. Dogs' livers, earthworms, hares' feet, live ants, human bones, doves' dung, wolves' entrails, and powdered mummy still rank high as remedies, while for patients who can afford it such precious products as dew from Mount Carmel are prescribed. Invocations, prayers, and superstitious practices form the stock in trade of the "Gabbetes," generally elderly persons who attend on the sick. They have a multitude of infallible cures in their repertoires. Powdered, freshly roasted earthworms in wine, or live grasshoppers in water, are given by them for biliousness. For bronchial complaints they write some Hebrew letters on a new plate, wash it off with wine, add three grains of a citron which has been used at the Tabernacle festival, and give this as a draught. Dogs' excrements made up with honey form a poultice for sore eyes, mummy or human bones ground up with honey is a precious tonic, and wolves' liver is a cure for fits. But the administration of these remedies must be accompanied by the necessary invocation, generally to the names of patriarchs, angels, or prophets, but often mere gibberish, such as "Adar, gar, vedar, gar," which is the formula for use with a toothache remedy.

The phylacteries still worn by modern Jews at certain parts of their services, now perhaps by most of them only in accordance with inveterate custom, have been in all ages esteemed by them as protecting them against evil and demoniac influences. They are leathern receptacles, which they bind on their left arms and on their foreheads in literal obedience to the Mosaic instructions in the passages transcribed, and contained in the cases, from Exodus c. 13, v. 1–10, and c. 13, v. 11–16, Deuteronomy c. 6, v. 4–9, and c. 9, v. 13–21. To a modern reader these passages appear to protest against superstitions and heathenish beliefs and practices, but the rabbis and scribes taught that these and the mesuza, the similar passages affixed to the doorposts, would avert physical and spiritual dangers, and they invented minute instructions for the preparation of the inscriptions. A scribe, for example, who had commenced to write one of the passages, was not to allow himself to be interrupted by any human distraction, not even if the king asked him a question.

All the eastern nations trusted largely to amulets of various kinds for the prevention and treatment of disease. Galen quotes from Nechepsus, an Egyptian king, who lived about 630 B.C., who wrote that a green jasper cut in the form of a dragon surrounded by rays, applied externally would cure indigestion and strengthen the stomach. Among the books attributed to Hermes was one entitled "The Thirty-six Herbs Sacred to Horoscopes." Of this book Galen says it is only a waste of time to read it. The title, however, as Leclerc has pointed out, rather curiously confirms the statement attributed to Celsus which is found in Origen's treatise, "Contra Celsum," to which allusion has already been made.

Amulets are still in general use in the East. Bertherand in "Medicine of the Arabs" says the uneducated Arab of to-day when he has anything the matter with him goes to his priest and pays him a fee for which the priest gives him a little paper about two inches square on which certain phrases are written. This is put up in a leathern case, and worn as near the affected part as is possible. The richer Arab women wear silver cases with texts from the Koran in them. But it is essential that the paper must have been written on a Friday, a little before sunset, and with ink in which myrrh and saffron have been dissolved.

In the Third Report of the Wellcome Research Laboratories at the Gordon Memorial College, Khartoum (London: Baillière, Tindall, & Cox, 1908), Dr. R. G. Anderson writes an interesting chapter on the medical superstitions of the people of Kordofan, and gives a number of illustrations of amulets and written charms actually in use by the Arabs of that country. "To the native," says Dr. Anderson, "no process is too absurd for belief, and often, within his limits, no price too high to accomplish a cure." Most of them wear talismans of some kind. Some of them spend a great part of their scanty earnings on charms to cure some chronic disease, stone in the bladder, for example. The son of the late Mahdi presented to Dr. Anderson a charm which his father wore round the arm above the elbow, designed against evil spirits and the evil eye. It consisted of a square case containing a written charm, and a bag filled with a preparation of roots. The charms worn by the natives generally consist of quotations from the Koran, often repeated many times and with signs of the great prophets interspersed. The principal of these signs are the following:—

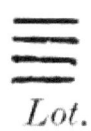

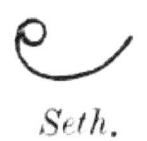

Solomon.

Enoch.

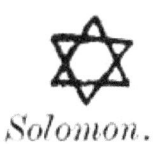

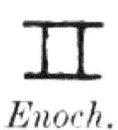

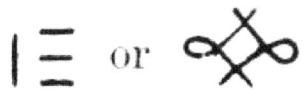

David.

Lot.

Seth.

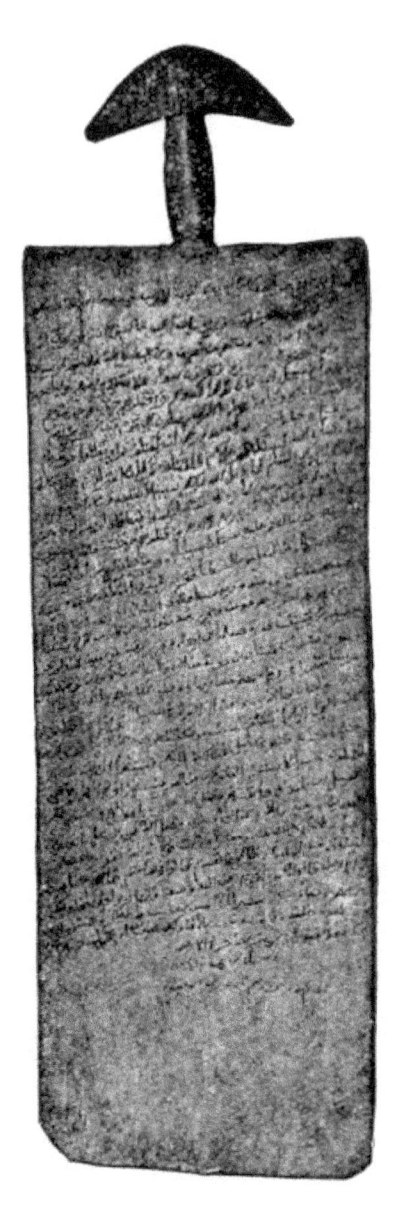

"Lohn" (or Writing Board).

The annexed illustration has been kindly lent by Mr. Wellcome (on behalf of the Gordon Memorial College) from the Report mentioned above. It represents a "Lohn," or writing board on which Koranic phrases or mystic inscriptions have been written by Fikis (holy men). When the writing is dry it is washed off and the fluid is taken internally or applied externally.

THE ABRACADABRA MYSTERY.

Abracadabra was the most famous of the ancient charms or talismans employed in medicine. Its mystic meaning has been the subject of much ingenious investigation, but even its derivation has not been agreed upon. The first mention of the term is found in the poem "De Medicina Praecepta Saluberrima," by Quintus Serenus Samonicus. Samonicus was a noted physician in Rome in the second and third centuries. He was a favourite with the Emperor Severus, and accompanied him in his expedition to Britain A.D. 208. Severus died at York in A.D. 211, and in the following year his son Caracalla had his brother Geta, and 20,000 other people supposed to be favourable to Geta's claims, assassinated. Among the victims was Serenus Samonicus. The poem, which is the only existing work of Serenus, consists of 1,115 hexameter lines which illustrate the medical practice and superstitions of the period when it was written. The lines in which the word "Abracadabra," and the way to employ it are introduced are these:—

> Inscribis chartae, quod dicitur Abracadabra,
>
> Saepius: et subter repetas, sed detrahe summae,
>
> Et magis atque magis desint elementa figuris
>
> Singula, quae semper rapies et coetera figes,
>
> Donec in angustam redigatur litera conum.
>
> His lino nexis collum redimire memento.

In a paper on Serenus Samonicus by Dr. Barnes of Carlisle, contributed to the *St. Louis Medical Review*, the following translation of the above passage is given. A semitertian fever of a particular character is the disease under discussion.

"Write several times on a piece of paper the word 'Abracadabra,' and repeat the word in the lines below, but take away letters from the complete word and let the letters fall away one at a time in each succeeding line. Take these away ever, but keep the rest until the writing is reduced to a narrow cone. Remember to tie these papers with flax and bind them round the neck."

The charm was written in several ways all in conformity with the instructions. Dr. Barnes gives these specimens:

```
ABRACADABRA    abracadabra
 ABRACADABR    abracadabr
  ABRACADAB    abracadab
   ABRACADA    abracada
    ABRACAD    abracad
     ABRACA    abraca     ABRACADABRA
      ABRAC    abrac       BRACADABR
       ABRA    abra         RACADAB
        ABR    abr           ACADA
         AB    ab             CAD
          A    a               A
```

After wearing the charm for nine days it had to be thrown over the shoulder into a stream running eastwards. In cases which resisted this talisman Serenus recommended the application of lion's fat, or yellow coral with green emeralds tied to the skin of a cat and worn round the neck.

Serenus Samonicus is believed to have been a disciple of a notorious Christian heretic named Basilides, who lived in the early part of the second century, and was himself the founder of a sect branching out of the gnostics. Basilides had added to their beliefs some fanciful notions based on the teachings of Pythagoras and Apollonius of Tyre, especially in regard to names and numbers. To him is attributed the invention of the mystic word "abraxas," which in Greek numeration represents the total 365, thus:—a—1, b—2, r—100, a—1, x—60, a—1, s—200. This word is supposed to have been a numeric representation of the Persian sungod, or if it was invented by Basilides, more likely indicated the 365 emanations of the infinite Deity. It has been generally supposed that abracadabra was derived from abraxas.

There are, however, other interpretations. Littré associates it with the Hebrew words, Ab, Ruach, Dabar; Father, Holy Ghost, Word. Dr. King, an authority on the curious gnostic gems well-known to antiquarians, regards this explanation as purely fanciful and suggests that Abracadabra is a modification of the term Ablathanabla, a word frequently met with on the gems alluded to, and meaning Our Father, Thou art Our Father. Others hold that Ablathanabla is a corruption of Abracadabra. An ingenious correspondent of *Notes and Queries* thinks that a more likely Hebrew origin of the term than the one favoured by Littré would be Abrai seda brai, which would signify Out, bad spirit, out. It is agreed that the word should be pronounced Abrasadabra. Another likely origin, suggested by Colonel C. R. Conder in "The Rise of Man" (1908), p. 314, is Abrak-ha-dabra, a Hebrew phrase meaning "I bless the deed." The triangular form of the charm was no doubt significant of the Trinity in Unity.

Greek and Roman Magic.

Pythagoras taught that holding dill in the left hand would prevent epilepsy. Serapion of Alexandria (B.C. 278) prescribed for epilepsy the warty excrescences on the forelegs of animals, camel's brain and gall, rennet of seal, dung of crocodile, blood of turtle, and other animal products. Pliny alludes to a tradition, that a root of autumnal nettle would cure a tertian fever, provided that when it is dug the patient's name and his parent's names are pronounced aloud; that the longest tooth of a black dog worn as an amulet would cure quartan fever; that the snout and tips of the ears of a mouse, the animal itself to run free, wrapped in a rose coloured patch, also worn as an amulet, would similarly cure the same disease; the right eye of a living lizard wrapped in a piece of goat's skin; and a herb picked from the head of a statue and tied up with red thread, are other specimens of the amulets popular in his time. But Pliny appears to doubt if all these treatments can be trusted. He mentions one, that is that the heart of a hen placed on a woman's left breast while she is asleep will make her tell all her secrets, and this he characterizes as a portentous lie. Mr. Cockayne quoting this, remarks dryly, "Perhaps he had tried it." Alexander of Tralles recommends a number of amulets, some of which he mentions he has proved. Thus for colic he names the dung of a wolf with some bits of bone in it in a closed tube worn on the right arm or thigh; an octagonal iron ring on which are engraved the words "Flee, flee, ho, ho, Bile, the lark was searching" good for bilious disorders; for gout, gather henbane when the moon is in Aquarius or Pisces before sunset with the thumb and third finger of the left hand, saying at the time an invocation inviting the holy herb to come to the house of blank and cure M. or N.; with a lot more.

The Greeks named the Furies Eumenides, good people, evidently with the idea of propitiating them. For a similar reason fairies were known as good folk by our ancestors.

English Folk-Lore Superstitions.

It would be as tedious as it would be useless to relate at any length the multitude of silly superstitions which make up the medicinal folk-lore of this and other countries. Methods of curing warts, toothache, ague, worms, and other common complaints are familiar to everyone. The idea that toothache is caused by tiny worms which can be expelled by henbane, is very ancient and still exists. A process from one of the Anglo-Saxon Leechdoms converted into modern English by the Rev. Oswald Cockayne may be quoted as a sample:—

"For tooth worms take acorn meal and henbane seed and wax, of all equally much, mingle them together, work into a wax candle and burn it, let it reek into the mouth, put a black cloth under, and the worms will fall on it."

Marcellus, a late Latin medical author whose work was translated into Saxon, gave a simpler remedy. It was to say "Argidam, Margidum, Sturdigum," thrice, then spit into a frog's mouth and set him free, requesting him at the same time to carry off the toothache.

Another popular cure for toothache in early England was to wear a piece of parchment on which the following charm was written:—"As St. Peter sat at the gate of Jerusalem our Blessed Lord and Saviour, Jesus Christ, passed by and said, What aileth thee? He said Lord, my teeth ache. He said, Arise and follow me and thy teeth shall never ache any more."

Sir Kenelm Digby's method was less tempting. He directed that the patient should scratch his gum with an iron nail until he made it bleed, and should then drive the nail with the blood upon it into a wooden beam. He will never have toothache again, says this sage.

For warts the cures are innumerable. They are all more or less like this: Steal a piece of meat from a butcher's stall or basket, bury it secretly at a gateway where four lanes meet. As the meat decays the warts will die away. An apple cut into slices and rubbed on the warts and buried is equally efficacious. So is a snail which after being rubbed on the warts is impaled on a thorn and left to die.

A room hung with red cloth was esteemed in many countries to be effective against certain diseases, small-pox especially. John of Gaddesden relates how he cured Edward II's son by this device. The prejudice in favour of red flannel which still exists, for tying a piece of it round sore throats is probably a remnant of the fancy that red was specially obnoxious to evil spirits. The Romans hung red coral round the necks of their infants to protect them from the evil eye. This practice, too, has come down to our day.

```
      er          |     hx
         ┌───┬───┐
         │ h │ h │
         ├───┼───┤
         │ δ │ δ │
  δ      └─n─┴─n─┘           δ
         ─────────
         xh      |     hx
```

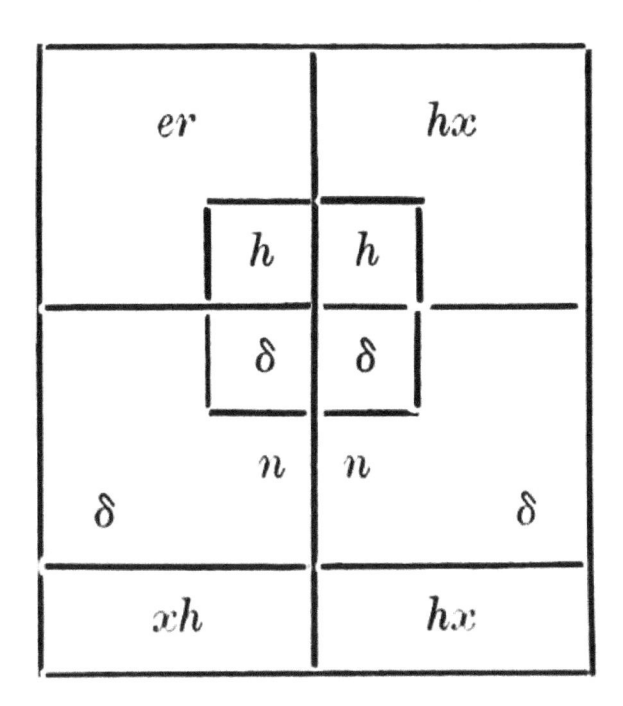

Among other charms and incantations quoted by Mr. Cockayne in his account of Saxon Leechdoms we find that for a baby's recovery "some would creep through a hole in the ground and stop it up behind them with thorns," "if cattle have a disease of the lungs, burn (something undeciphered) on midsummer's day; add holy water, and pour it into their mouths on midsummer's morrow; and sing over them: Ps. 51, Ps. 17, and the Athanasian Creed." "If anything has been stolen from you write a copy of the annexed diagram and put it into thy left shoe under the heel. Then thou shalt soon hear of it."

TRANSFERRING DISEASES.

It was widely believed that disease could be transferred by means of certain silly formalities. This was a very ancient notion. Pliny explains how pains in the stomach could be transferred to a duck or a puppy. A prescription of about two hundred years ago for the cure of convulsions was to take parings of the sick man's nails, some hair from his eyebrows, and a halfpenny, and wrap them all in a clout which had been round his head. This package must be laid in a gateway where four lanes meet, and the first person who opened it would take the sickness and relieve the patient of it. A certain John Dougall was prosecuted in Edinburgh in 1695 for prescribing this treatment. A more gruesome but less unjust proceeding was to transfer the disease to the dead. An example is the treatment of boils quoted from Mr. W. G. Black's "Folk Medicine." The boil was to be poulticed three days and nights, after which the poultices and cloths employed were to be placed in the coffin with a dead person and buried with the corpse. In Lancashire warts could be transferred by rubbing each with a cinder which must be wrapped in paper and laid where four roads meet. As before, the person who opens this parcel will take the warts from the present owner. In Devonshire a child could be cured of whooping cough by putting one of its hairs between slices of bread and butter and giving these to a dog. If the dog coughed, as was probable, the whooping cough was transferred.

WITCHES' POWERS.

The powers of witches were extensive but at the same time curiously restricted. When Agnes Simpson was tried in Scotland in 1590 she confessed that to compass the death of James VI she had hung up a black toad for nine days and caught the juice which dropped from it. If she could have obtained a piece of linen which the king had worn she could have killed him by applying to it some of this venom, which would have caused him such pain as if he had lain on sharp thorns or needles.

Another means they had of inflicting torture was to make an effigy in wax or clay of their victim and then to stick pins into it or beat it. This would cause the person represented the pain which it was desired to inflict.

THE UNIVERSAL TENDENCY.

It would merely try the patience of the reader to enumerate even a tithe of the absurd things which have been and are being used by people, civilised and savage, as charms, talismans, and amulets. The teraphim which Rachel stole from her father Laban, the magic knots of the Chaldeans, the gold and stone ornaments of the Egyptians, which they not only wore themselves but often attached to their mummies—a multitude of these going back as far as the flint amulets of the predynastic period, are to be seen in the British Museum—the precious stones whose virtues were discovered by Orpheus, the infinite variety of gold and silver ornaments adopted by the Romans with superstitious notions, the fish, ichthys, being the initials of the Greek words for Jesus Christ, the Lord, our Saviour, engraved on stones and worn by the early Christians, the Gnostic gems, the coral necklaces, the bezoar stones, the toad ashes, the strands of the ropes used for hanging criminals, the magnets of the middle ages and of modern times, and a thousand other things, credited with magical curative properties, might be cited. Besides these there are myriads of forms of words written or spoken, some pious, some gibberish, which have been used and recommended both with and without drugs.

Schelenz in "Geschichte der Pharmacie" (1904) quotes from Jakob Mærlant of Bruges, "the Father of Flemish science" (born about 1235) the recommendation of an "Amulettring" on the stone of which the figure of Mercury was engraved, and which would make the wearer healthy, "die mæct sinen traghere ghesont." (See Cramp Rings, p. 305.)

How widespread has been the belief in the power of amulets and charms may be gathered from a few instances of such superstitions among famous persons. Lord Bacon was convinced that warts could be cured by rubbing lard on them and transferring the lard to a post. The warts would die when the lard dried. Robert Boyle attributed the cure of a hæmorrhage to wearing some moss from a dead man's skull. The father of Sir Christopher Wren relates that Lord Burghley, the Lord Treasurer of England in Queen Elizabeth's reign, kept off the gout by always wearing a blue ribbon studded with a particular kind of snail shells round his leg. Whenever he left it off the pain returned violently. Burton in the "Anatomy of Melancholy" (1621) says St. John's Wort gathered on a Friday in the horn of Jupiter, when it comes to his effectual operation (that is about full moon in July), hung about the neck will mightily help melancholy and drive away fantastical spirits.

Pepys writing on May 28, 1667, says, "My wife went down with Jane and W. Hewer to Woolwich in order to get a little ayre, and to lie there to-night and so to gather May Dew to-morrow morning, which Mrs. Turner hath taught her is the only thing to wash her face with; and I am content with it." But Mrs. Turner ought to have explained to Mrs. Pepys that to preserve beauty it was necessary to collect the May Dew on the first of the month.

Catherine de Medici wore a piece of an infant's skin as a charm, and Lord Bryon presented an amulet of this nature to Prince Metternich. Pascal died with some undecipherable inscription sewn into his clothes. Charles V always wore a sachet of dried silkworms to protect him from vertigo. The Emperor Augustus wore a piece of the skin of a sea calf to keep the lightning from injuring him, and the Emperor Tiberius wore laurel round his neck for the same reason when a thunderstorm seemed to be approaching. Thyreus reports that in 1568 the Prince of Orange condemned a Spaniard to be shot, but that the soldiers could not hit him. They undressed him and found he was wearing an amulet bearing certain mysterious figures. They took this from him, and then killed him without further difficulty. The famous German physician, Frederick Hoffman, tells seriously of a gouty subject he knew who could tell when an attack was approaching by a stone in a ring which he wore changing colour.

X
DOGMAS AND DELUSIONS.

> See skulking Truth to her old cavern fled,
>
> Mountains of casuistry heap'd o'er her head;
>
> Philosophy that lean'd on Heav'n before
>
> Shrinks to her Second Cause and is no more.
>
> Physic of Metaphysic begs defence,
>
> And Metaphysic calls for aid on Sense.
>
> See Mystery to Mathematics fly;
>
> In vain! they gaze, turn giddy, rave, and die.
>
> POPE—"The Dunciad" (641–648).

ELEMENTS AND PHLOGISTON.

The ancient idea that earth, air, fire, and water were the elements of Nature was held by chemists in the 18th century. Empedocles appears to have been the author of this theory, which was adopted by Aristotle. Some speculative philosophers, however, taught that all of these were derived from one original first principle; some held that this was water, some earth, some fire, and others air. Paracelsus, who does not seem to have objected to this idea, contributed another fantastic one to accompany it. According to him everything was composed of sulphur, salt, and mercury; but he did not mean by these the material sulphur, salt, and mercury as we know them, but some sort of refined essence of these. These three essentials came to be tabulated thus:—

SALT.	SULPHUR.	MERCURY.
Unpleasant and bitter.	Sweet.	Acid.
Body.	Soul.	Spirit.
Matter.	Form.	Idea.
Patient.	Agent.	Informant or movent.
Art.	Nature.	Intelligence.

Sense.	Judgment.	Intellect.
Material.	Spiritual.	Glorious.

This is taken from Beguin, who explains that the mercury, sulphur, and salt of this classification are not those "mixt and concrete bodies such as are vulgarly sold by merchants. Mercury, which combines the elements of air and water, Sulphur represents Fire, and Salt, Earth." "But the said principles, to speak properly, are neither bodies; because they are plainly spiritual, by reason of the influx of celestial seeds, with which they are impregnated: nor spirits, because corporeal, but they participate of either nature; and have been insignized by Phylosophers with various names, or at the least unto them they have alluded these."

Instances of the combination of these principles are given. If you burn green woods, you first have a wateriness, mercury; then there goes forth an oleaginous substance easily inflammable, sulphur; lastly, a dry and terrestrial substance remains, salt. Milk contains a sulphurous buttery substance; mercurial, whey; saline, cheese. Eggs: white, mercury, yolk, sulphur, shell, salt. Antimony regulus, mercury, red sulphur conceiving flame; a salt which is vomitive.

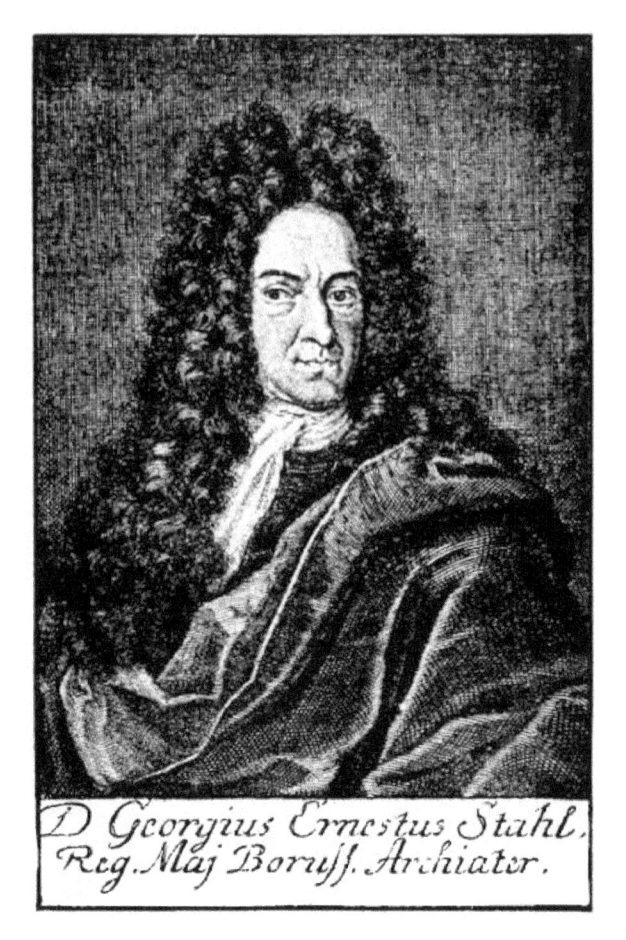

George Ernest Stahl.

> Born at Anspach, 1660; died at Berlin, 1734. Stahl was the originator of the "phlogiston theory" which generally prevailed in chemistry until Lavoisier disproved it in the last quarter of the 18th century.

Nowhere do you get these principles pure. Mercury (the metal) contains both sulphur and salt; so with the others.

Becker, the predecessor of Stahl, was not quite satisfied with the orthodox opinion, and improved upon it by limiting the elements to water and earth; but he recognised three earths, vitrifiable, inflammable, and mercurial. The last yielded the metals. Stahl was inclined to go back to the four elements again, but he had his doubts about their really elementary character. He, however, concentrated his attention on fire, out of which he evolved his well-known phlogiston theory. This substance, if it was a substance, was conceived as floating about all through the atmosphere, but only revealing itself by its effects when it came into contact with material bodies. There was some doubt whether it possessed the attribute of weight at all; but its properties were supposed to be quiescent when it became united with a substance which thereby became phlogisticated. It needed to be excited in some special way before it could be brought again into activity. When combined it was in a passive condition.

The amusing features of the phlogiston theory only developed when it came to be realised that when the phlogiston was driven out of a body, as in the case of the calcination of a metal, the calx remaining was heavier than the metal with the phlogiston had been. The first explanation of this phenomenon was that phlogiston not only possessed no heaviness, but was actually endowed with a faculty of lightness. This hypothesis was, however, a little too far-fetched for even the seventeenth century. Boerhaave thereupon discovered that as the phlogiston escaped it attacked the vessel in which the metal was calcined, and combined some of that with the metal. This notion would not stand experiment, but Baume's explanation of what happened was singularly ingenious. He insisted that phlogiston was appreciably ponderable. But, he said, when it is absorbed into a metal or other substance it does not combine with that substance, but is constantly in motion in the interstices of the molecules. So that as a bird in a cage does not add to the weight of the cage so long as it is flying about, no more does phlogiston add to the weight of the metal in which it is similarly flying about. But when the calcination takes place the dead phlogiston, as it may be called, does actually combine with the metal, and thus the increase of weight is accounted for.

Humours and Degrees.

The doctrine of the "humours," or humoral pathology, as it is generally termed, is usually traced to Hippocrates. It is set forth in his book on the Nature of Man, which Galen regarded as a genuine treatise of the Physician of Cos, but which other critics have supposed to have been written by one or more of his disciples or successors. At any rate, it is believed to represent his views. Plato elaborated the theory, and Galen gave it dogmatic form.

The human body was composed not exactly of the four elements, earth, air, fire, and water, but of the essences of these elements. The fluid parts, the blood, the phlegm, the bile, and the black bile, were the four humours. There were also three kinds of spirits, natural, vital, and animal, which put the humours in motion.

The blood was the humour which nourished the various parts of the body, and was the source of animal heat. The bile kept the passages of the body open, and served to promote the digestion of the food. The phlegm kept the nerves, the muscles, the cartilages, the tongue, and other organs supple, thus facilitating their movements. The black bile (the melancholy, Hippocrates termed it) was a link between the other humours and sustained them. The proportion of these humours occasioned the temperaments, and it is hardly necessary to remark that this fancy still prevails in our language; the sanguine, the bilious, the phlegmatic, and the atrabilious or melancholy natures being familiar descriptions to this day.

The humours had different characters. The blood was naturally hot and humid, the phlegm cold and humid, the bile hot and dry, and the black bile cold and dry. Alterations of the humours would cause diseased conditions; distempers was the appropriate term. There might be a too abundant provision of one or more of the humours. A plethora of blood would cause drowsiness, difficulty of breathing, fatty degeneration. A plethora of either of the other humours would have the effect of causing corruption of the blood; plethora of bile, for example, would result in a jaundiced condition, bad breath, a bitter taste in the mouth, and other familiar symptoms. Hæmorrhoids, leprosy, and cancer might result from a plethora of the melancholic humour; colds, catarrhs, rheumatisms were occasioned by a superabundance of the phlegm.

It must not be supposed that Galen or any other authority pretended that the humours were the sole causes of disease. Ancient pathology was a most complicated structure which cannot be even outlined here. The theory of the humours is only indicated in order to show how these explained the action of drugs. To these were attributed hot, humid, cold, and dry qualities to a larger or less extent. Galen classifies them in four degrees—that is to say, a drug might be hot, humid, cold, or dry in the first, second, third, or fourth degree. Consequently the physician had to estimate first which humour was predominant, and in what degree, and then he had to select the drug which would counteract the disproportionate heat, cold, humidity, or dryness. Of course he had his manuals to guide him. Thus Culpepper tells us that horehound, for example, is "hot in the second degree, and dry in the third"; herb Trinity, or pansies, on the other hand, "are cold and moist, both herbs and flowers"; and so forth. Medicines which applied to the skin would raise a blister, mustard, for example, are hot in the fourth degree; those which provoke sweat abundantly, and thus "cut tough and compacted humours" (Culpepper) are hot in the third degree. Opium was cold in the fourth degree, and therefore should only be given alone to mitigate violent pain. In ordinary cases it is wise to moderate the coldness of the opium by combining something of the first degree of cold or heat with it.

An amusing illustration of the reverence which this doctrine of the temperatures inspired is furnished by Sprengel in the second volume of his History of Medicine. Dealing with the Arab period, he tells us that Jacob-Ebn-Izhak-Alkhendi, one of the most celebrated authors of his nation, who lived in the ninth century, and cultivated mathematics, philosophy, and astrology as well as medicine, wrote a book on the subject before us, extending Galen's theory to compound medicines, explaining their action in accordance with the principles of harmony in music. The degrees he explains progress in geometric ratio, so that the fourth degree counts as 16 compared with unity. He sets out his proposition thus: $x = b^{n-1}a$; a being the first, b the last, x the exponent, and n the number of the terms. Sprengel has pity on those of us who are not familiar with mathematical manipulations, and gives an example to make the formula clear.

Medicament.	Weight.	Hot.	Cold.	Humid.	Dry.
CARDAMOMS	ʒi	1	½	½	1
SUGAR	ʒii	2	1	1	2
INDIGO	ʒi	½	1	½	1
MYROBALANS	ʒii	1	2	1	2
	ʒvi	4½	4½	3	6

This preparation therefore forms a mixture exactly balanced in hot and cold properties, but twice as dry as it is humid; the mixture is therefore dry in the first degree. If the total had shown twelve of the dry to three of the humid qualities, it would have been dry in the second degree. When it is remembered that in addition to these calculations the physician had to realise that drugs adapted for one part of the body might be of no use for another, it will be perceived that the art of prescribing was a serious business under the sway of the old dogmas.

THE ROSICRUCIANS.

It has never been pretended, so far as I am aware, that the Rosicrucian mystics of the middle ages did anything for the advancement of pharmacy. They are only mentioned here because they claimed the power of curing disease, and also because it happens that the fiction which created the legends concerning them was almost contemporaneous with the not unsimilar one (if the latter be a fiction) which made a historical figure of Basil Valentine. Between 1614 and 1616 three works were published professing to reveal the history of the brethren of the Rosy Cross. The first was known as Fama Fraternitatis, the second was the Confessio Fraternitatis, and the third and most important was the "Chymical Marriage of Christian Rosencreutz." The treatises are written in a mystic jargon, and have been interpreted as alchemical or religious parables, though vast numbers of learned men adopted the records as statements of facts. It was asserted that Christian Rosencreutz, a German, born in 1378, had travelled in the East, and from the wise men of Arabia and other countries had learnt the secrets of their knowledge, religious, necromantic, and alchemical. On his return to Germany he and seven other persons formed this fraternity, which was to be kept secret for a hundred years. The brethren, it is suggested, communicated to each other their discoveries and the knowledge which had been transmitted to them to communicate with each other. They were to treat the sick poor free, were to wear no distinctive dress, but they used the letters C.R. They knew how to make gold, but this was not of much value to them, for they did not seek wealth. They were to meet once a year, and each one appointed his own successor, but there were to be no tombstones or other memorials. Christian Rosencreutz himself is reported to have died at the age of 106, and long afterwards his skeleton was found in a house, a wall having been built over him. Their chief business being to heal the sick poor, they must have known much about medicine, but the books do not reveal anything of any use. They acquired their knowledge, not by study, but by the direct illumination of God. The theories—such as they were—were Paracelsian, and the fraternity, though mystic, was Protestant.

The most curious feature of the story is that the almost obviously fictitious character of the documents which announced it should have been so widely believed. Very soon after their publication German students were fiercely disputing concerning the authenticity of the revelations, and the controversy continued for two hundred years. Much learned investigation into the origin of the first treatises has been made, and the most usual conclusion has been that they were written by a German theologian, Johann Valentin Andreas, of Württemberg, b. 1586, d. 1654. He is said to have declared before his death that he wrote the alleged history expressly as a work of fiction.

The Doctrine of Signatures

was at least intelligible. It associated itself, too, with the pious utterances so frequent among the mediæval teachers and practitioners of medicine. The theory was that the Creator in providing herbs for the service of man had stamped on them, at least in many instances, an indication of their special remedial value. The adoption of ginseng root by the Chinese as a remedy for impotence, and of mandrake by the Hebrews and Greeks in the treatment of sterility, those roots often resembling the male form, have been often cited as evidence of the antiquity of the general dogma.... But isolated instances of that kind are very far from proving the existence of systematic belief. Hippocrates states that diseases are sometimes cured by the use of "like" remedies; but he was not the founder of homœopathy.

It is likely that the belief in a special indication of the virtues of remedies grew up slowly in the monasteries, and was originated, perhaps, by noticing some curious coincidences. It found wide acceptance in the sixteenth century, largely owing to the confident belief in the doctrine expressed in the writings of Paracelsus. Oswald Crollius and Giovanni Batista Porta, both mystical medical authors, taught the idea with enthusiasm. But it can hardly be said that it maintained its influence to any appreciable extent beyond the seventeenth century. Dr. Paris describes the doctrine of signatures as "the most absurd and preposterous hypothesis that has disgraced the annals of medicine"; but except that it may have led to experiments with a few valueless herbs, it is difficult to see sufficient reason for this extravagant condemnation of a poetic fancy.

The signatures of some drugs were no doubt observed after their virtues had been discovered. Poppy, for instance, under the doctrine was appropriated to brain disorders, on account of its shape like a head. But its reputation as a brain soother was much more ancient than the inference.

It is only necessary to give a few specimens of the inductive reasoning involved in the doctrine of signatures as revealed by the authors of the old herbals. The saxifrages were supposed to break up rocks; their medicinal value in stone in the bladder was therefore manifest. Roses were recommended in blood disorders, rhubarb and saffron in bilious complaints, turmeric in jaundice, all on account of their colour. Trefoil "defendeth the heart against the noisome vapour of the spleen," says William Coles in his "Art of Simpling," "not only because the leaf is triangular like the heart of a man, but because each leaf contains the perfect icon of a heart and in the proper flesh colour." Aristolochia Clematitis was called birthwort, and from the shape of its corolla was believed to be useful in parturition. Physalis alkekengi, bladder wort, owed its reputation as a cleanser of the bladder and urinary passages to its inflated calyx. Tormentilla officinalis, blood root, has a red root, and would therefore cure bloody fluxes. Scrophularia nodosa, kernel wort, has kernels or tubers attached to its roots, and was consequently predestined for the treatment of scrofulous glands of the neck. Canterbury bells, from their long throats, were allocated to the cure of sore throats. Thistles, because of their prickles, would cure a stitch in the side. Scorpion grass, the old name of the forget-me-not, has a spike which was likened to the tail of a scorpion, and was therefore a remedy for the sting of a scorpion. [The name forget-me-not was applied in England, until about a century ago, to the Ground Pine (Ajuga Chamœpitys), for the unpoetical reason that it left a nauseous taste in the mouth.]

Oswald Crollius, who describes himself as Medicus et Philosophus Hermeticus, in his "Tractatus de Signatures," writes a long and very pious preface explaining the importance of the knowledge of signatures. It is the most useful part of botany, he observes, and yet not a tenth part of living physicians have fitted themselves to practise from this study to the satisfaction of their patients. His inferences from the plants and animals he mentions are often very far-fetched, but he gives his conclusions as if they had been mathematically demonstrated. Never once does he intimate that a signature is capable of two interpretations. A few illustrations not mentioned above may be selected from his treatise.

Walnuts have the complete signature of the head. From the shell, therefore, a salt can be made of special use for wounds of the pericranium. The inner part of the shell will make a decoction for injuries to the skull; the pellicle surrounding the kernel makes a medicine for inflammation of the membrane of the brain; and the kernel itself nourishes and strengthens the brain. The down on the quince shows that a decoction of that fruit will prevent the hair falling out. So will the moss that grows on trees. The asarum has the signature of the ears. A conserve of its flowers will therefore help the hearing and the memory. Herb Paris, euphrasia, chamomile, hieracium, and many other herbs yield preparations for the eyes. Potentilla flowers bear the pupil of the eye, and may similarly be employed. The seed receptacle of the henbane resembles the formation of the jaw. That is why these seeds are good for toothache. The lemon indicates the heart, ginger the belly, cassia fistula the bowels, aristolochia the womb, plantago the nerves and veins, palma Christi and fig leaves the hands.

The signatures sometimes simulate the diseases themselves. Lily of the valley has a flower hanging like a drop; it is good for apoplexy. The date, according to Paracelsus, cures cancer; dock seeds, red colcothar, and acorus palustris will cure erysipelas; red santal, geraniums, coral, blood stones, and tormentilla, are indicated in hæmorrhage; rhubarb in yellow bile; wolves' livers in liver complaints, foxes' lungs in pulmonary affections, and dried worms powdered in goats' milk to expel worms. The fame of vipers as a remedy was largely due to the theory of the renewal of their youth. Tartarus, or salt of man's urine, is good against tartar and calculi.

Colour was a very usual signature. Red hangings were strongly advocated in medical books for the beds of patients with small-pox. John of Gaddesden, physician to Edward II, says, "When I saw the son of the renowned King of England lying sick of the small-pox I took care that everything round the bed should be of a red colour, which succeeded so completely that the Prince was restored to perfect health without the vestige of a pustule."

METALS AND PRECIOUS STONES.

It will be noticed that parts of animals are credited in the examples just quoted with remedial properties. This was a natural extension of the doctrine. Metals, too, were credited with medicinal virtues corresponding with their names or with the deities and planets with which they had been so long associated. The sun ruled the heart, gold was the sun's metal, therefore gold was especially a cordial. The moon, silver, and the head were similarly associated. Iron was a tonic because Mars was strong.

"Have a care," says Culpepper, "you use not such medicines to one part of your body which are appropriated to another; for if your brain be overheated and you use such medicines as cool the heart or liver you may make mad work."

But it was not quite so simple a thing as it may seem to be to select the proper remedy, because there were conditions which made it necessary to follow an antipathetical treatment. For instance, Saturn ruling the bones caused toothache; but if Jupiter happened to be in the ascendant, the proper drug to employ was one in the service of the opposing planet. Modern astronomy has removed the heavenly bodies so far from us that we have ceased to regard them in the friendly way which once characterised our relations with them. To quote Culpepper again: "It will seem strange to none but madmen and fools that the stars should have influence upon the body of man, considering he being an epitomy of the Creation must needs have a celestial world within himself; for ... if there be an unity in the Godhead there must needs be an unity in all His works, and a dependency between them, and not that God made the Creation to hang together like a rope of sand."

SYMPATHETIC REMEDIES.

Among the strange theories which have found acceptance in medical history, mainly it would seem by reason of their utter baselessness and absurdity, none is more unaccountable than the belief in the so-called sympathetic remedies. There is abundant material for a long chapter on this particular manifestation of faith in the impossible, but a few prominent instances of the remarkable method of treatment comprised in the designation will suffice to prove that it was seriously adopted by men capable of thinking intelligently.

The germ of the idea goes back to very early ages. Dr. J. G. Frazer, the famous authority on primitive beliefs, traces the commandment in the Pentateuch, "Thou shalt not seethe a kid in its mother's milk," to an ancient prejudice against the boiling of milk in any circumstances, on the ground that this would cause suffering to the animal which yielded the milk. If the suffering could be thus conveyed, it was logical to believe that healing was similarly capable of transference.

Pliny (quoted by Cornelius Agrippa) says: "If any person shall be sorry for a blow he has given another, afar off or near at hand, if he shall presently spit into the middle of the hand with which he gave the blow, the party that was smitten shall presently be free from pain."

Paracelsus developed the notion with the confidence which he was wont to bestow on theories which involved far-fetched explanations. This was his formula for "Unguentum Sympatheticum":—

Take 4 oz. each of boar's and bear's fat, boil slowly for half an hour, then pour on cold water. Skim off the floating bit, rejecting that which sinks. (The older the animals yielding the fat, the better.)

Take of powdered burnt worms, of dried boar's brain, of red sandal wood, of mummy, of bloodstone, 1 oz. of each. Then collect 1 drachm of the moss from the skull of a man who died a violent death, one who had been hanged, preferably, and had not been buried. This should be collected at the rising of the moon, and under Venus if possible, but certainly not under Mars or Saturn. With all these ingredients make an ointment, which keep in a closed glass vessel. If it becomes dry on keeping it can be softened with a little fresh lard or virgin honey. The ointment must be prepared in the autumn.

Paracelsus describes the methods of applying this ointment, the precautions to be taken, and the manner in which it exerts its influence. It was the weapon which inflicted the wound which was to be anointed, and it would be effective no matter how far away the wounded person might be. It would not answer if an artery had been severed, or if the heart, the brain, or the liver had suffered the lesion. The wound was to be kept properly bandaged, and the bandages were to be first wetted with the patient's urine. The anointment of the weapon was to be repeated every day in the case of a serious wound, or every second or third day when the wound was not so severe, and the weapon was to be wrapped after anointment in a clean linen cloth, and kept free from dust and draughts, or the patient would experience much pain. The anointment of the weapon acted on the wound by a magnetic current through the air direct to the healing balsam which exists in every living body, just as the heat of the sun passes through the air.

Paracelsus also prescribed the leaves of the Polygonum persicaria to be applied to sores and ulcers, and then buried. One of his disciples explains that the object of burying the leaves was that they attracted the evil spirits like a magnet, and thus drew these spirits from the patient to the earth.

The sympathetic egg was another device to cheat diseases, attributed to the same inventive genius. An empty chicken's egg was to be filled with warm blood from a healthy person, carefully sealed and placed under a brooding hen for a week or two, so that its vitality should not be impaired. It was then heated in an oven for some hours at a temperature sufficient to bake bread. To cure a case this egg was placed in contact with the affected part and then buried. It was assumed that it would inevitably take the disease with it, as healthy and concentrated blood must have a stronger affinity for disease than a weaker sort.

Robert Fludd, M.D., the Rosicrucian, who fell under the displeasure of the College of Physicians on account of his unsound views from a Galenical standpoint, was a warm advocate of the Paracelsian Weapon Salve. In reply to a contemporary doctor who had ridiculed the theory he waxes earnest, and at times sarcastic. He explains that "an ointment composed of the moss of human bones, mummy (which is the human body combined with balm), human fat, and added to these the blood, which is the beginning and food of them all, must have a spiritual power, for with the blood the bright soul doth abide and operateth after a hidden manner. Then as there is a spiritual line protracted or extended in the Ayre between the wounded person and the Box of Ointment like the beam of the Sun from the Sun, so this animal beam is the faithful conductor of the Healing nature from the box of the balsam to the wounded body. And if it were not for that line which conveys the wholesome and salutiferous spirit, the value of the ointment would evaporate or sluce out this way or that way and so would bring no benefit to the wounded persons."

Van Helmont, Descartes, Batista Porta, and other leaders of science, in the seventeenth century, espoused the theory cordially enough. Van Helmont's contribution to the evidence on which it was founded is hard to beat. In his "De Magnetica Vulnerum Curatione," written about 1644, he relates that a citizen of Brussels having lost his nose in a combat in Italy, repaired to a surgeon of Bologna named Tagliacozzi, who provided him with another, taking the required strip of flesh from the arm of a servant. This answered admirably, and the Brussels man returned home. But thirteen months later he found his nose was getting cold; and then it began to putrefy. The explanation, of course, was that the servant from whom the flesh had been borrowed had died. Van Helmont adds, "Superstites sunt horum testes oculati Bruxellae"; there are still eye-witnesses of this case at Brussels.

Moss from a dead man's skull is a principal ingredient in all the sympathetic ointments, and the condition that the dead man should have died a violent death is generally insisted on. But Van Helmont, quoting from one

Goclenius, adds another condition still more absurd. It is that the dead man's name should only have three letters. Thus, for example, Dod would do, but not Dodd.

Sir Gilbert Talbot (in the time of Charles II) communicated to the Royal Society particulars of a cure he had made with Sympathetic Powder. An English mariner was stabbed in four places at Venice, and bled for three days without intermission. Sir Gilbert, who happened to be at Venice at the same time, was told of this disaster. He sent for some of the man's blood and mixed Sympathetic Powder with it. At the same time he sent a man to bind up the patient's wounds with clean linen. Soon after he visited the mariner and found all the wounds closed, and the man much comforted. Three days later the poor fellow was able to call on Sir Gilbert to thank him, but even then "he appeared like a ghost with noe blood left in his body."

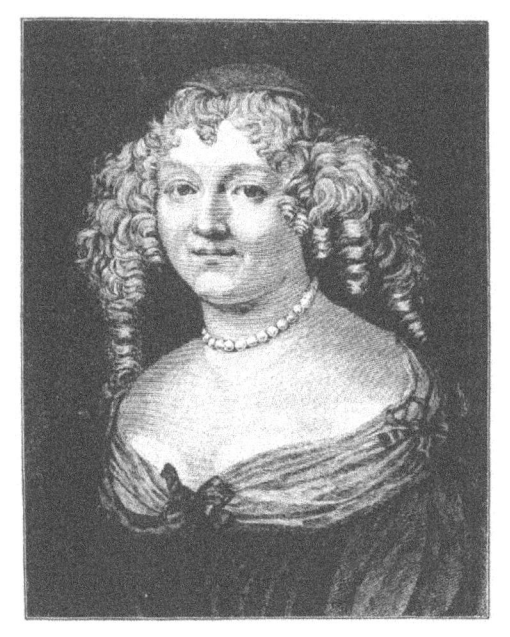

Marquise de Sévigné.

> Born 1626, died 1696, whose famous "letters" are of great historical importance, frequently introduces references to the medicine of the period, and was herself a faithful disciple of many of its quackeries.

Madame de Sévigné, an experienced amateur in medical matters, provides interesting evidence of the popularity of the powder of sympathy. Writing to her daughter on January 28th, 1685, she tells her that "a little wound which was believed to have been healed had shown signs of revolt; but it is only for the honour of being cured by your powder of sympathy. The Baume Tranquille is of no account now; your powder of sympathy is a perfectly divine remedy. My sore has changed its appearance and is now half dried and cured." On February 7th, 1685, she writes again:—"I am afraid the powder of sympathy is only suitable for old standing wounds. It has only cured the least troublesome of mine. I am now using the black ointment, which is admirable." Even the black ointment proved unfaithful, for in June of the same year the marchioness writes that she has gone to the Capucins of the Louvre. They did not believe in the powder of sympathy; they had something much better. They gave her certain herbs which were to be applied to the affected part and removed twice a day. Those removed are to be buried; "and laugh if you like, as they decay so will the wound heal, and thus by a gentle and imperceptible transpiration I shall cure the most ill-treated leg in the world."

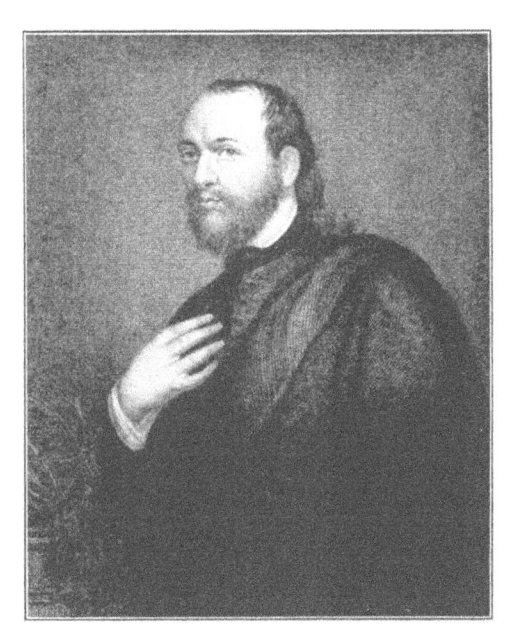

Sir Kenelm Digby.

(From a painting by Vandyke in the Bodleian Gallery, Oxford.)

The name of Sir Kenelm Digby is more closely associated with the "powder of sympathy" than that of any other person, and indeed he is often credited with the invention of the idea; but this was not the case. He was an extraordinary man who played a rather prominent part in the stirring days of the Stuarts. His father, Sir Everard Digby, was implicated in the Gunpowder Plot, and was duly executed. Kenelm must have been gifted with unusual attractions or plausibility to have overcome this unfortunate stain on his pedigree, but he managed it, and history introduces him to us at the court of that suspicious monarch,

James I., while he was quite a young man. He had inherited an income of £3,000 a year, and seems to have been popular with the King and with his fellow courtiers. But he was not contented to lead an idle life, so he pressed James to give him a commission to go forth and steal some Spanish galleons, which was the gentlemanly thing to do in those days. James consented, but at the last moment it was discovered that the commission would not be in order unless it was countersigned by the Lord High Admiral, who was away from England at the time. James therefore simply granted the buccaneer a licence to undertake a voyage "for the increase of his knowledge." Digby scoured the Mediterranean for a year or two, captured some French, Spanish, and Flemish ships, and won a rather severe engagement with French and Venetian vessels at Scanderoon in the Levant. This exploit was celebrated by Digby's friend, Ben Jonson, in verse, which can only be termed deathless on account of its particularly imbecile ending:—

> Witness his action done at Scanderoon
>
> Upon his birthday, the eleventh of June.

The writer of Digby's epitaph plagiarised the essence of this brilliant strophe in the following lines:—

> Born on the day he died, the eleventh of June,
>
> And that day bravely fought at Scanderoon.
>
> It's rare that one and the same day should be
>
> His day of birth and death and victory.

On his return home after thus distinguishing himself, Digby was knighted, changed his religion occasionally, was imprisoned and banished at intervals, and dabbled in science between times, or shone in society in London, Paris, or Rome, visiting the two last-named cities frequently on real or pretended diplomatic missions.

During his residence in France, in 1658, he lectured to the University of Montpellier on his sympathetic powder, and the fame of this miraculous compound soon reached England. When he came back he professed to be shy of using it lest he should be accused of wizardry. But an occasion soon occurred when he was compelled to take the risk for the sake of a friend. Thomas Howel, the Duke of Buckingham's secretary, was seriously wounded in trying to prevent a duel between two friends of his, and the doctors prognosticated gangrene and probably death. The friends of the wounded man appealed to Sir Kenelm, who generously consented to do his best. He told the attendants to bring him a rag on which was some of the sufferer's blood. They brought the garter which had been used as a bandage and which was still thick with blood. He soaked this in a basin of water in which he had dissolved a handful of his sympathetic powder. An hour later the patient said he felt an agreeable coolness. The fever and pain rapidly abated, and in a few days the cure was complete. It was reported that the Duke of Buckingham testified to the genuineness of the cure and that the king had taken a keen interest in the treatment.

Digby asserted that the secret of the powder was imparted to him by a Carmelite monk whom he met at Florence. His laboratory assistant, George Hartman, published a "Book of Chymicall Secrets," in 1682, after Sir Kenelm's death, and therein explained that the Powder of Sympathy, which was then made by himself (Hartman), and "sold by a bookseller in Cornhill named Brookes" was prepared "by dissolving good English vitriol in as little warm water as will suffice, filter, evaporate, and set aside until fair, large, green crystals are formed. Spread these in the sun until they whiten. Then crush them coarsely and again dry in the sun." Other recipes say it should be dried in the sun gently (a French formula says "amoureusement") for 365 days.

Sir Kenelm's scientific explanation of the action of his sympathetic powder is on the same lines as the others I have quoted. Briefly it was that the rays of the sun extracted from the blood and the vitriol associated with it the spirit of each in minute atoms. At the same time the inflamed wound was exhaling hot atoms and making way for a current of air. The air charged with the atoms of blood and vitriol were attracted to it, and acted curatively.

In a letter written by Straus to Sir Kenelm, it is related that Lord Gilborne had followed the system, but his method was described as "the dry way." A carpenter had cut himself severely with an axe. The offending axe still bespattered with blood was smeared with the proper ointment and hung up in a cupboard. The wound was going on well, but one day it suddenly became violently painful again. On investigation it was found that the axe had fallen from the nail on which it was hung.

Inscribed on the plate attached to the portrait of Sir Kenelm Digby in the National Portrait Gallery, it is stated that "His character has been summed up as a prodigy of learning, credulity, valour, and romance." Although this appreciation is quoted the author is not named. Other testimonials to his character and reliability are to be found in contemporary literature. Evelyn alludes to him as "a teller of a strange things." Clarendon describes him as "a person very eminent and notorious throughout the whole course of his life from his cradle to his grave. A man of very extraordinary person and presence; a wonderful graceful behaviour, a flowing courtesy, and such a volubility of language as surprised and delighted." Lady Fanshawe met him at Calais with the Earl of Strafford and others and says, "much excellent discourse passed; but, as was reason, most share was Sir Kenelm Digby's who had enlarged somewhat more in extraordinary stories than might be averred." At last he told the company about the barnacle goose he had seen in Jersey; a barnacle which changes to a bird, and at this they all laughed incredulously. But Lady Fanshawe says this "was the only thing true he had declaimed with them. This was his infirmity, though otherwise of most excellent parts, and a very fine-bred gentleman." In John Aubrey's "Brief Lives" ("set down between 1669 and 1696") Digby is described as "such a goodly person, gigantique and great voice, and had so graceful elocution and noble address, etc., that had he been drop't out of the clowdes in any part of the world he would have made himself respected."

It may be of interest to add that a daughter of Sir Kenelm Digby's second son married a Sir John Conway, of Flintshire. Her granddaughter, Honora, married a Sir John Glynne whose great-grandson, Sir Stephen Glynne, was the father of the late Mrs. W. E. Gladstone.

In 1690, Lemery had the courage to express some doubts about this powder of sympathy, and in 1773 Baumé declared its pretensions to be absolutely illusory.

To conclude the account of this curious delusion, a few quotations from English literature may be added.

There are several allusions to sympathetic cures in Hudibras. For instance,

> For by his side a pouch he wore
>
> Replete with strange hermetick powder
>
> That wounds nine miles point blank would solder,
>
> By skilful chemist at great cost
>
> Extracted from a rotten post.

And again,

> 'Tis true a scorpion's oil is said
>
> To cure the wounds the vermin made;
>
> And weapons dress'd with salves restore

> And heal the wounds they made before.

In Dryden's *Tempest*, the sympathetic treatment is referred to. Hippolito has been wounded by Fernando, and Miranda instructed by Ariel, visits him. Ariel says, "Anoint the sword which pierced him with this weapon salve, and wrap it close from air." The following is the next scene between Hippolito and Miranda.

> *Hip.* Oh! my wound pains me.
>
> *Mir.* I am come to ease you.[*Unwrapping the sword.*
>
> *Hip.* Alas! I feel the cold air come to me.
>> My wound shoots worse than ever.
>
>> [*Miranda wipes and anoints the sword.*
>
> *Mir.* Does it still grieve you?
>
> *Hip.* Now, methinks, there's something laid just upon it.
>
> *Mir.* Do you find no ease?
>
> *Hip.* Yes, yes; upon the sudden all the pain
>> Is leaving me; Sweet heaven, how I am eased.

Lastly, in the *Lay of the Last Minstrel*, Scott alludes to this same superstition in the lines

> But she has ta'en the broken lance
>
> And washed it from the clotted gore
>
> And salved the splinter o'er and o'er.

It would appear from the explanations already given that by washing the gore away she destroyed the communication between the wound and the remedy.

Animal Magnetism.

The first allusion to the application of the magnet as a cure for disease is found in the works of Aetius, who wrote in the early part of the sixth century. He mentions that holding a magnet in the hand is said to give relief in gout. He does not profess to have tested this treatment himself. Writers of the fifteenth and sixteenth centuries recommend it strongly for toothache, headache, convulsions, and nerve disorders. About the end of the seventeenth century magnetic tooth-picks and earpicks were sold. To these were attributed the virtues of preventing and healing pains in those organs.

Paracelsus originated the theory of animal magnetism. The mysterious properties possessed by the loadstone and transferable from that body to iron, were according to Paracelsus an influence drawn directly from the stars and possessed by all animate beings. It was a fluid which he called Magnale. By it he explained the movements of certain plants which follow the course of the sun, and it was on the basis of this hypothesis that he composed his sympathetic ointment and explained the action of talismans. Paracelsus applied the magnet in epilepsy, and also prepared a magisterium magnetis.

Glauber professed to have a secret magnet which would draw only the essence or tincture from iron, leaving the gross body behind. With this he made a tincture of Mars and Venus, thus "robbing the dragon of the golden fleece which it guards." This is understood to mean that he dissolved iron and copper in aqua fortis. And as Jason restored his aged father to youth again, so would this tincture prove a wonderful restorative. He commenced to test it on one occasion and very soon black curly hair began to grow on his bald head. But he had not enough of the tincture to permit him to carry on the experiment, and though he had a great longing to make some more, he apparently put off doing so until it was too late.

Van Helmont, Fludd, and other physicians of mystic instincts, were among the protagonists of animal magnetism, and physicians administered pulverised magnet in salves, plasters, pills and potions. But in 1660 Dr. Gilbert, of Colchester, noted that, when powdered, the loadstone no longer possessed magnetic properties. Ultimately, therefore, it was understood that the powder of magnet was not capable of producing any other effects than any other ferruginous substance. But the belief in magnets applied to the body was by no means dissipated. The theory was exploited by various practitioners, but notably towards the latter part of the eighteenth century, when the Viennese doctor, F. A. Mesmer, excited such a vogue in Paris that the Court, the Government, the Academy of Sciences, and aristocratic society generally were ranged in pro-and anti-Mesmer sections. Franklin stated that at one time Mesmer was taking more money in fees than all the regular physicians of Paris put together. And yet Mesmer's explanations of the phenomena attending his performances were only an amplification of the doctrines which Paracelsus had first imagined.

The excitement did not spread to England to any great extent, but about the same time an American named Perkins created a great deal of stir with his metallic tractors, which sent the nation tractor-mad for the time. Dr. Haygarth, of Bath, contributed to the failure of this delusion by a series of experiments on patients with pieces of wood painted to resemble the tractors from which equally wonderful relief was felt, proving that the cures such as they were, could only have been the consequence of faith.

The Treatment of Itch.

The history of the treatment of itch is such a curious instance of the blind acceptance of authority through many centuries, in the course of which the true explanation lay close at hand, that it is worth narrating briefly.

It is stated in some histories that the disease was known to the Chinese some thousands of years ago, and the name they gave it, Tchong-kiai, which means pustules formed by a worm, indicates that at least when that term was adopted they had some acquaintance with the character of the disease.

Some writers have supposed that certain of the uncleannesses alluded to in the Book of Leviticus have reference to this complaint; and it is quite possible that in old times it acquired a much more severe character than it ever has now, owing to neglect or improper treatment. Psora, in Greek, and the equivalent term Scabies, in Latin, are supposed to have at least included the itch, though in all probability those words comprehended a number of skin diseases which are now more exactly distinguished. Hippocrates mentions psora, and apparently treated it solely by the internal administration of diluents and purgatives. Aristotle mentions not only the disease but the insects found, he said, in the blisters. Celsus advocated the application of ointments composed of a miscellaneous lot of drugs, such as verdigris, myrrh, nitre, white lead, and sulphur. Galen hints at the danger of external applications which might drive the disease inwards. In Cicero, Horace, Juvenal, and other of the classical writers, the word scabies is used to indicate something unnatural; showing that it had come to be adopted metaphorically.

The Arab writers are much more explicit. Rhazes, Haly Abbas, and Avicenna are very definite in their descriptions of the nature of the complaint, and how it is transmitted from one person to another; but Avicenna's mode of treatment was directed to the expulsion of the supposed vicious humours from the body by bleeding and purgatives, especially by a purgative called Hamech. At the same time he advised that the constitution should be reinforced by suitable diet and astringent medicines.

Avenzoar of Seville, a remarkable observer, who lived in the twelfth century, alludes to a malady of the skin, common among the people, and known as Soab. This, he says, is caused by a tiny insect, so small that it can scarcely be seen, which, hidden beneath the epidermis, escapes when a puncture has been made.

One would have supposed that the doctors were at that time on the eve of understanding the itch correctly, and in fact the writers of the next few centuries were at least quite clear about the acarus. Ambrose Paré, for example, who lived through the greater part of the sixteenth century, uses this language:—"Les cirons sont petits animaux cachés dans le cuir, sous lequel ils se trainent, rampent, et rongent petit par petit, excitant une facheuse demangeaison et gratelle;" and elsewhere "Ces cirons doivent se tirer avec espingles ou aiguilles."

All this time, however, the complaint was regarded as a disturbance of the humours which had to be treated by suitable internal medicines. In a standard work, *De Morbis Cutaneis*, by Mercuriali, published at Venice in 1601, the author attributes the disease to perverted humours, and says it is contagious because the liquid containing the contagious principle is deposited on or in the skin.

This view, or something like it, continued to be the orthodox opinion at least up to the seventeenth century. Van Helmont's personal experience of the itch is referred to in dealing with that eccentric genius who was converted from Galenism to Paracelsianism as a consequence of his cure; but he never got beyond the idea that the cause of the complaint was a specific ferment.

The earliest really scientific contribution to the study of this disorder may be credited to Thomas Mouffet, of London, who, in a treatise published in 1634, entitled *Insectorum sive Minimorum Animalium Theatrum*, showed not only that the animalculæ were constantly associated with the complaint, but made it clear that they were not to be found in the vesicles, but in the tunnels connected with these. For this was the stumbling block of most of the investigators. It had been so often stated that the parasites were to be found in the vesicles, that when they were not there the theory failed. Mouffet's exposition ought to have led to a correct understanding of the cause of the complaint, but it was practically ignored.

About this time the microscope was invented, and in 1657 a German naturalist named Hauptmann published a rough drawing of the insect magnified. A better, but still imperfect, representation of it was given a few years later by Etmuller.

In 1687 a pharmacist of Leghorn, named Cestoni, induced a Dr. Bonomo of that city to join him in making a series of experiments to prove that the acarus was the cause of itch. They had both observed the women of the city extracting the insects from the hands of their children by the aid of needles, and the result of their research was a treatise in which the parasitic nature of the complaint was maintained, and the uselessness of internal remedies was insisted on. These intelligent Italians recommended sulphur or mercury ointment as the essential application.

Even with this evidence before them the doctors went on faithful to their theory of humours. Linnæus supported the view of Bonomo and Cestoni, but made the mistake of identifying the itch parasite with the cheese mite. The great medical authorities of the eighteenth century, such as Hoffmann and Boerhaave, still recommended general treatment, and a long list of drugs might be compiled which were supposed to be suitable in the treatment of itch. Among these, luckily, some parasiticides were included, and, consequently, the disease did get cured by these, but the wrong things got the credit. About the end of the eighteenth century Hahnemann promulgated the theory that the "psoric miasm" of which the itch eruption was the symptomatic manifestation, was the cause of a large proportion of chronic diseases.

Some observers thought there were two kinds of itch, one caused by the acarus, the other independent of it. Bolder theorists held that the insect was the product of the disease. The dispute continued until 1834, in which year Francois Renucci, a native of Corsica, and at the time assistant to the eminent surgeon d'Alibert at the Hôpital St. Louis, Paris, undertook to extract the acarus in any genuine case of itch. As a boy he had seen the poor women extract it in Corsica, as Bonomo and Cestoni had seen others do it at Leghorn, though his learned master at the hospital remained sceptical for some years. It was near the middle of the nineteenth century before the parasitic character of itch was universally acknowledged.

XI
MASTERS IN PHARMACY

> We are guilty, we hope, of no irreverence towards those great nations to which the human race owes art, science, taste, civil and intellectual freedom, when we say that the stock bequeathed by them to us has been so carefully improved that the accumulated interest now exceeds the principal.
>
> MACAULAY: "Essay on Lord Bacon" (1837).

DIOSCORIDES.

It has been a subject of lively dispute whether Dioscorides lived before or after Pliny. It seems certain that one of these authors copied from the other on particular matters, and in neither case is credit given. Pliny was born A.D. 23 and died A.D. 79, and would therefore have lived under the Emperors Tiberius, Caligula, Claudius, Nero, Galba, Otho, Vitellius, and Vespasian. Suidas, the historian, who probably wrote in the tenth century, dates Dioscorides as contemporary with Antony and Cleopatra, about B.C. 40, and some Arab authorities say he wrote at the time of Ptolemy VII, which would be still a hundred years earlier. But Dioscorides dedicates his great work on materia medica to Areus Asclepiades, who is otherwise unknown, but mentions as a friend of his patron the consul Licinius Bassus. There was a consul Lecanius Bassus in the reign of Nero, and it is therefore generally supposed that Dioscorides was in his prime at that period, and would consequently be a contemporary of Pliny's. It is possible that both authors drew from another common source.

Dioscorides was a native of Anazarbus in Cilicia, a province where the Greek spoken and written was proverbially provincial. Our word solecism is believed to have been derived from the town of Soloe in the same district. The Greek of Dioscorides is alleged to have been far from classical. He himself apologises for it in his preface, and Galen remarks upon it. Nevertheless Dioscorides maintained for at least sixteen centuries the premier position among authorities on materia medica. Galen complains that he was sometimes too indefinite in his description of plants, that he does not indicate exactly enough the diseases in which they are useful, and that he does not explain the degrees of heat, cold, dryness, and humidity which characterise them. He will often content himself with saying that a herb is hot or cold, as the case may be. As an illustration of one of his other criticisms Galen mentions the Polygonum, of which he notes that Dioscorides says "it is useful for those who urinate with difficulty." But Galen adds that he does not particularise precisely the cases of which this is a symptom and which the Polygonum is good for. But these defects notwithstanding, Galen recognises that Dioscorides is the best authority on the subject of the materials of medicine.

It is generally stated that Dioscorides was a physician; but of this there is no certain evidence. According to his own account he was devoted to the study and observation of plants and medical substances generally, and in order to see them in their native lands he accompanied the Roman armies through Greece, Italy, and Asia Minor. This was the easiest method of visiting foreign countries in those days. It is not unlikely that he went as assistant to a physician, perhaps to the one to whom he dedicated his book. That is to say, he may have been an army compounder. Suidas says of him that he was nicknamed Phocas, because his face was covered with stains of the shape of lentils.

In his treatise on materia medica, "Peri Ules Iatrikes," or, according to Photius, originally "Peri Ules," On Matter, only, he describes some six hundred plants, limiting himself to those which had or were supposed to have medicinal virtues. He mentions, besides, the therapeutic properties of many animal substances. Among these are roasted grasshoppers, for bladder disorders; the liver of an ass for epilepsy; seven bugs enclosed in the skin of a bean to be taken in intermittent fever; and a spider applied to the temples for headache.

Dioscorides also gives a formula for the Sal Viperum, which was a noted remedy in his time and for long afterwards. His process was to roast a viper alive in a new earthen pot with some figs, common salt, and honey, reducing the whole to ashes. A little spikenard was added to the ashes. Pliny only adds fennel and frankincense to the viper, but Galen and later authors make the salt a much more complicated mixture.

His botany is very defective. He classifies plants in the crudest way; often only by a similarity of names. Of many his only description is that it is "well-known," a habit which has got him into much trouble with modern investigators who have looked into his work for historical evidence verifying the records of herbs named in other works. Hyssop is an example. As stated in the section entitled "The Pharmacy of the Bible," it has not been found possible to identify the several references to hyssop in the Bible. Dioscorides contents himself by saying that it is a well-known plant, and then gives its medicinal qualities. But that his hyssop was not the plant known to us by that name is evident from the fact that in the same chapter he describes the "Chrysocome," and says of it that it flowers in racemes like the hyssop. He also speaks of an origanum which has leaves arranged like an umbel, similar to that of the hyssop. It is evident, therefore, that his hyssop and ours are not the same plant.

The mineral medicines in use in his time are also included in the treatise of Dioscorides. He mentions argentum vivum, cinnabar, verdigris, the calces of lead and antimony, flowers of brass, rust of iron, litharge, pompholix, several earths, sal ammoniac, nitre, and other substances.

Other treatises, one on poisons and the bites of venomous animals, and another on medicines easy to prepare, have been attributed to Dioscorides, but it is not generally accepted that he was the author. The best known translation of Dioscorides into Latin was made by Matthiolus of Sienna in the sixteenth century. The MS. from which Matthiolus worked is still preserved at Vienna and is believed to have been written in the sixth century.

The very competent authority Kurt Sprengel, while recognising the defects in the Materia Medica of Dioscorides, credits him with the record of many valuable observations. His descriptions of myrrh, bdellium, laudanum, asafoetida, gum ammoniacum, opium, and squill are selected as particularly useful; the accounts he gives of treatments since abandoned (some of which are mentioned above, but to these Sprengel adds the application of wool fat to wounds which has been revived since he wrote), are of special interest; and the German historian further justly points out that many remedies rediscovered in modern times were referred to by Dioscorides. Among these are castor oil, though Dioscorides only alludes to the external application of this substance; male fern against tape worms; elm bark for eruptions; horehound in phthisis; and aloes for ulcers. He describes many chemical processes very intelligently, and was the first to indicate means of discovering the adulterations of drugs.

Galen.

No writer of either ancient or modern times can compare with Claudius Galenus probably in the abundance of his output, but certainly in the influence he exercised over the generations that followed him. For fifteen hundred years the doctrines he formulated, the compound medicines he either introduced or endorsed, and the treatments he recommended commanded almost universal submission among medical practitioners. In Dr. Monk's Roll of the College of Physicians, mention is made of a Dr. Geynes who was admitted to the Fellowship of the College in 1560, "but not until he had signed a recantation of his error in having impugned the infallibility of Galen."[2] This was at the time when to deny Galen meant to follow Paracelsus, and the contest was fiercer just then than at any time before or since.

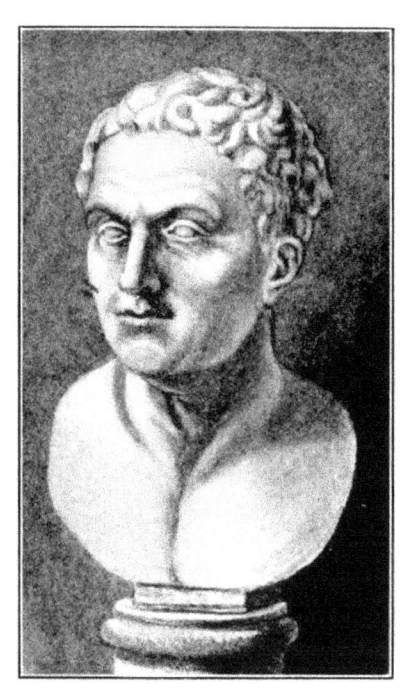

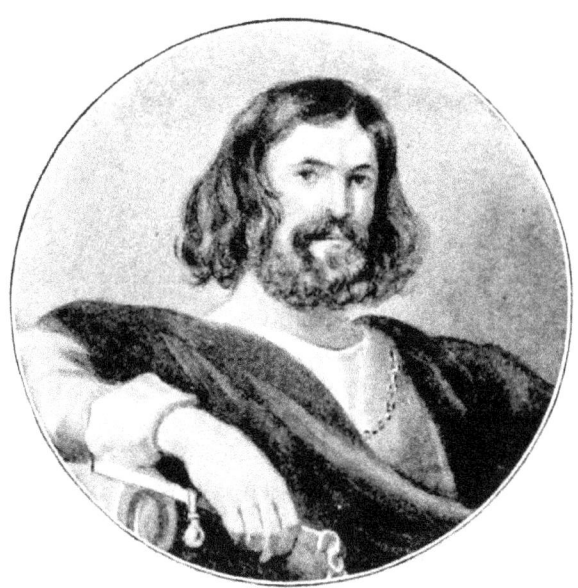

There is of course no authentic likeness of Galen in existence. The Royal College of Physicians possesses an unquestionably antique bust, copied in Pettigrew's Medical Portraits (and illustrated in the margin), which is traditionally credited with being a representation of the

- 157 -

Physician of Pergamos. It was presented to the College by Lord Ashburton, to whom it was presented by Alexander Adair, who had acquired it from his relative Robert Adair, principal surgeon to the British forces at the siege of Quebec. This Robert Adair was a man of considerable eminence in his profession, and is described as a man of character and a scholar. Beyond this very slight evidence there is no authority for the presumption that the bust was intended for Galen. The other portrait is copied from the diploma of the Pharmaceutical Society, but this is not said to have any history. With these may be compared the portrait given on the title page of the first London Pharmacopœia. The conclusion will probably be reached that we have no idea what manner of man the eminent physician was.

Galen was born at Pergamos, in Asia Minor, A.D. 131, and died in the same city between A.D. 200 and 210. His father was an architect of considerable fortune, and the son was at first destined to be a philosopher, but while he was going through his courses of logic, Nicon (the father) was advised in a dream to direct the youth's studies in the direction of medicine. It will be seen directly that Galen's career was a good deal influenced by dreams.

Nothing was spared to obtain for the youth the best education available, though his father died when he was 21. After exhausting the Pergamos teachers, Galen studied at Smyrna, Corinth, and Alexandria. Then he travelled for some years through Cilicia, Phœnicia, Palestine, Scyros, and the Isles of Crete and Cyprus. He commenced practice at Pergamos when he was 29 and was appointed Physician to the School of Gladiators in that city. At 33 he removed to Rome and soon acquired the confidence and friendship of many distinguished persons, among them Septimus Severus, the Consul and afterwards Emperor, Sergius Paulus, the Prætor, the uncle of the reigning Emperor, Lucius Verus, many of whom he cured of various illnesses.

His success caused bitter jealousy among the other Greek physicians then practising in Rome. They called him Paradoxologos, and Logiatros, which meant that he was a boaster and a master of phrases. It appears that he was able to hold his own in this wordy warfare. Some of his opponents he described as Asses of Thessaly, and he also made allegations against their competence and probity. However, he quitted Rome in the year 167, and as at a later time he left Aquilea, both movings being coincident with the occurrence of serious plagues, his reputation for courage has suffered. It was at this period of his life that he visited Palestine to see the shrub which yielded Balm of Gilead, and then proceeded to Armenia to satisfy himself in regard to the preparation of the Terra Sigillata. He was able to report that the general belief that blood was used in the process was incorrect.

It was to Aquilea that Galen was sent for by the Emperor Marcus Aurelius, who was there preparing a campaign against the Marcomans, a Germanic nation dwelling in what is now called Bohemia. Marcus Aurelius was in the habit of taking Theriaca, and would have none but that which had been prepared by Galen. He urged Galen to accompany him on his expedition, but the physician declined the honour and the danger, alleging that Æsculapius had appeared to him in a dream, and had forbidden him to take the journey. The Emperor therefore sent him to Rome and charged him with the medical care of his son Commodus, then 11 years of age. Galen is said to have done the world the ill-service of saving the life of this monster. Galen retained the favour of Marcus Aurelius till the death of the Emperor, and continued to make Theriaca for his successors, Commodus, Pertinax, and Septimus Severus. He died during the reign of the last named Emperor.

Galen is sometimes said to have kept a pharmacy in the Via d'Acra at Rome, but his "apotheca" there appears to have been a house where his writings were kept and where other physicians came to consult them. This house was afterwards burned, and it is supposed that a number of the physician's manuscripts were destroyed in that fire.

His medical fame began to develop soon after his death. In about a hundred years Eusebius, Bishop of Cæsarea, reproaches the world with treating Galen almost as a divinity. Nearly all the later Roman medical writers drew freely from his works, and some seemed to depend entirely on them. Arabic medicine was largely based on Galen's teaching, and it was the Arabic manuscripts translated into Latin which furnished the base of the medical teaching of Europe from the eleventh and twelfth centuries to the eighteenth.

Galen aimed to create a perfect system of physiology, pathology, and treatment. He is alleged to have written 500 treatises on medicine, and 250 on other subjects, philosophy, laws, grammar. Nothing like this number remains, and the so-called "books" are often what we should call articles. His known and accepted medical works number eighty-five. All his writings were originally in Greek.

ORIBASIUS.

Oribasius, like Galen, was a native of Pergamos, and was physician to and friend of the Emperor Julian. He is noted for having compiled seventy-two books in which he collected all the medical science of preceding writers. This was undertaken at the instance of Julian. Only seventeen of these books have been preserved to modern times. Oribasius adds to his compilation many original observations of his own, and in these often shows remarkable good sense. He was the originator of the necklace method of treatment, for he recommends a necklace of beads made of peony wood to be worn in epilepsy, but does not rely on this means alone.

AETIUS.

Aetius, who lived either in the fifth or sixth century, was also a compiler, but he was besides a great authority on plasters, which he discusses and describes at enormous length. He was a Christian, and gives formulas of words to be said when making medicinal compounds, such as "O God of Abraham, of Isaac, and of Jacob, give to this remedy the virtues necessary for it." In the works of Aetius, mention is made of several nostrums famous in his time for which fabulous prices were charged. The Collyrium of Danaus was sold in Constantinople for 120 numismata. If this means the nummus aureus of Roman money it would be equal to nearly £100 of our money. At this price, Aetius says, the Collyrium could only be had with difficulty. He also mentions a Colical Antidote of Nicostratus called very presumptuously Isotheos (equal to God), which sold for two talents.

The remedy devised by Aetius for gout was called Antidotos ex duobus Centaureae generibus, and was the same as the compound which became popular in this country under the title of Duke of Portland's Powder. (See page 309). Aetius prescribed a regimen along with his medicine extending over a year. In September the patient was to take milk; in October, garlic; in November to abstain from baths; December, no cabbage; in January to take a glass of pure wine every morning; in February to eat no beet; in March to be allowed sweets in both food and drink; in April, no horse radish; in May, no Polypus (a favourite dish); in June, to drink cold water in the morning; in July, no venery; in August, no mallows.

ALEXANDER OF TRALLES.

This writer, who acquired considerable celebrity as a medical authority, lived a little later than Aetius, towards the end of the sixth century. He was a native of Tralles, in Lydia, and is much esteemed by the principal medical historians, Sprengel, Leclerc, Freind, and others who have studied his writings. Especially notable is his independence of opinion; he does not hesitate occasionally to criticise even Galen. He impresses strongly on his readers the danger of becoming bound to a particular system of treatment. The causes of each disease are to be found, and the practitioner is not to be guided exclusively by symptoms. Among his favourite drugs were castorum, which he gave in fevers and many other maladies; he had known several persons snatched from the jaws of death by its use in lethargy (apoplexy); bole Armeniac, in epilepsy and melancholia; grapes and other ripe fruits instead of astringents in dysentery; rhubarb appeared as a medicine for the first time in his writings, but only as an astringent; and he was the first to use cantharides for blisters in gout instead of soothing applications. His treatment of gout by internal remedies and regimen recalls that of Aetius and is worth quoting. He prescribed an electuary composed of myrrh, coral, cloves, rue, peony, and aristolochia. This was to be taken regularly every day for a hundred days. Then it was to be discontinued for fifteen days. After that it was to be recommenced and continued during 460 days, but only taking a dose every other day; then after another interval thirty-five more doses were to be taken on alternate days, making 365 doses altogether in the course of nearly two years. Meanwhile the diet was strictly regulated, and it may well be that Alexander only provided the medicine to amuse his patient while he cured the gout by a calculated reduction of his luxuries. Alexander of Tralles was the author who recommended hermodactyls, supposed to be a kind of colchicum in gout; a remedy which was forgotten until its use was revived in a French proprietary medicine. His prescription compounded hermodactyls, ginger, pepper, cummin seeds, anise seeds, and scammony. He says it will enable sufferers who take it to walk immediately. He is supposed to have been the first to advocate the administration of iron for the removal of obstructions.

Mesuë and Serapion.

These names are often met with in old medical and pharmaceutical books, and there is an "elder" and a "younger" of each of them, so that it may be desirable to explain who they all were. The elder and the younger of each are sometimes confused. Serapion the Elder, or Serapion of Alexandria, as he is more frequently named in medical history, lived in the Egyptian city about 200 B.C., and was the recognised leader of the sect of the Empirics in medicine. He is credited with the formula that medicine rested on the three bases, Observation, History, and Analogy. No work of his has survived, but he is alleged to have violently attacked the theories of Hippocrates, and to have made great use of such animal products as castorum, the brain of the camel, the excrements of the crocodile, the blood of the tortoise, and the testicles of the boar.

Serapion the Younger was an Arabian physician who lived towards the end of the tenth century and wrote a work on materia medica which was much used for some five or six hundred years.

Mesuë the Elder was first physician at the court of Haroun-al-Raschid in the ninth century. He was born at Khouz, near Nineveh, in 776, and died at Bagdad in 855. Under his superintendence the School of Medicine of Bagdad was founded by Haroun. Although a Nestorian Christian, Mesuë retained his position as first physician to five Caliphs after Haroun. To his teaching the introduction of the milder purgatives, such as senna, tamarinds, and certain fruits is supposed to be due. His Arabic name was Jahiah-Ebn-Masawaih.

Mesuë the Younger is the authority generally meant when formulas under his name, sometimes quaintly called Dr. Mesuë in old English books, are quoted. He lived at Cairo about the year 1000. He was a Christian, like his earlier namesake, and is believed to have been a pupil or perhaps a companion of Avicenna; at all events, when the latter got into disgrace it is alleged that both he and Mesuë took refuge in Damascus. At Damascus Mesuë wrote his great work known in Latin as Receptarium Antidotarii. From the time of the invention of printing down to the middle of the seventeenth century, when pharmacopœias became general, more than seventy editions of this work, mostly in Latin, but a few in Italian, have been counted. In some of the Latin translations he is described as "John, the son of Mesuë, the son of Hamech, the son of Abdel, king of Damascus." This dignity has been traced to a confusion of the Arabic names, one of which was very similar to the word meaning king. Nearly half of the formulæ in the first London Pharmacopœia were quoted from him.

NICOLAS MYREPSUS.

For several centuries before the era of modern pharmacopœias the Antidotary of Nicolas Myrepsus was the standard formulary, and from this the early dispensatories were largely compiled. This Nicolas, who was not the Nicolas Praepositus of Salerno, is sometimes named Nicolas Alexandrinus. He appears to have been a practising physician at Constantinople, and as he bore the title of Actuarius, it is supposed that he was physician to the Emperor. He is believed to have lived in the thirteenth century. Myrepsus, which means ointment maker, was a name which he assumed or which was applied to him, probably in allusion to his Antidotary.

This was the largest and most catholic of all the collections of medical formulas which had then appeared. Galen and the Greek physicians, the Arabs, Jews, and Christians who had written on medicine, were all drawn upon. A Latin translation by Leonard Fuchs, published at Nuremberg in 1658, contains 2,656 prescriptions, every possible illness being thus provided against. The title page declares the work to be "Useful as well for the medical profession and for the seplasarii." The original is said to have been written in barbarous Greek.

Sprengel, who has hardly patience to devote a single page to this famous Antidotary, tells us that the compiler was grossly ignorant and superstitious.

He gives an instance of his reproduction of some Arab formulæ. One is the use of arsenic as a spice to counteract the deadly effects of poisons. This advice was copied, he says, down to the seventeenth century. It was Nicolas's rendering of the Arabic word Darsini, which meant cannella, and which they so named because it was brought from China.

The compounds collected in this Antidotary are of the familiar complicated character of which so many specimens are given in this volume. Many of the titles are curious and probably reminiscent of the pious credulity of the period when Myrepsus lived. There is, for example, the Salt of the Holy Apostles, which taken morning and evening with meals, would preserve the sight, prevent the hair from falling out, relieve difficulty of breathing, and keep the breath sweet. It was obtained by grinding together a mixture of herbs and seeds (hyssop, wild carrot, cummin, pennyroyal, and pepper) with common salt. The Salt of St. Luke was similar but contained a few more ingredients.

A Sal Purgatorius prescribed for the Pope Nicholas consisted of sal ammoniac, 3 oz., scammony, 3 drachms, poppy seeds, 2 drachms, orris root, 3 drachms, pepper, 13 grains, one date, pine nut 25 grains, and squill 2 drachms. This might be made into an electuary with honey.

Antidotus Acharistos, which means unthanked antidote, is stated to be so named because it cured so quickly that patients were not sufficiently grateful. They did not realise how bad they might have been without it.

An electuary said to have been prescribed for King David for his melancholy was composed of aloes, opium, saffron, lign-aloes, myrrh, and some other spices, made up with honey. A Sal Sacerdotale (salt combined with a few spices) stated to have been used by the prophets in the time of Elijah had come down to this Antidotary through St. Paul.

RAYMOND LULLY.

The life of Raymond Lully is so romantic that it is worth telling, though it only touches pharmaceutical history occasionally. Born at Palma, in the island of Majorca, in 1235, in a good position of life, he married at the age of twenty-two, and had two sons and a daughter. But home life was not what he desired, and he continued to live the life of a gallant, serenading young girls, writing verses to them, and giving balls and banquets, to the serious derangement of his fortune. Ultimately he conceived a violent passion for a beautiful and virtuous married woman named Ambrosia de Castello who was living at Majorca with her husband. She, to check this libertine's ardour, showed him her breast, ravaged by cancer. This so afflicted him that he set himself to study medicine with the object of discovering a cure for the cruel disease. With the study of medicine and of alchemy he now associated an insatiable longing for the deliverance of the world from Mohammedan error. He renounced the world, including it would seem his wife and children (though it is recorded that he first shared his possessions with his wife), and went to live on a mountain in a hut which he built with his own hands. This career, however, did not promise an early enough extirpation of infidels, so before long Lully is found travelling, and residing at Paris, Rome, Vienna, Genoa, Tunis, and in other cities, preaching new crusades, importuning the Pope to establish new orders of missionary Christians, and at intervals writing books on medicine. He had invented a sort of mathematical scheme which in his opinion absolutely proved the truth of Christianity, and by the use of diagrams he hoped to convert the Saracens. His ideas are set forth, if not explained, in his *Ars Magna*. In the course of his strange life he visited Palestine and Cyprus, and at Naples in 1293 he made the acquaintance of Arnold de Villanova. This learned man taught Lully much, and found a fervent disciple in him. He was more than seventy when, according to tradition, he travelled to London with the object of urging on Edward III a new war against the Saracens. Edward alleged his want of means, but Lully was prepared to meet the difficulty, and some of the historians of the science of the period assert that he coined a lot of gold for the purpose of the new crusade. Edward promptly used this money for the war with France, in which he was more interested. Disappointed and disgusted, Lully left England, and some time after, at the age of seventy-eight, set out to visit Jerusalem. Having accomplished that journey he visited several of the cities of North Africa on his way back, and at Bougia, after preaching with his usual vehemence against the Mohammedan heresy, he was stoned by the Moors and left for dead. Some friendly merchants took his body on their ship bound for his native Majorca. He revived, but died on the voyage in his eightieth year, A.D. 1415. His tomb is still shown in the church of San Francisco in the City of Palma.

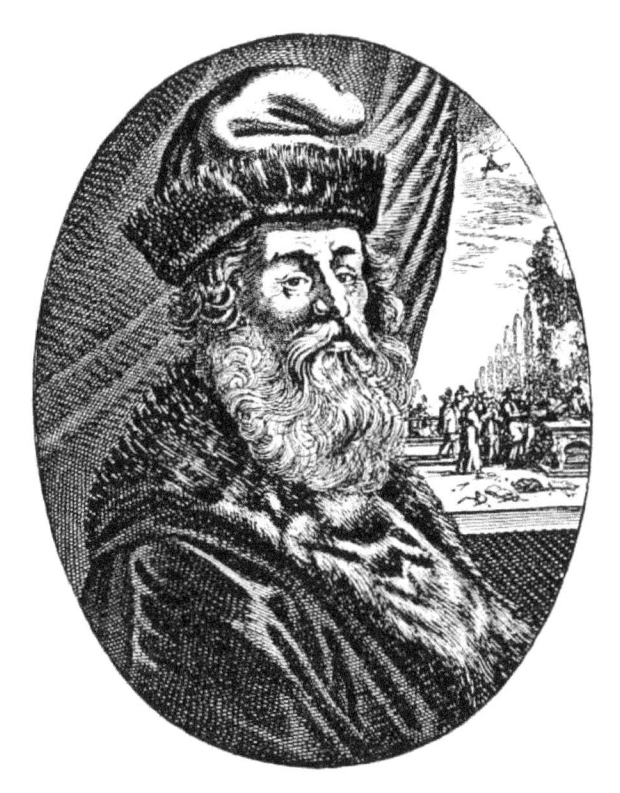

Raymond Lully.

(From a portrait in the Royal Court and State Library, Munich.)

Raymond Lully is particularly famous in pharmaceutical history for the general use of the aqua vitae or aqua ardens which he introduced. He had learned the process of distilling it from wine from Arnold of Villanova, who had himself probably acquired it from the Arab chemists of Spain, but Lully discovered the art of concentrating the spirit by means of carbonate of potash. Of the aqua vitae which he made he declared that "the taste of it exceedeth all other tastes, and the smell of it all other smells."

FRASCATOR.

Hieronymo Frascatoro, generally known as Jerome Frascator, was a physician and poet of high repute in the early part of the sixteenth century. Frascator was born at Verona in 1483 and died near that city in 1553. As a physician he aided the Pope, Paul III, to get the Council of Trent removed from Germany to Italy by alarming the delegates into believing that they were in imminent danger of an epidemic. They therefore adjourned to Bologna. Frascator especially studied infectious diseases, and his celebrated Diascordium, which is described in the section entitled "The Four Officinal

Capitals," was invented as a remedy for the Plague. His great literary fame depended principally on a Latin poem he wrote with the now repellent title of "Syphillides, sive Morbi Gallici," in three books. This was published in 1530. The author did not accept the view that this disease had been imported from America. He held that it had been known in ancient times, and that it was caused by a peculiar corruption of the air. His hero, Syphilis, had given offence to Apollo, who, in revenge, had poisoned the air he breathed. Syphilis is cured by plunging three times in a subterraneous stream of quicksilver. The best classical scholars of the age regarded the poem as the finest Latin work written since the days when that language was in its full life, and they compared it appreciatively with the poems of Virgil. The following lines will serve as a specimen:—

> ... nam saepius ipsi
>
> Carne sua exutos artus, squallentia ossa
>
> Vidimes, et foedo rosa era dehiscere hiatu
>
> Ora, atque exiles renentia guttura voces.

The name of the disease was acquired from this poem, and though it has a Greek form and appearance, no ancient derivative for it can be suggested. Frascator also wrote a poem on hydrophobia.

BASIL VALENTINE.

The name and works of Basil Valentine are inseparably associated with the medical use of antimony. His "Currus Triumphalis Antimonii" (the Triumphal Chariot of Antimony) is stated in all text-books to have been the earliest description of the virtues of this important remedy, and of the forms in which it might be prescribed. And very wonderful indeed is the chemical knowledge displayed in this and other of Valentine's writings.

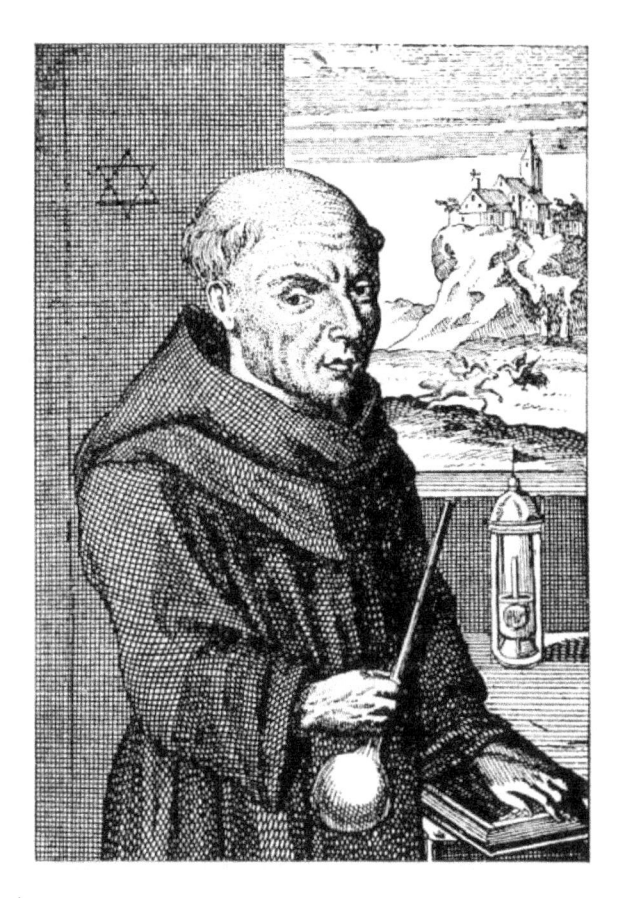

Basil Valentine.

(From the Collection of Etchings in the Royal Gallery, Munich.)

Basil Valentine explains the process of fusing iron with this stibium and obtaining thereby "by a particular manipulation a curious star which the wise men before me called the signet star of philosophy." He commences the treatise already mentioned by explaining that he is a monk of the Order of St. Benedict, which (I quote from an English translation by Theodore Kirkringius, M.D., published at London in 1678) "requires another manner of Spirit of Holiness than the common state of mortals exercised in the profane business of this World."

After thus introducing himself he proceeds to mingle chemistry, piety, and abuse of the physicians and apothecaries of his day with much repetition though with considerable shrewdness for about fifty pages. At last, after many false starts, he expounds the origin and nature of antimony, thus:—

"Antimony is a mineral made of the vapour of the Earth changed into water, which spiritual syderal Transmutation is the true Astrum of Antimony; which water, by the stars first, afterwards by the Element of Fire which resides in the Element of Air, is extracted from the Elementary Earth, and by coagulation formally changed into a tangible essence, in which tangible essence is found very much of Sulphur predominating, of Mercury not so much, and of Salt the least of the three. Yet it assumes so much Salt as it thence acquires an hard and unmalleable Mass. The principal quality of it is dry and hot, or rather burning; of cold and humidity it hath very little in it, as there is in common Mercury; in corporal Gold also is more heat than cold. These may suffice to be spoken of the matter, and three fundamental principles of Antimony, how by the Archeus in the Element of Earth it is brought to perfection."

It needs some practice in reading alchemical writings to make out the drift of this rhapsody, and no profit would be gained by a clear interpretation of the mysticism. It may, however, be noted that the Archeus was a sort of friendly demon who worked at the formation of metals in the bowels of the earth; that all metals were supposed to be compounds of sulphur, mercury, and salt in varying proportions, the sulphur and the salt, however, being refined spiritual essences of the substances we know by these names; and that it was a necessary compliment to pay to any product which it was intended to honour to trace its ancestry to the four elements.

As the author goes on to deal with the various compounds or derivatives from antimony, it is abundantly clear that he writes from practical experience. He describes the Regulus of Antimony (the metal), the glass (an oxy-sulphide), a tincture made from the glass, an oil, an elixir, the flowers, the liver, the white calx, a balsam, and others.

Basil Valentine's scathing contempt for contemporary medical practitioners calls for quotation. "The doctor," he says, "knows not what medicines he prescribes to the sick; whether the colour of them be white, black, grey, or blew, he cannot tell; nor doth this wretched man know whether the medicament he gives be dry or hot, cold or humid.... Their furnaces stand in the Apothecaries' shops to which they seldom or never come. A paper scroll in which their usual Recipe is written serves their purpose to the full, which Bill being by some Apothecary's boy or servant received, he with great noise thumps out of his mortar every medicine, and all the health of the sick."

Valentine concludes his "Triumphal Chariot" by thus apostrophising contemporary practitioners:—"Ah, you poor miserable people, physicians without experience, pretended teachers who write long prescriptions on large sheets of paper; you apothecaries with your vast marmites, as large as may be seen in the kitchens of great lords where they feed hundreds of people; all you so very blind, rub your eyes and refresh your sight that you may be cured of your blindness."

In the same treatise Basil Valentine describes spirit of salt which he had obtained by the action of oil of vitriol on marine salt; brandy, distilled from wine; and how to get copper from pyrites by first obtaining a sulphate, then precipitating the metal by plunging into the solution a blade of iron. This operation was a favourite evidence with later alchemists of the transmutation of iron into copper.

According to some of his biographers Basil Valentine was born in 1393; others are judiciously vague and variously suggest the twelfth, thirteenth, or fourteenth century. That he was a Benedictine monk, he tells us himself, and several monasteries of the order have been named where he is supposed to have lived and laboured.

Many medical historians have doubted whether such a person as Basil Valentine ever existed. His writings are said to have been circulated in manuscript, but no one has ever pretended to have seen one of those manuscripts, and the earliest known edition of any of Basil Valentine's works was published about 1601, by Johann Thölde, a chemist, and part owner of salt works at Frankenhausen in Thuringia. It is rather a large claim on our credulity, or incredulity, to assume that Thölde was himself the author of the works attributed to the old monk, and that he devised the entire fiction of the alleged discoveries, chemistry and all. It was not an uncommon thing among the alchemists and other writers of the middle ages to represent their books as the works of someone of acknowledged fame, just as the more ancient theologians were wont to credit one of the apostles or venerated fathers with their inventions. But it was not common for a discoverer to hide himself behind a fictitious sage whose existence he had himself invented. This theory is, however, held by some chemical critics.

It is certain that the real Basil Valentine could not have been so ancient as he was generally believed to be. Syphilis is referred to in the "Triumphal Chariot" as the new malady of soldiers (Neue Krankheit der Kriegsleute), as morbus Gallicus, and lues Gallica. It was not known by these names until the invasion of Naples by the French in 1495. Another allusion in the same treatise is to the use of antimony in the manufacture of type metal, which was certainly not adopted at any time at which Basil Valentine could have lived. Another reason for questioning his actual existence is that the most diligent search has failed to discover his name either on the provincial list or on the general roll of the Benedictine monks preserved in the archives of the order at Rome. Boerhaave asserted that the Benedictines had no monastery at Erfurt, which was generally assigned as the home of Valentine.

A curious item of evidence bearing on the allegation that Thölde was the fabricator of Basil Valentine's works, or at least of part of them, has been indicated by Dr. Ferguson, of Glasgow, in his notes on Dr. Young's collection of alchemical works. Thölde, it appears, had written a book in his own name entitled "Haliographia." This is divided into four sections, namely: 1. Various kinds of Salts. 2. Extraction of Salts. 3. Salt Springs. 4. Salts obtained from metals, minerals, animals, and vegetables. This Part 4 of the work was subsequently published by Thölde among Basil Valentine's writings. One of two things therefore is obvious. Either Thölde adopted a work by Valentine and issued it as his own, or one at least of the pieces alleged to have been by Valentine was really by Thölde.

Basil Valentine, meaning the valiant king, has assuredly an alchemical ring about it. It is exactly such a name as might be invented by one of the scientific fictionists of the middle ages. It is impossible, too, to read the "Triumphal Chariot," at least when suspicion has been awakened, without feeling that the character of the pious monk is a little overdone. A really devout monk would hardly be proclaiming his piety on every page with so much vehemence. Then there is the legend which accounts for the long lost manuscripts. It is explained that they were revealed to someone, unnamed, when a pillar in a church at Erfurt was struck and split open by lightning, the manuscripts having been buried in that pillar. When this happened is not recorded.

In Kopp's "Beitrage zur Geschichte der Chemie" the learned author argued that Thölde could only be regarded as an editor of Basil Valentine's works, because when they were published they gave so many new chemical facts and observations that it was impossible to think that Thölde would have denied himself the credit of the discoveries if they had been his in fact. That book was published in 1875. In "Die Alchemie," which Kopp published in 1886, he refers to Basil Valentine, and says that there is reason to think that the works attributed to him were an intentional literary deception perpetrated by Thölde.

Paracelsus: His Career.

No one man in history exercised such a revolutionary influence on medicine and pharmacy as the erratic genius Philipus Aureolus Theophrastus Bombast von Hohenheim. The name Paracelsus is believed to have been coined by himself, probably with the intention of somewhat Latinising his patronymic, von Hohenheim, and also perhaps as claiming to rank with the famous Roman physician and medical writer, Celsus. The family of Bombast was an old and honourable one from Württemberg, but the father of the founder of the iatro-chemists was a physician who had settled at Maria-Einsiedeln, a small town in Switzerland, not far from Zurich. He (the father) died at Villach, in Carinthia, in 1534, aged 71.

Theophrastus was an only child. He was born in 1490 or 1491, and owed to his father the first inclination of his mind towards medicine and alchemy. Later he was taught classics at a convent school, and at 16 went to the University of Basel. Apparently he did not stay there long. Classical studies, and the reverence of authorities, which the Universities taught, never attracted him. He is found next at Wurzburg, in the laboratory of Trithemius, an abbot of that city, and a famous adept in alchemy, astrology, and magic generally. He must have acquired much chemical skill in that laboratory, and, doubtless, many of his mystic views began to shape themselves under the instruction of the learned abbot. But Paracelsus was not content with the artificial ideas of the alchemists. By some means he became acquainted with the wealthy Sigismund Fugger, a mine owner in the Tyrol, and either as assistant or friend he joined him. The Fuggers were the Rothschilds of Germany at that time, and one of them entertained Charles V at Augsburg, when the famous diet at which the Emperor was to crush the Reformation was held in that city. On that occasion the wealthy merchant made a cinnamon fire for the Emperor, and lighted it with a bond representing a large sum which Charles owed him.

In the Tyrolese mines Paracelsus learned much about minerals, about diseases, and about men. Then he travelled through various parts of Europe, paying his way by his medical and surgical skill, or, as his enemies said, by conjuring and necromancy. He states that he was in the wars in Venice, Denmark, and the Netherlands; it is supposed as an army surgeon, for he afterwards declared that he then learned to cure forty diseases of the body. He boasted that he learned from gypsies, physicians, barbers, executioners, and from all kinds of people. He claims also to have been in Tartary, and to have accompanied the Khan's son to Constantinople. Van Helmont tells us that it was in this city that he met an adept who gave him the philosopher's stone. Other chroniclers relate that this adept was a certain Solomon Trismensinus, who also possessed the elixir of life, and had been met with some two hundred years later.

Although Paracelsus in his writings appears to hold the current belief in the transmutation of metals, and in the possibility of producing medicines capable of indefinitely prolonging life, he wasted no energy in dreaming about these, as the alchemists generally did. The production of gold does not seem to have interested him, and his aims in medicine were always eminently practical. It is true that he named his compounds catholicons, elixirs, and panaceas, but they were all real remedies for specific complaints; and in the treatment of these he must have been marvellously successful.

Whether he ever went to Tartary or not, and whether he served in any wars or not, may be doubtful. His critics find no evidence of acquaintance with foreign languages or customs in his works, and they do find indications of very elementary notions of geography. But it is certain that for ten years he was peregrinating somewhere; if his travels were confined to Germany the effect was the same. Germany was big enough to teach him. Passionately eager to wrest from Nature all her secrets, gifted with extraordinary powers of observation and imagination, with unbounded confidence in himself, and bold even to recklessness as an experimenter, this was a man who could not be suppressed. Armed with his new and powerful drugs, and not afraid to administer them, cures were inevitable; other consequences also, in all probability.

When, therefore, Paracelsus arrived at Basel, in the year 1525, in the thirty-second year of his age, his fame had preceded him. Probably he was backed by high influence. According to his own account he had cured eighteen princes during his travels, and some of these may have recommended him to the University authorities. It is to the credit of Paracelsus that he was warmly supported by the saintly priest Œcolampadius (Hausschein), who subsequently threw in his lot with the reformers. Besides being appointed to the chair of medicine and surgery, Paracelsus was made city physician.

His lectures were such as had never been heard before at a university. He began his course by burning the works of Galen and Avicenna in a chafing dish, and denouncing the slavish reliance on authority which at that time characterised medical teaching and practice. He taught from his own experience, and he gave his lectures in German. Many quotations of his boastful utterance have been handed down to us, and they match well with what we know of him from his recognised writings. All the universities had less experience than he, and the very down on his neck was more learned than all the authors. He likened himself to Hippocrates, the one ancient whom he esteemed. He contrasted himself with the doctors in white gloves who feared to soil their fingers in the laboratory. "Follow me," he cried; "not I you, Avicenna, Galen, Rhazes, Montagnana, Mesuë, and ye others. Ye of Paris, of Montpellier, of Swabia, of Cologne, of Vienna; from the banks of the Danube, of the Rhine, from the islands of the seas, from Italy, Dalmatia, Sarmatia, and Athens, Greeks, Arabs, Israelites. I shall be the monarch, and mine shall be the monarchy."

In his capacity as city physician he naturally created many enemies among his fellow practitioners. His friends said he cured the cases which they found hopeless; they said he only gave temporary relief at the best, and that his remedies often killed the patients. He fell foul, too, of the apothecaries. He denounced their drugs and their ignorance. The three years he spent in Basel must have been lively both for him and his opponents.

"In the beginning," he says, "I threw myself with fervent zeal on the teachers. But when I saw that nothing resulted from their practice but killing, laming, and distorting; that they deemed most complaints incurable; and that they administered scarcely anything but syrups, laxatives, purgatives, and oatmeal gruel, with everlasting clysters, I determined to abandon such a miserable art and seek truth elsewhere." Again he says: "The apothecaries are my enemies because I will not empty their boxes. My recipes are simple and do not call for forty or fifty ingredients. I seek to cure the sick, not to enrich the apothecaries."

His career at Basel was brought to a close by a dispute with a prebendary of the cathedral named Lichtenfels, whom he had treated. The canon, in pain, had promised him 200 florins if he would cure him. The cure was not disputed, but as Paracelsus had only given him a few little pills, the clergyman relied on the legal tariff. Paracelsus sued him, and the court awarded the legal fee, which was six florins. The doctor published his comments on the case, and it can readily be supposed that they were of such a character as to amount to contempt of court. He found it advisable to leave Basel hurriedly.

Between 1528 and 1535 he lived and practised at Colmar, Esslingen, Nuremberg, Noerdlingen, Munich, Regensburg, Amberg, Meran, St. Gall, and Zurich. From Switzerland he again set forth, and records of him are to be traced in Carinthia and Hungary. Lastly, the Prince Palatine, Duke Ernst of Bavaria, took him under his protection, and settled him at Salzburg. There a few months afterwards he died. From dissipation and exhaustion, say his enemies; by assassination, say his friends. A German surgeon who examined his skull when the body was exhumed thirty years after death, found in it a fracture of the temporal bone, which, he declared, could only have been produced during life, because the bones of a solid but desiccated skull could not have separated as was the case here. It was suggested that some hirelings of the local doctors whose prospects were endangered by this formidable invader had "accidentally" pushed him down some rocks, and that it was then that the fracture was caused. A monument to this great medical revolutionist is still to be seen by the chapel of St. Philip Neri, at Salzburg. It is a broken pyramid of white marble, with a cavity in which is his portrait, and a Latin inscription which commemorates his cures of diseases, and his generosity to the poor in the following terms:—

> "Conditur hic Philippus Theophrastus, insignis Medicinæ
> Doctor, qui dira illa vulnera, lepram, podagram,
> hydroposim, aliaque insanabilia contagia mirificu arte

sustulit; ac bona sua in pauperes distribuenda collocandaque honoravit. Anno 1541, die 24 Septembr. vitam cum morte mutavit."

("Here lies Philippus Theophrastus, the famous Doctor of Medicine, who by his wonderful art cured the worst wounds, leprosy, gout, dropsy, and other diseases deemed incurable and to his honour, shared his possessions with the poor.")

Among the contemporaries of Paracelsus were Luther, Columbus, and Copernicus. Their names alone are sufficient to show how the long-suppressed energy of the human intellect was at that period bursting forth. These four men were perhaps the greatest emancipators of the human race from the chains of slavish obedience to authority in the past thousand years. Paracelsus was not, so far as is known, a Lutheran Protestant. But he could not help sympathising with his heroic countryman. "The enemies of Luther," he wrote, "are to a great extent fanatics, knaves, bigots, and rogues. You call me a medical Luther, but you do not intend to honour me by giving me that name. The enemies of Luther are those whose kitchen prospects are interfered with by his reforms. I leave Luther to defend what he says, as I will defend what I say. That which you wish for Luther you wish for me; you wish us both to the fire." There was, indeed, much in common between these two independent souls.

Columbus landed in the Western world the year before Paracelsus was born. Luther burnt the Pope's Bull at Wittenberg in 1520, and it was this action of his which at the time at least thrilled the German nation more than any other event in the history of the Reformation. It is evident that Paracelsus, in imitating the conduct of his famous contemporary, was only demonstrating his conviction that scientific, no less than religious, thought needed to free itself from the shackles of tyrannic tradition.

His Character.

Such details of the personality of Paracelsus as have come down to us were written by his enemies. Erastus, a theologian as well as a physician, who may have met Paracelsus, and who fiercely attacked his system, depreciates him on hearsay. But Operinus, a disciple who had such reverence for him that when Paracelsus left Basel, he accompanied him and was with him night and day for two years, wrote a letter about him after his death to which it is impossible not to attach great importance.

In this letter Operinus expresses the most unbounded admiration of Paracelsus's medical skill; of the certainty and promptitude of his cures; and especially of the "miracles" he performed in the treatment of malignant ulcers. But, adds Operinus, "I never discovered in him any piety or erudition." He had never seen him pray. He was as contemptuous of Luther as he was of the Pope. Said no one had discovered the true meaning or got at the kernel of the Scriptures.

During the two years he lived with him, Operinus declares Paracelsus was almost constantly drunk. He was scarcely sober two hours at a time. He would go to taverns and challenge the peasantry to drink against him. When he had taken a quantity of wine, he would put his finger in his throat and vomit. Then he could start again. And yet Operinus also reports how perpetually he worked in his laboratory. The fire there was always burning, and something was being prepared, "some sublimate or arsenic, some safran of iron, or his marvellous opodeldoch." Moreover, however drunk he might be he could always dictate, and Operinus says "his ideas were as clear and consecutive as those of the most sober could be."

According to this same letter Paracelsus had been an abstainer until he was 25. He cared nothing for women. Operinus had never known him undress. He would lie down with his sword by his side, and in the night would sometimes spring up and slash at the walls and ceiling. When his clothes got too dirty he would take them off and give them to the first passer, and buy new ones. How he got his money Operinus did not know. At night he often had not an obolus; in the morning he would have a new purse filled with gold.

It is not easy to form a fair judgment of Paracelsus from this sketch. Many writers conclude that Operinus was spiteful because Paracelsus would not tell him his secrets. More likely Operinus left his master because his religious sentiments were shocked by him. Paracelsus was evidently a born mocker, and it may be that he took a malicious delight in making his disciple's flesh creep. Operinus gives an instance of the levity with which his master treated serious subjects. He was sent for one day to see a poor person who was very ill. His first question was whether the patient had taken anything. "He has taken the holy sacrament," was the reply. "Oh, very well," said Paracelsus, "if he has another physician he has no need of me." I think Operinus wrote in good faith, but the stories of the doctor's drunkenness must have been exaggerated. It is inconceivable that he could have been so constantly drunk, and yet always at work. Operinus, it may be added, returned to Basel and set up as a printer, but failed and died in poverty.

Robert Browning's dramatic poem of "Paracelsus" has been much praised by the admirers of the poet. It was written when Browning was 23, and represents in dramatic form the ambitious aspirations of a youth of genius who believes he has if mission in life; has intellectual confidence in his own powers; and the assurance that it is the Deity who calls him to the work.

> In some time, His good time, I shall arrive;
>
> He guides me.

His bitter disappointment with his professorship at Basel, and his contempt for those who brought about his fall there, are depicted, and the effect which the realisation that his aims had proved impossible had on his habits and character is suggested; and at last, on his death-bed in a cell in the Hospital of St. Sebastian at Salzburg, he tells his faithful friend, Festus, who has all his life sought to restrain the ambitions which have possessed him—

> You know the obstacles which taught me tricks
>
> So foreign to my nature, envy, hate,
>
> Blind opposition, brutal prejudice,
>
> Bald ignorance—what wonder if I sank
>
> To humour men the way they most approved.

"A study of intellectual egotism," this poem has been called. Paracelsus was an egotist, without doubt. Indeed, egotism seems a ludicrously insignificant term to apply to his gorgeous self-appreciation. But it is, perhaps, a little difficult to recognise the wild untameable energy of this astonishing medical reformer in the prolix preacher represented in the poem.

Butler's verse (in "Hudibras") may be taken to represent the popular view held about Paracelsus after the first enthusiasm of his followers had cooled down

> Bombastus kept a Devil's bird,
>
> Shut in the pommel of his sword,
>
> That taught him all the cunning pranks
>
> Of past and future mountebanks.

German studies of Paracelsus have been very numerous during the past fifty years, and the general tendency has been greatly to enhance his fame.

After the death of Paracelsus, the Archbishop of Cologne desired to collect his works, many of which were in manuscript and scattered all over Germany. By this time there were many treatises attributed to him which he never wrote. It was a paying business to discover a new document by the famous doctor. It is believed that the fraudulent publications were far more numerous than the genuine ones, and it is quite possible that injustice has been done to his memory by the association with his name of some other peoples' absurdities.

His Mysticism.

The mystic views of Paracelsus, or those attributed to him, are curious rather than useful. He seemed to have had as much capacity for belief as he had disbelief in other philosophers' speculations. He believed in gnomes in the interior of the earth, undines in the seas, sylphs in the air, and salamanders in fire. These were the Elementals, beings composed of soul-substance, but not necessarily influencing our lives. The Elementals know only the mysteries of the particular element in which they live. There is life in all matter. Every mineral, vegetable, and animal has its astral body.

That of the minerals is called Stannar or Trughat; of the vegetable kingdom, Leffas; while the astral bodies of animals are their Evestra. The Evestrum may travel about apart from its body; it may live long after the death of the body. Ghosts are, in fact, the Evestra of the departed. If you commit suicide the Evestrum does not recognise the act; it goes on as if the body were going on also until its appointed time.

Man is a microcosm; the universe is the macrocosm. Not that they are comparable to each other; they are one in reality, divided only by form. If you are not spiritually enlightened you may not be able to perceive this. Each plant on earth has its star. There is a stella absinthii, a stella rorismarini. If we could compile a complete "herbarium spirituale sidereum" we should be fully equipped to treat disease. Star influences also form our soul-essences. This accounts for our varying temperaments and talents.

The material part of man, the living body, is the Mumia. This is managed by the Archæus, which rules over everybody; it is the vital principle. It provides the internal balsam which heals wounds or diseases, and controls the action of the various organs.

His theories of mercury, sulphur, and salt, as the constituents of all things, seem at first likely to lead to something conceivable if not credible. But before we grasp the idea we are switched off into the spiritual world again. It is the sidereal mercury, sulphur, and salt, spirit, soul, and body, to which he is alluding.

His Chemical and Pharmaceutical Innovations.

These fantastic notions permeate all the medical treatises of Paracelsus. But every now and then there are indications of keen insight which go some way towards explaining his success as a physician; for it cannot be doubted that he did effect many remarkable cures. His European fame was not won by mere boasting. His treatise, *De Morbis ex Tartare oriundus*, is admittedly full of sound sense.

Some of his chemical observations are startling for their anticipations of later discoveries. If there were no air, he says, all living beings would die. There must be air for wood to burn. Tin, calcined, increases in weight; some air is fixed on the metal. When water and sulphuric acid attack a metal there is effervescence; that is due to the escape of some air from the water. He calls metals that have rusted, dead.

Saffron of Mars (the peroxide) is dead iron. Verdigris is dead copper. Red oxide of mercury is dead mercury. But, he adds, these dead metals can be revivified, "reduced to the metallic state," are his exact words (and it is to be noted that he was the first chemist to employ the term "reduce" in this sense), by means of coal. Elsewhere he describes digestion as a solution of food; putrefaction as a transmutation. He knew how to separate gold from silver by nitric acid. It is quite certain that the writer of Paracelsus's works was a singularly observant and intelligent chemist. He had "a wolfish hunger after knowledge," says Browning.

"Have you heard," wrote Gui Patin to a friend a hundred years after the death of the famous revolutionary, "that 'Paracelsus' is being printed at Geneva in four volumes in folio? What a shame that so wicked a book should find presses and printers which cannot be found for better things. I would rather see the Koran printed. It would not deceive so many people. Chemistry is the false money of our profession."

HIS PHARMACY.

The composition of Paracelsus's laudanum, the name of which he no doubt invented, has never been satisfactorily ascertained. Paracelsus himself made a great secret of it, and probably used the term for several medicines. It was generally, at least, a preparation of opium, sometimes opium itself. He is believed to have carried opium in the pommel of his sword, and this he called the "stone of immortality."

Next to opium he believed in mercury, and was largely influential in popularising this metal and its preparations for the treatment of syphilis. It was principally employed externally before his time. He mocked at "the wooden doctors with their guaiacum decoctions," and at the "waggon grease with which they smeared their patients." He used turpith mineral (the yellow sulphate), and alembroth salt (ammonio-chloride), though he did not invent these names, and it is possible that he did not mean by them the same substances as the alchemists did. Operinus states that he always gave precipitated mercury (red precipitate, apparently) as a purgative. He gave it in pills with a little theriaca or cherry juice. This he also appears to have designated laudanum. It is certain that he gave other purgatives besides.

It must be admitted that if Basil Valentine is a mythical character, the reputation of Paracelsus is greatly enhanced. Nowhere does the latter claim to have been the first to introduce antimony into medical practice, but it is certain that it could not have been used to any great extent before his time. If we suppose that the works attributed to Basil Valentine were fictitious, so far, that is, as their authorship is concerned, they were compiled about fifty years after the death of Paracelsus, and at the time when his fame was at its zenith. Many of the allusions to antimony contained in those treatises might have been collected from the traditions of the master's conversations and writings, much from his immediate disciples, and the whole skilfully blended by a literary artist.

Paracelsus praises highly his magistery of antimony, the essence, the arcanum, the virtue of antimony. Of this, he says, you will find no account in your books of medicine. This is how to prepare it. Take care at the outset that nothing corrupts the antimony; but keep it entire without any change of form. For under this form the arcanum lies concealed. No deadhead must remain, but it must be reduced by a third cohobation into a third nature. Then the arcanum is yielded. Dose, 4 grains taken with quintessence of melissa.

His "Lilium," or tinctura metallorum, given as an alterative and for many complaints, was formulated in a very elaborate way by his disciples, but simplified it consisted of antimony, 4, tin 1, copper 1, melted together in a crucible, the alloy powdered, and combined (in the crucible) with nitre 6, and cream of tartar 6, added gradually. The mixture while still hot was transferred to a matrass containing strong alcohol 32, digested, and filtered.

Besides mercury and antimony, of which he made great use, iron, lead, copper, and arsenic were among the mineral medicines prescribed by him. He made an arseniate of potash by heating arsenic with saltpetre. He had great faith in vitriol, and the spirit which he extracted from it by distillation. This "spirit" he again distilled with alcohol and thereby produced an ethereal solution. His "specificum purgans" was afterwards said to be sulphate of potash. He recommended sublimed sulphur in inflammatory maladies, saffron of Mars in dysentery, and salts of tin against worms.

Whether his formulas were purposely obscure in so many cases, or whether mystery is due to the carelessness or ignorance of the copyists cannot be known. Much of his chemical and pharmaceutical advice is clear enough.

Honey he extols as a liquor rather divine than human, inasmuch as it falls from heaven upon the herbs. To get its quintessence you are to distil from it in a capacious retort a liquid, red like blood. This is distilled over and over again in a bain mariæ until you get a liquid of the colour of gold and of such pleasant odour that the like cannot be found in the world. This quintessence is itself good for many things, but from it the precious potable gold may be made. The juice of a lemon with this quintessence will dissolve leaf gold in warm ashes in forty-eight hours. With this Paracelsus says he has effected many wonderful cures which people thought he accomplished by enchantment. Elsewhere he speaks of an arcanum drawn from vitriol which is so excellent that he prefers it to that drawn from gold.

He refers with great respect to alchemy and the true alchemists, but with considerable shrewdness in regard to their professions of transmuting other metals into gold. He considered it remarkable that a man should be able to convert one substance into another in a few short days or weeks, while Nature requires years to bring about a similar result; but he will not deny the possibility. What he insists on, however, is that from metals and fire most valuable remedies can be obtained; and the apothecary who does not understand the right way of producing these is but a servant in the kitchen, and not a master cook.

Hellebore was an important medicine with Paracelsus. The white, he said, was suitable for persons under 50, the black for persons over 50. Physicians ought to understand that Nature provides different medicines for old and for young persons, for men and for women. The ancient physicians, although they did not know how to get the essence of the hellebore, had discovered its value for old persons. They found that people who took it after 50 became younger and more vigorous. Their method was to gather the hellebore when the moon was in one of the signs of conservation, to dry it in an east wind, to powder it and mix with it its own weight of sugar. The dose of this powder was as much as could be taken up with three fingers night and morning. The vaunted essence was simply a spirituous tincture. It was more effective if mistletoe, pellitory and peony seeds were combined with it. It was a great remedy for epilepsy, gout, palsy and dropsy. In the first it not merely purges out the humours, but drives away the epileptic body itself. The root must be gathered in the waning of the moon, when it is in the sign Libra, and on a Friday.

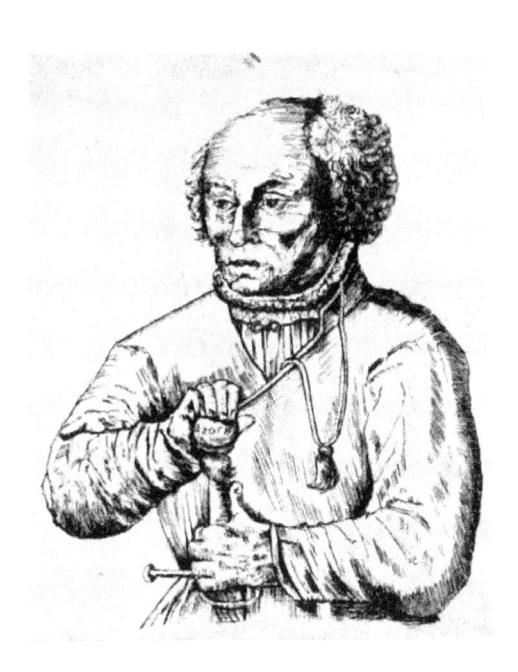

Paracelsus (a).

Paracelsus made balsam from herbs by digesting them in their own moisture until they putrefied, and then distilling the putrefied material. He obtained a number of essential oils and used them freely as quintessences. He defines quintessences thus:—Every substance is a compound of various elements, among which there is one which dominates the others, and impresses its own character on the compound. This dominating element, disengaged, is the quintessence. This term he obtained from Aristotle.

His oil of eggs was obtained by boiling the eggs very hard, then powdering them, and distilling until an oil rose to the surface. This he recommended against scalds and burns. Oil of aniseed he prescribed in colds to be put in the nostrils and applied to the temples on going to bed. Oil of tartar rectified in a sand-bath until it acquires a golden colour will cure ulcers and stone. Coral would quicken fancy, but drive away vain visions, spectres, and melancholy. Oil of a man's excrements, twice distilled, is good to apply in fistulas, and also in baldness. Oil of a man's skull which had never been buried got by distillation was given in 3 grain doses for epilepsy.

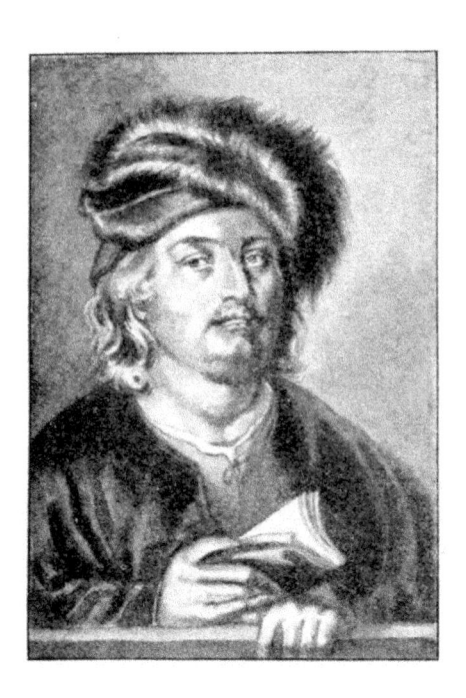

Paracelsus (b).

He had abundant faith in animal remedies. His "Confectio Anti-Epileptica," formulated by his interpreter, Oswald Crollius, is as follows:—First get three human skulls from men who have died a violent death and have not been buried. Dry in the air and coarsely crush. Then place in a retort and apply a gradually increasing heat. The liquor that passed over was to be distilled three times over the same fæces. Eight ounces of this liquor were to be slowly distilled with 3 drachms each of species of diamusk, castorum, and anacardine honey. To the distilled liquor 4 scruples of liquor of pearls and one scruple of oil of vitriol were to be added. Of the resulting medicine one teaspoonful was to be taken in the morning, fasting, by epileptic subjects, for nine days consecutively.

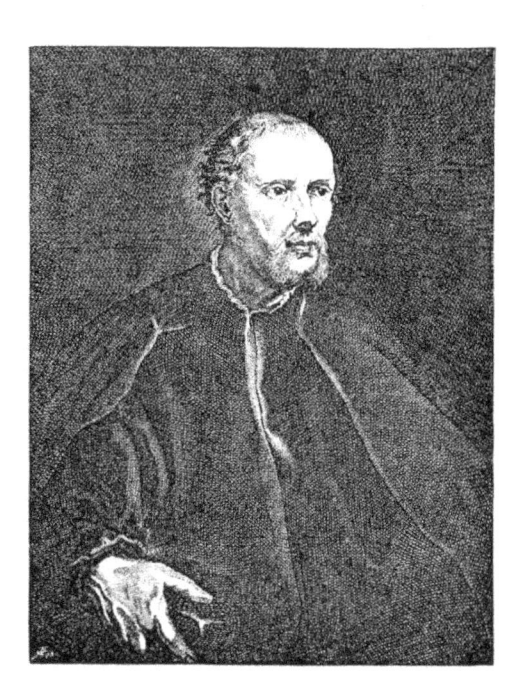

Paracelsus (c).

An Arcanum Corallinum of Paracelsus which was included in some of the earlier London Pharmacopœias, was simply red precipitate prepared in a special manner. The Committee of the College of Physicians which sat in 1745 to revise that work rejected this product with the remark that an arcanum was not a secret known only to some adept, but was simply a medicine which produces its effect by some hidden property. (This might be said of many medicines now as well as then.) They recognised, however, that "Paracelsus, whose supercilious ignorance merits our scorn and indignation," did use the term in the sense of a secret remedy.

The Pharmacy of Paracelsus is so frequently referred to in other sections of this book that it is not necessary to deal with it here at greater length. It is evident, however, that some of the formulas he devised, some of the names he coined, and some of the theories he advanced have entered into our daily practice; and even the dogmas now obsolete which are sometimes quoted to show how superior is our knowledge to his, served to quicken thought and speculation.

Portraits of Paracelsus.

The portraits of Paracelsus to be found in old books, as well as some celebrated paintings, are curiously various as likenesses. The oldest and by far the most frequent representation of him on title pages of his works is more or less similar to the portrait marked A, p. 247. This particular drawing was copied from one in the print room of the British Museum. Portrait B is copied from a painting attributed to Rubens which was for a long time in the Duke of Marlborough's collection at Blenheim. It was sold publicly in 1886 in London for £125 and is now in the "Collection Kums" at Antwerp. There is a similar painting, believed to be a copy of this one, in the Bodleian Library at Oxford.

In the year 1875, at an exhibition of historical paintings held at Nancy (France), a painting "attributed to Albert Dürer," and bearing his name in a cartouche, was exhibited and described as "Portrait presumé de Paracelse." It was not a copy but was unmistakably the same person as the one shown in the painting of Rubens. It came from a private collection and was sold to a local dealer for 2,000 francs, and afterwards disposed of to an unknown stranger for 3,000 francs. It has not been traced since. Dürer died in 1528 (thirteen years before the date of the death of Paracelsus). There is no mention of this likeness in any of his letters. It may have been the work of one of his pupils.

The third portrait (C) which is unlike either of the others professes to have been painted from life ("Tintoretto ad vivum pinxit") by Jacope Robusti, more commonly known as Tintoretto. The original has not been found, and the earliest print from it was a copper-plate engraving in a collection issued by Bitiskius of Geneva in 1658. The picture here given is a reduced copy of that engraving from a phototype made by Messrs. Angerer and Göschl, of Vienna, and published in a valuable work by the late Dr. Carl Aberle in 1890 entitled "Grabdenkmal, Schadel, und Abbildungen des Theophrastus Paracelsus." The publisher of that book, Mr. Heinrich Dieter, has kindly permitted me to use this picture.

Tintoretto scarcely left Venice all his life, and it has been supposed that he may have become acquainted with Paracelsus when the latter was, as he said he was, an army surgeon in the Venetian army in the years 1521–1525. Dr. Aberle points out that if Tintoretto was born in 1518, as is generally supposed, the painting from life was impossible; even if he was born in 1512, as has also been asserted, it was unlikely. Moreover, the gentle-looking person represented, whose amiable "bedside manner" is obviously depicted in the portrait, could not possibly have been the untamable Paracelsus if any reliance can be placed on the art of physiognomy.

NICHOLAS CULPEPPER.

This well-known writer, whose "Herbal" has been familiar to many past generations as a family medicine book, deserves a place among our Masters in Pharmacy for the freedom, and occasional acuteness with which he criticised the first and second editions of the London Pharmacopœia. One specimen of his sarcastic style must suffice. The official formula for Mel Helleboratum was to infuse 3 lbs. of white hellebore in 14 lbs. of water for three days; then boil it to half its bulk; strain; add 3 lbs. of honey and boil to the consistence of honey. This is Culpepper's comment (in his "Physicians' Library"):—

> "What a *monstrum horrendum*, horrible, terrible recipe have we got here:—A pound of white hellebore boiled in 14 lbs. of water to seven. I would ask the College whether the hellebore will not lose its virtue in the twentieth part of this infusion and decoction (for it must be infused, forsooth, three days to a minute) if a man may make so bold as to tell them the truth. A Taylor's Goose being boiled that time would make a decoction near as strong as the hellebore, but this they will not believe. Well, then, be it so. Imagine the hellebore still remaining in its vigour after being so long tired out with a tedious boiling (for less boiling would boil an ox), what should the medicine do? Purge melancholy, say they. But from whom? From men or beasts? The devil would not take it unless it were poured down his throat with a horn. I will not say they intended to kill men, *cum privilegio*; that's too gross. I charitably judge them. Either the virtue of the hellebore will fly away in such a martyrdom, or else it will remain in the decoction. If it evaporate away, then is the medicine good for nothing; if it remain in it is enough to spoil the strongest man living. (1.) Because it is too strong. (2.) Because it is not corrected in the least. And because they have not corrected that, I take leave to correct them."

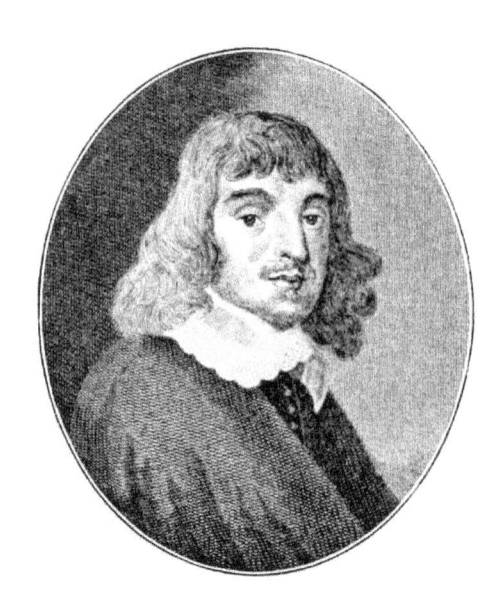

Culpepper.

(From an old book of his.)

This passage is not selected as a favourable specimen of Culpepper's pharmaceutical skill, but as a sample of the manner in which he often rates "the College." His own opinions are open to quite as severe criticism. A large part of his lore is astrological; and he is very confident about the doctrine of signatures. But he knew herbs well, and his general advice is sound.

Perhaps many of those who have studied his works have formed the idea that he was a bent old man with a long grey beard, who busied himself with the collection of simples. He was, in fact, a soldier, and died at the early age of 38. His portraits and the descriptions of him by his astrological friends represent him as a smart, brisk young Londoner, fluent in speech and animated in gesture, gay in company, but with frequent fits of melancholy, an extraordinarily good conceit of himself, and plenty of reason for it.

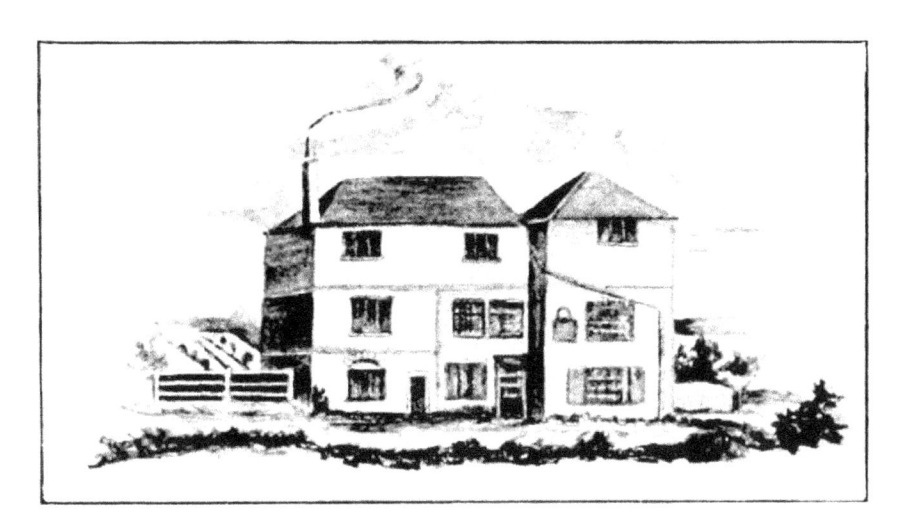

Culpepper's House.

(From an old book of his.)

Culpepper lived in the stirring times of the Civil War, and fought on one side or the other, it is not certain which. Most likely, judging from the frequent pious expressions in his works, he was a Parliamentarian. He was severely wounded in the chest in one of the battles, but it is not known in which. It is probable that it was this wound which caused the lung disease from which he died.

Such information as we have of Culpepper's career is gathered from his own works, and from some brutal attacks on him in certain public prints. He describes himself on the title-pages of some of his big books as "M.D.," but there is no evidence that he ever graduated. He lived, at least during his married life, at Red Lion Street, Spitalfields, and there he carried on his medical practice. Probably it was a large one, for he evidently understood the art of advertising himself. He claims to have been the only doctor in London at the time who gave advice gratis to the poor, and his frequent comments on the cost of the pharmacopœia preparations suggest that the majority of his patients were not of the fashionable class.

Nicholas Culpepper was apprenticed to an apothecary in Great St. Helen's, Bishopsgate, and at the same time a certain Marchmont Nedham was a solicitor's clerk in Jewry Street. Nedham became the most notorious journalist in England, and founded and edited in turn the *Mercurius Britannicus*, an anti-royalist paper, the *Mercurius Pragmaticus*, violently anti-Commonwealth, and the *Mercurius Politicus*, subsidised by Cromwell's government, and supervised by Mr. John Milton. This publication, amalgamated with the *Public Intelligencer*, its principal rival, has descended to us as the *London Gazette*. Probably Nedham and Culpepper were friends in their early days, and they may have been comrades in arms when the war broke out. But evidently they became fierce enemies later. In *Mercurius Pragmaticus* Nedham, pretending to review Culpepper's translation of the official Dispensatory, takes the opportunity of pouring on him a tirade of scurrilous abuse. The translation, he says, "is filthily done," which was certainly not true. This is the only piece of criticism in the article. The rest deals with the author personally. Nedham informs his readers that Culpepper was the son of a Surrey parson, "one of those who deceive men in matters belonging to their most precious souls." That meant that he was a Nonconformist. Nicholas himself, according to Nedham, had been an Independent, a Brownist, an Anabaptist, a Seeker, and a Manifestationist, but had ultimately become an Atheist. During his apprenticeship "he ran away from his master upon his lewd debauchery"; afterwards he became a compositor, then a "figure-flinger," and lived about Moorfields on cozenage. After making vile insinuations about his wife, Nedham states that by two years' drunken labour Culpepper had "gallimawfred the Apothecaries' Book into nonsense"; that he wore an old black coat lined with plush which his stationer (publisher) had got for him in Long Lane to hide his knavery, having been till then a most despicable ragged fellow; "looks as if he had been stued in a tanpit; a frowzy headed coxcomb." He was aiming to "monopolise to himself all the knavery and cozenage that ever an apothecary's shop was capable of."

Culpepper's works answer this spiteful caricature, for at any rate he must have been a man of considerable attainments, and of immense industry. That his writings acquired no little popularity is best proved by the fact that after his death it was good business to forge others somewhat resembling them and pass them off as his.

Turquet de Mayerne.

Sir Theodore Turquet de Mayerne, Baron Aulbone of France, was born at Geneva in 1573, of a Calvinistic family and studied for the medical profession first at Heidelberg and afterwards at Montpellier. Moving to Paris he acquired popularity as a lecturer on anatomy to surgeons, and on pharmacy to apothecaries. His inclination towards chemical remedies brought him to the notice of Rivierus, the first physician to Henri IV, and he was appointed one of the king's physicians. But his medical heterodoxy offended the faculty, and his Protestantism raised enemies for him at court. The king, who valued Turquet, did his best to persuade him to conform to the Church of Rome as he himself had done, and to moderate the rancour of his professional foes. But he was unsuccessful in both efforts. Still Henri tried to keep him, ignoring his heresies, and perhaps rather sympathising with them. But the queen, Marie de Medici, insisted on Turquet's dismissal, and the Faculty of

Paris was no whit behind the queen in intolerance. Coupling him with a quack named Pierre Pena, a foreigner then practising medicine illicitly at Paris, they issued a decree forbidding all physicians who acknowledged their control to consult with De Turquer, and exhorting practitioners of all nations to avoid him and all similar pests, and to persevere in the doctrines of Hippocrates and Galen.

Turquet de Mayerne came to England evidently with a high reputation, for he was soon appointed first physician to the king (James I) and queen, and held the same position under Charles I and Charles II. He seems to have kept in retirement during the Commonwealth, though in 1628 it appears from his manuscript records ("Ephemerides Anglicæ," he called them) that he was consulted by a "Mons. Cromwell" whom he describes as "Valde melancholicus." He died at Chelsea in 1655 at the age of 82. It was in England that he used the name of Mayerne.

De Mayerne exercised a considerable influence on English pharmacy. The Society of Apothecaries owed to him their separate incorporation, and the first London Pharmacopœia was compiled and authorised probably to some extent at his instigation. He certainly wrote the preface to it. Paris quotes him as prescribing among absurd and disgusting remedies "the secundines of a woman in her first labour of a male child, the bowels of a mole cut open alive, and the mummy made of the lungs of a man who had died a violent death." But such remedies were common to all practitioners in England and France at the time. The principal ingredient in a gout powder which he composed was the raspings of an unburied human skull. He devised an ointment for hypochondria which was called the Balsam of Bats. It contained adders, bats, sucking whelps, earthworms, hog's grease, marrow of a stag, and the thigh bone of an ox. On the other hand, Mayerne is credited with the introduction of calomel and black wash into medical practice.

VAN HELMONT.

Jean Baptiste Van Helmont, born at Brussels in 1577, and died at Vilvorde near that city in 1644, was an erratic genius whose writings and experiments sometimes astonish us by their lucidity and insight, and again baffle us by their mysticism and puerility.

Van Helmont was of aristocratic Flemish descent, and possessed some wealth. He was a voracious student and a brilliant lecturer. At the University of Louvain, however, where he spent several years, he refused to take any degree because he believed that such academic distinctions only ministered to pride. He resolved at the same time to devote his life to the service of the poor, and with this in view he made over his property to his sister, and set himself to study medicine. His gift of exposition was so great that the authorities of the University insisted on his acceptance of the chair of

Surgery, though that was the branch of medical practice he knew least about, and though it was contrary to the statutes of the faculty to appoint a person as Professor not formally qualified.

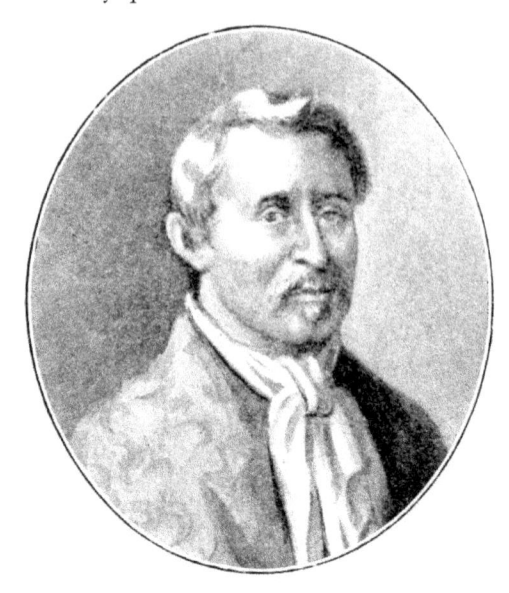

J. B. VAN HELMONT. 1577–1644.

(From an engraving in the Bibliothèque Nationale, Paris.)

For a time things went well, but Van Helmont got tired of medical teaching before the University became tired of him. The particular occasion which disgusted him with medical science was that he contracted the itch, and though he consulted many eminent physicians could not get cured of it. He came to the conclusion that the pretended art of healing was a fraud, and he consequently resolved to shake the dust of it from his feet, after he had recovered from the weakening effects of the purgatives which had been prescribed for his complaint.

Then he set forth on his travels, and in the course of them he met with a quack who cured him of his itch by means of sulphur and mercury. After this he became a violent anti-Galenist. He studied the works of Paracelsus, and after some years came back to his native country full of ideas and phantasies.

By marrying a wealthy woman Van Helmont became independent, and his scientific career now commenced. He erected and fitted a laboratory at Vilvorde, and devoted his time and skill to the study of chemistry, medicine, and philosophy. He described himself as "Medicus per Ignem," and was one of the most earnest believers in the possibility of discovering the philosopher's stone, and the elixir of life. Indeed he claimed that he had actually transmuted mercury into gold, and by his medical compounds it is alleged that he performed such miraculous cures that the Jesuits actually brought him before the Inquisition.

The advance in chemistry for which he is most famous was the discovery of carbonic acid gas, and the first steps in the recognition of the various kinds of gases. Previous to his discovery chemists had no clear perception of a distinction between the various gases; they reckoned them all as air. Geber and other predecessors of Van Helmont had observed that certain vapours were incorporated in material bodies, and they regarded these as the spirits, or souls, of those bodies. Van Helmont was the first actually to separate and examine one of these vapours. He tracked this gas through many of the compounds in which it is combined or formed: he got it from limestone, from potashes, from burning coal, from certain natural mineral waters, and from the fermentation of bread, wine, and beer. He found that it could be compressed in wines and thus yield the sparkling beverages we know so well. He also observed that it extinguished flame, and asphyxiated animals. He alludes to other kinds of vapour, but does not precisely define them. The carbon dioxide he named "gas sylvestre."

This was the first use of the term gas. "Hunc spiritum, hactenus ignotum, novo nomine gas voco." (I call this spirit, heretofore unknown, by the new name gas.) What suggested this name to him is not certain. Some have supposed that it was a modification of the Flemish, *geest*, spirit; by others it is traced to the verb *gaschen*, to boil, or ferment; and by many its derivation from chaos is assumed.

His physiology was a modification of that of Paracelsus. An Archeus within ruled the organism with the assistance of sub-archei for different parts of the body. Ferments stirred these archei into activity. In this way the processes of digestion were accounted for. The vital spirit, a kind of gas, causes the pulsation of the arteries. The Soul of Man he assigned to the stomach. The exact locality of this important adjunct was a subject of keen discussion among the philosophers of that age. Van Helmont's conclusive argument for the stomach as its habitation was the undoubted fact that trouble or bad news had the effect of destroying the appetite.

GLAUBER

John Rudolph Glauber, who was born at Carlstadt, in Germany, in 1603, contributed largely to pharmaceutical knowledge, and deserves to be remembered by his many investigations, and perhaps even more for the clear common sense which he brought to bear on his chemical work. For though he retained a confident belief in the dreams of alchemy, he does not appear to have let that belief interfere with his practical labour; and some of his processes were so well devised that they have hardly been altered from his day to ours.

Not much is known of his history except what he himself wrote or what was related of him by his contemporaries. According to his own account he took to chemistry when as a young man he got cured of a troublesome stomach complaint by drinking some mineral waters. Eager to discover what was the essential chemical in those waters to which he owed his health he set to work on his experiments. The result was the discovery of sulphate of soda, which he called "Sal mirabile," but which all subsequent generations have known as Glauber's Salts. This, it happens, was the one of his discoveries of which he was not particularly vain, for he supposed that he had only obtained from another source Paracelsus's sal enixon, which was in fact sulphate of potash. His own account of this discovery is necessarily of pharmaceutical interest. He gives it in his work *De Natura Salium*, as follows:—

> In the course of my youthful travels I was attacked at Vienna with a violent fever known there as the Hungarian disease, to which strangers are especially liable. My enfeebled stomach rejected all food. On the advice of several friends I dragged myself to a certain spring situated about a league from Newstadt. I had brought with me a loaf of bread, but with no hope of being able to eat it. Arrived at the spring I took the loaf from my pocket and made a hole in it so that I could use it as a cup. As I drank the water my appetite returned, and I ended by eating the improvised cup in its turn. I made several visits to the spring and was soon miraculously cured of my illness. I asked what was the nature of the water and was told it was "salpeter-wasser."

Glauber was twenty-one at that time, and knew nothing of chemistry. Later he analysed the water and got from it, after evaporation, long crystals, which, he says, a superficial observer might confuse with saltpetre; but he soon satisfied himself that it was something quite different. Subsequently he obtained an identical salt from the residue in his retort after distilling marine salt and vitriol to obtain spirit of salt. As already stated, he believed he had produced the "sal enixon" of Paracelsus. But in memory of the benefit he had himself experienced from its use he gave it the title of "sal mirabile."

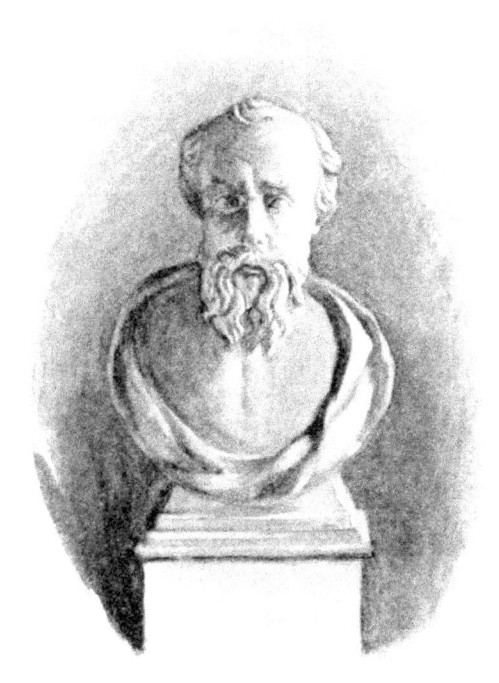

In the seventeenth and eighteenth centuries the sign of "Glauber's Head" appears to have been used in this country by some chemical manufacturers. The picture annexed is from one of these signs which was used more than a hundred years ago by Slinger and Son, of York, and is now in the possession of Messrs. Raimes and Co., of that city, who have kindly given me a photograph of it. It is a wooden bust which was once gilded, and presumably presents the traditional likeness of the famous German chemist.

This distillation of sulphuric acid with sea-salt, which yielded spirit of salt, or as it is now called hydrochloric acid, was probably Glauber's principal contribution to the development of chemistry. He observed the gas given off from the salt, and it is a wonder that with his acuteness he did not isolate and describe the element chlorine. He called it the spirit of rectified salt, and described it as a spirit of the colour of fire, which passed into the receiver, and which would dissolve metals and most minerals. He noted that if digested with dephlegmated (concentrated) spirit of wine his spirit of salt formed a layer of oily substance, which was the oil of wine, "an excellent cordial and very agreeable." He distilled ammonia from bones, and showed how to make sal ammoniac by the addition of sea salt. His sulphate of ammonia, now so largely used as a fertiliser and in the production of other ammonia salts, was known for a long time as "Sal ammoniacum secretum Glauberi." He made sulphate of copper, and his investigation of the acetum lignorum, now called pyroligneous acid, though he did not claim to have discovered this substance, was of the greatest value. He produced artificial gems, made chlorides of arsenic and zinc, and added considerably to the chemistry of wine and spirit-making.

Glauber worked at many subjects for manufacturers, and sold his secrets in many cases. His enemies asserted that he sold the same secret several times, and that he not unfrequently sold secrets which would not work. It is impossible now to test the truth of these accusations. Probably some of the allegations made against him were due to the fact that those who bought his processes were not as skilful as he was. One secret which he claimed to have discovered he would neither sell nor publish. It was that of the Alkahest, or universal solvent. To make this known might, he feared, "encourage the luxury, pride, and godlessness of poor humanity."

Oliver Cromwell wrote in an old volume of Glauber's Alchemy: "This Glauber is an errant knave. I doe bethinke me he speaketh of wonders which cannot be accomplished; but it is lawful for man too the endeavour."

Glauber complained that he was not appreciated, which was probably true. "I grieve over the ignorance of my contemporaries," he wrote, "and the ingratitude of men. Men are always envious, wicked, ungrateful. For myself, faithful to the maxim, *Ora et Labora*, I fulfil my career, do what I can, and await my reward." Elsewhere he writes, "If I have not done all the good in the world that I should have desired, it has been the perversity of men that has hindered me." His employees, he says, were unfaithful. Having learned his processes, they became inflated with pride, and left him. Apparently there was a good business to be done in chemical secrets at that time. But Glauber did not give away all he knew, and he found it best to do all his important work himself. "I have learnt by expensive experience," he wrote, "the truth of the proverb, 'Wer seine Sachen will gethan haben recht, Muss selbsten seyn Herr und Knecht.'"

Although all Glauber's books appeared with Latin titles they were written in German.

GOULARD.

Thomas Goulard was a surgeon of Montpellier with rather more than a local reputation. He was counsellor to the king, perpetual mayor of the town of Alet, lecturer and demonstrator royal in surgery, demonstrator royal of anatomy in the College of Physicians, fellow of the Royal Academies of Sciences in Montpellier, Toulouse, Lyons, and Nancy, pensioner of the king and of the province of Languedoc for lithotomy, and surgeon to the Military

Hospital of Montpellier. His treatise on "The Extract of Saturn" was published about the middle of the eighteenth century, and his name and the preparations he devised were soon spread all over Europe. White lead and sugar of lead, and litharge as the basis of plasters had been familiar in medical practice for centuries; and Galen and other great authorities had highly commended lead preparations for eye diseases and for general lotions. The preparation of sugar of lead is indicated in the works attributed to Basil Valentine. Goulard's special merit consisted in the care which he gave to the production of his "Extract of Saturn," and in his intelligent experiments with it, and its various preparations in the treatment of external complaints.

Goulard made his extract of Saturn by boiling together golden litharge and strong French wine vinegar at a moderate heat for about an hour, stirring all the while, and after cooling drawing off for use the clear supernatant liquor. Diluting this extract by adding 100 drops to a quart of river water with four teaspoonfuls of brandy, made what he called his Vegeto-Mineral Water, which he used for lotions. His cerate of Saturn was made by melting 4 oz. of wax in 11 oz. of olive oil, and incorporating with this 6 lbs. of vegeto-mineral water (containing 4 oz. of extract of Saturn). A cataplasm was made by gently boiling the vegeto-mineral water with crumb of bread. A pomatum was prepared by combining 4 oz. of the extract with a cerate composed of 8 oz. of wax in 18 oz. of rose ointment. This was made stronger or milder as the case might need. There was another pomatum made with the extract of Saturn, sulphur, and alum, for the treatment of itch; and several plasters for rheumatic complaints. Goulard gave full details of the various uses of these applications in inflammations, bruises, wounds, abscesses, erysipelas, ophthalmia, ulcers, cancers, whitlows, tetters, piles, itch, and other complaints. His own experience was supported by that of other practitioners.

In giving the results of his experience thus freely and completely, Goulard was aware of the sacrifice he was making. "I flatter myself," he says, "that the world is in some measure indebted to me for publishing this medicine, which, if concealed in my own breast, might have turned out much more to my private emolument"; at the same time he did not object to reap some profit from his investigations, if this could be done. At the end of the English translation of his book, a copy of a document is printed addressed to his fellow student of fifty years before, Mr. G. Arnaud, practising as a surgeon in London, engaging to supply to him, and to him only, a sufficient quantity of extract of Saturn made by himself, to be distributed by the said Mr. Arnaud, or by those commissioned by him, over all the dominions of his British Majesty.

SCHEELE.

Karl Wilhelm Scheele is the most famous of pharmacists, and has few equals in scientific history. He was the seventh child of a merchant at Stralsund, then in the possession of Sweden, and was born on December 9th, 1742. He had a fair education and at school was diligent and apt in acquiring knowledge. If he was born with a gift, if his genius was anything more than an immense capacity for taking pains, this aptness was the faculty which distinguished Scheele from other men. He made thousands of experiments and never forgot what he had learned from any one of them; he read such scientific books as he could get, and never needed to refer to them again. His friend Retsius, a pharmacist like himself as a young man, but subsequently Director of the Museum of Lund, has recorded Scheele's remarkable power in this respect. "When he was at Malmö," he writes (this was when Scheele was about twenty-four years of age), "he bought as many books as his small pay enabled him to procure. He would read these once or twice, and would then remember all that interested him, and never consulted them again."

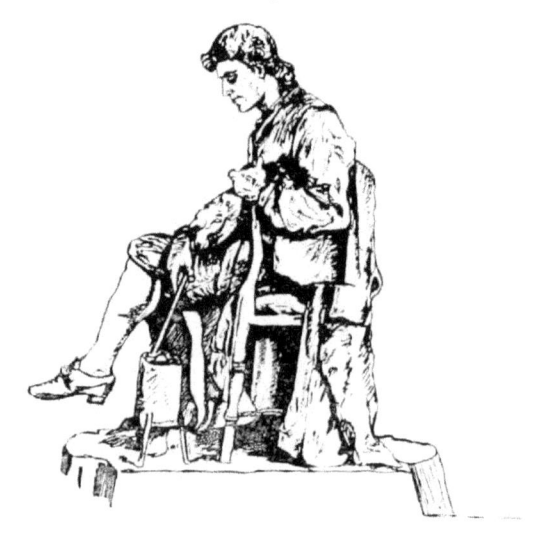

Karl Wilhelm Scheele.

An elder brother of Karl had been apprenticed to an apothecary at Gothenburg, but had died during his apprenticeship. Karl went to this apothecary, a Mr. Bauch, as apprentice at the age of fourteen, and remained there till Bauch sold his business in 1765. Then he went to another apothecary named Kjellström at Malmö. Three years later he was chief assistant to a Mr. Scharenberg at Stockholm. His next move was to Upsala with a Mr. Lokk, who appreciated his assistant and gave him plenty of time for his scientific work.

Lastly, he took the management of a pharmacy at Köping for a widow who owned it, and after an anxious time in clearing the business from debt, he bought the business in 1776 and for the rest of his short life was in fairly comfortable circumstances. Ill-health then pursued him, rheumatism and attacks of melancholy. In the spring of 1786, in the forty-fourth year of his age, after suffering for two months from a slow fever, he died. Two days before his death he married the widow of his predecessor, whose business he had rescued from ruin, so that she might repossess it. A few months later she married again.

That was Scheele's life as a pharmacist; patient, plodding, conscientious, only moderately successful, and shadowed by many disappointments. The work he accomplished as a scientific chemist would have been marvellous if he had had all his time to do it in; under the actual circumstances in which it was performed it is simply incomprehensible. A bare catalogue of his achievements is all that can be noted here, but it must be remembered that he never announced any discovery until he had checked his first conclusions by repeated and varied tests.

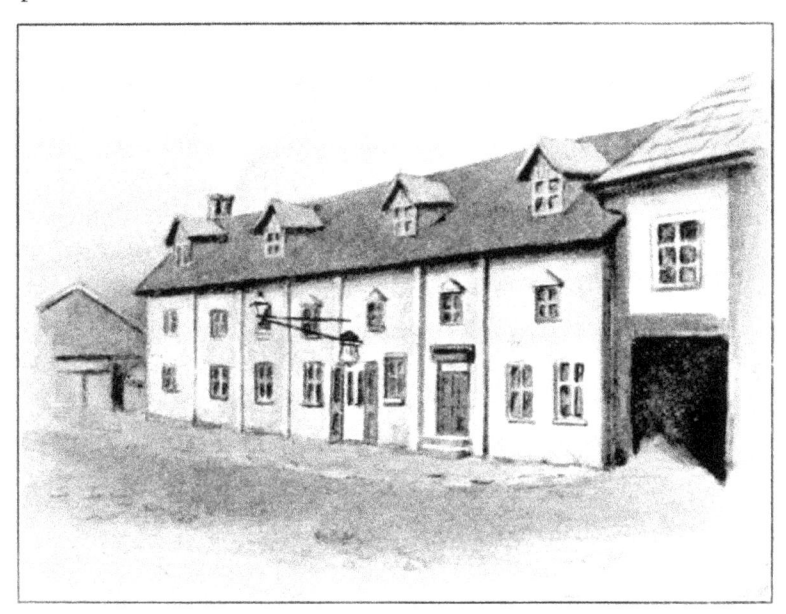

Scheele's Pharmacy at Köping.

An account of an investigation of cream of tartar resulting in the isolation of tartaric acid was his first published paper. He next made an examination of fluor-spar from which resulted the separation of fluoric acid. From this on the suggestion of Bergmann he proceeded to a series of experiments on black oxide of manganese which besides showing the many important combinations of the metal led the chemist direct to his wonderful discoveries of oxygen, chlorine, and barytes. This work put him on the track of the observations set forth in his famous work on "Air and Fire." In this he explained the composition of the atmosphere, which, he said, consisted of two gases, one of which he named "empyreal" or "fire-air," the same as he had obtained from black oxide of manganese, and other substances. He realised and described with much acuteness the part this gas played in nature, and the rest of the book contained many remarkable observations which showed how nearly Scheele approached the new ideas which Lavoisier was to formulate only a few years later. "Air and Fire" was not issued till 1777, three years after Priestley had demonstrated the separate existence and characteristics of what he termed "dephlogisticated air." But it is well known that the long delay of Scheele's printer in completing his work was one of the disappointments of his life, and there is evidence that his discovery of oxygen was actually made in 1773, a year before Priestley had isolated the same element. Both of these great experimenters missed the full significance of their observations through the confusing influence of the phlogiston theory, which neither of them questioned, and which was so soon to be destroyed as the direct result of their labours.

Among the other investigations which Scheele carried out were his proof that plumbago was a form of carbon, his invention of a new process for the manufacture of calomel, his discovery of lactic, malic, oxalic, citric, and gallic acids, of glycerin, and his exposition of the chemical process which yielded Prussian blue, with his incidental isolation of prussic acid, a substance which he described minutely though he gives no hint whatever to show that he knew anything of its poisonous nature.

The subjects mentioned by no means exhaust the mere titles of the work which Scheele accomplished; they are only the more popular of his results. The value of his scientific accomplishments was appreciated in his lifetime, but not fully until the advance of chemistry set them out in their true perspective. Then it was realised how completely and accurately he had finished the many inquiries which he had taken in hand.

A PHARMACEUTICAL PANTHEON.

The School of Pharmacy of Paris, built in 1880, honours a number of pharmacists of historic fame by placing a series of medallions on the façade of the building, as well as statues of two specially eminent representatives of the profession in the Court of Honour. These two are Vauquelin and Parmentier.

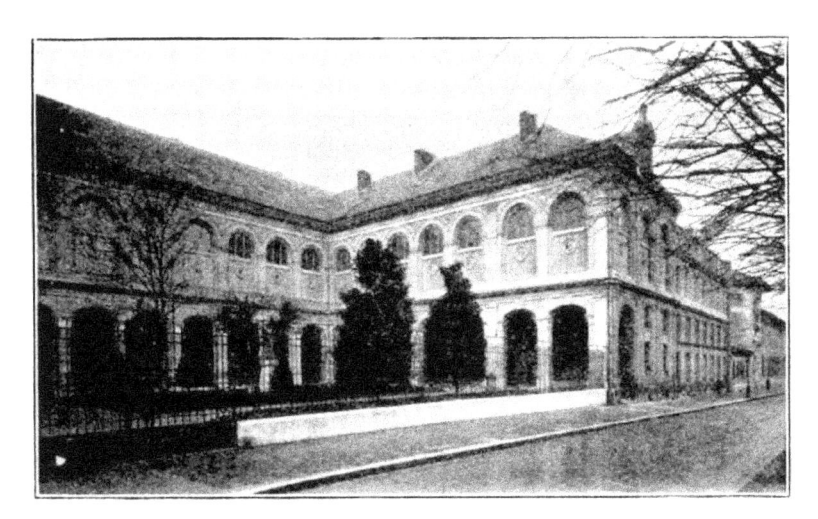

École de Pharmacie, Paris.

(From photo sold at School.)

Louis Nicolas Vauquelin was director of the School from its foundation in 1803 until his death in 1829. He also held professorships at the School of Mines, at the Polytechnic School, and with the Faculty of Medicine. He began his career as a boy in the laboratory of a pharmacist at Rouen, and later got a situation with M. Cheradame, a pharmacist in Paris. Cheradame was related to Fourcroy, to whom he introduced his pupil. Fourcroy paid him £12 a year with board and lodging, but he proved such an indefatigable worker that in no long time he became the colleague, the friend, and the indispensable substitute of his master in his analyses as well as in his lectures. He is cited as the discoverer of chromium, of glucinium, and of several animal products; but his most important work was a series of chemical investigations on belladonna, cinchona, ipecacuanha, and other drugs, which it is recognised opened the way for the definite separation of some of the most valuable of the alkaloids accomplished afterwards by Pelletier, Caventou, Robiquet, and others. Vauquelin published more than 250 scientific articles.

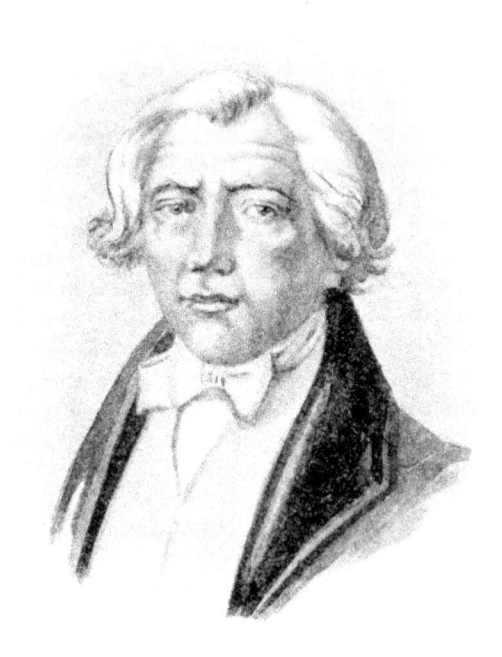

Vauquelin.

(Origin unknown.)

Antoine Augustin Parmentier (born 1737, died 1813), after serving an apprenticeship with a pharmacist at Montpellier, joined the pharmaceutical service in the army, and distinguished himself in the war in Germany, especially in the course of an epidemic by which the French soldiers suffered seriously. He was taken prisoner five times, and at one period had to support himself almost entirely on potatoes. On the last occasion he obtained employment with a Frankfort chemist named Meyer, who would have gladly kept him with him. But Parmentier preferred to return to his own country, and obtained an appointment in the pharmacy of the Hotel des Invalides, rising to the post of chief apothecary there in a few years. A prize offered by the Academy of Besançon for the best means of averting the calamities of famine was won by him in 1771, his German experience being utilised in his advocacy of the cultivation of potatoes. These tubers, though they had been widely cultivated in France in the sixteenth century, had gone entirely out of favour, and were at that time only given to cattle. The people had come to believe that they occasioned leprosy and various fevers. Parmentier worked with rare perseverance to combat this prejudice. He cultivated potatoes on an apparently hopeless piece of land which the Government placed at his disposal, and when the flowers appeared he made a bouquet of them and presented it to Louis XVI, who wore the blossoms in his button-hole. His triumph was complete, for very soon the potato was again cultivated all through France. The royalist favour that he had enjoyed put him in some danger during the Revolution; but in the latter days of the Convention, which had deprived him of his official position and salary, he was employed to organise the pharmaceutical service of the army. He also invented a syrup of grapes which he proposed to the Minister of War as a substitute for sugar during the continental blockade.

The medallions, in the order in which they appear on the façade of the École de Pharmacie, represent the following French and foreign pharmacists:—

Antoine Jerome Balard, the discoverer of bromine (born 1802, died 1876), was a native of Montpellier, where he qualified as a pharmacist and commenced business. As a student he had worked with the salts deposited from a salt marsh in the neighbourhood, and had been struck with a coloration which certain tests gave with a solution of sulphate of soda obtained from the marsh. Pursuing his experiments, he arrived at the discovery of bromine, the element which formed the link between chlorine and iodine. This early success won for him a medal from the Royal Society of London and a professorship of chemistry at Montpellier, and subsequently raised him to high scientific positions in Paris. Balard did much more scientific work, among which was the elaboration of a process for the production of potash salts from salt marshes. He had worked at this for some twenty years, and had taken patents for his methods, when the announcement of the discovery of the potash deposits at Stassfurt effectually destroyed all his hope of commercial success.

Joseph Bienaimé Caventou (born at St. Omer 1795, died 1877) carried on for many years an important pharmaceutical business in Paris. His fame rests on his association with Pelletier in the discovery of quinine in 1820.

Joseph Pelletier (born 1788, died 1842) was the son of a Paris pharmacist, and was one of the most brilliant workers in pharmacy known to us. He is best known for his isolation of quinine. Either alone, or in association with others, he investigated the nature of ipecacuanha, nux vomica, colchicum, cevadilla, hellebore, pepper, opium, and other drugs, and a long series of alkaloids is credited to him. He also contributed valuable researches on cochineal, santal, turmeric, and other colouring materials. To him and his associate, Caventou, the Institute awarded the Prix Monthyon of 10,000 francs for their discovery of quinine, and this was the only reward they obtained for their cinchona researches, for they took out no patents.

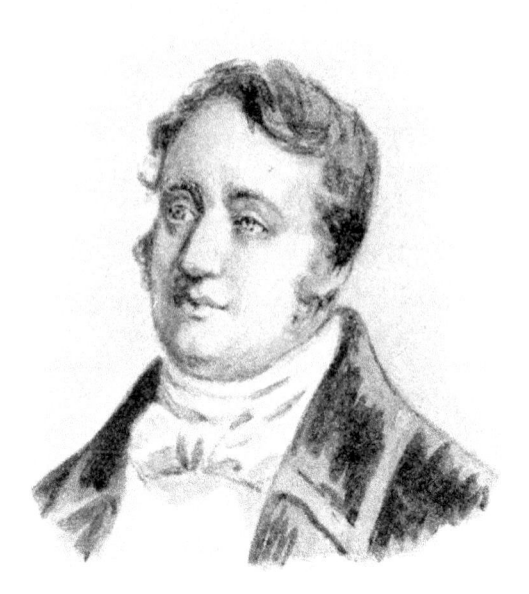

JOSEPH PELLETIER. 1788–1842.

(Discoverer—with Caventou—of Quinine.)

Pierre Robiquet (born at Rennes in 1780, died at Paris, 1840) served his apprenticeship to pharmacy at Lorient, and afterwards studied under Fourcroy and Vauquelin at Paris. His studies were interrupted by the conscription, which compelled him to serve under Napoleon in the Army of Italy. Returning to pharmacy after Marengo, he ultimately became the proprietor of a pharmacy, and to that business he added the manufacture of certain fine chemicals. His first scientific work was the separation of asparagin, accomplished in association with Vauquelin, in 1805. His later studies were in connection with opium (from which he extracted codeine), on liquorice, cantharides, barytes, and nickel.

André Constant Dumeril (born at Amiens, 1774, died 1860) was a physician, but distinguished himself as a naturalist and anatomist. He had been associated with Cuvier in early life. Latterly he was consulting physician to Louis Philippe.

Antoine Louis Brongniart (born 1742, died 1804) was the son of a pharmacist of Paris, and became himself pharmacien to Louis XVI. He also served the Convention as a military pharmacist, and was placed on the Council of Health of the Army. In association with Hassenfratz who was one of the organisers of the insurrection of August 10th, 1792, and himself a professor at the School of Mines, Brongniart edited a "Journal des Sciences, Arts, et Metiers" during the Revolution.

The next medallion memorialises Scheele, the great Swedish pharmacist and chemist, of whose career details have already been given.

Pierre Bayen (born at Chalons s/Marne, 1725, died 1798) was an army pharmacist for about half of his life, and to him was largely due the organisation of that service. He was with the French Army in Germany all through the Seven Years' War, 1757–1763. Among his scientific works were examinations of many of the natural mineral waters of France, and a careful investigation into the alleged danger of tin vessels used for cooking. Two German chemists, Margraff and Henkel, had reported the presence of arsenic in tin utensils generally, and the knowledge of this fact had produced a panic among housekeepers. Bayen went into the subject thoroughly and was able to publish a reassuring report. To him, too, belongs the glory of having been one of the chemists before Lavoisier to prove that metals gain and do not lose weight on calcination in the air.

Pierre Joseph Macquer, Master of Pharmacy and Doctor of Medicine (born 1718, died 1784), came of a noble Scotch family who had settled in France on account of their adherence to the Catholic faith, made some notable chemical discoveries, and became director of the royal porcelain factory at Sèvres. He worked on kaolin, magnesia, arsenic, gold, platinum, and the diamond. The bi-arseniate of arsenic was for a long time known as Macquer's arsenical salt. Macquer was not quite satisfied with Stahl's phlogiston theory, and tried to modify it; but he would not accept the doctrines of Lavoisier. He proposed to substitute light for phlogiston, and regarded light as precipitated from the air in certain conditions. These notions attracted no support.

Guillaume François Rouelle (born near Caen, 1703, died 1770) was in youth an enthusiastic student of chemistry, the rudiments of which he taught himself in the village smithy. Going to Paris he obtained a situation in the pharmacy which had been Lemery's, and subsequently established one of his own in the Rue Jacob. There he commenced courses of private lectures which were characterised by such intimate knowledge, and flavoured with such earnestness and, as appears from the stories given by pupils, by a good deal of eccentricity, that they became the popular resort of chemical students. Lavoisier is believed to have attended them. Commencing his lectures in full professional costume, he would soon become animated and absorbed in his subject, and throwing off his gown, cap, wig and cravat, delighted his hearers with his vigour. Rouelle was offered the position of apothecary to the king, but declined the honour as it would have involved the abandonment of his lectures. His chief published work was the classification of salts into neutral, acid, and basic. He also closely investigated medicinal plants, and got so near to the discovery of alkaloids as the separation of what he called the immediate principles, making a number of vegetable extracts.

Etienne François Geoffrey (born 1672, died 1731), the son of a Paris apothecary, himself of high reputation, for it was at his house that the first meetings were held which resulted in the formation of the Academy of Sciences, studied pharmacy at Montpellier, and qualified there. Returning to Paris he went through the medical course and submitted for his doctorate three theses which show the bent of his mind. The first examined whether all diseases have one origin and can be cured by one remedy, the second aimed to prove that the philosophic physician must also be an operative chemist, and the third dealt with the inquiry whether man had developed from a worm. Geoffrey was attached as physician to the English embassy for some time and was elected to the Royal Society of London. Afterwards he became professor of medicine and pharmacy at the College of France. His chief works were pharmacological researches on iron, on vitriol, on fermentation, and on some mineral waters. He wrote a notable treatise on Materia Medica.

Albert Seba was an apothecary of Amsterdam, who spent some part of his early life in the Dutch Indies. He was born in 1668 and died in 1736. He was particularly noted for a great collection illustrating all the branches of natural history, finer than any other then known in Europe. Peter the Great having seen this collection bought it for a large sum and presented it to the Academy of Sciences of St. Petersburg, where it is still preserved.

Anxious to pay due honour to the distinguished pharmacists of other nations, the authorities of the School of Pharmacy introduce the medallions of Dante and Sir Isaac Newton. The Italian poet's connection with pharmacy was the entirely nominal inscription of his name in the guild of apothecaries of the city of Florence; there are almost slighter grounds to the right of claiming the English philosopher among pharmacists, his immediate association with the business having been that as a schoolboy he lodged at Grantham with an apothecary of the name of Clark. In his later years he worked with Boyle on ether.

Moses Charas figures between these two. Living between the years 1618 and 1698, Charas attained European celebrity. He was the first French pharmacist to prepare the famous Theriaca. This he did in the presence of a number of magistrates and physicians. He also wrote a treatise on the compound. For nine years he was demonstrator of chemistry at the King's Garden at Paris, but he was a Protestant, and the Revocation of the Edict of Nantes in 1685 drove him from France. Charles II received him cordially in London, and made him a doctor. Afterwards he went to Holland, and from there the King of Spain sent for him to attend on him in a serious illness. While at Toledo he got into trouble with the ecclesiastics in a singular manner. An archbishop of Toledo being canonised, his successor announced that snakes in that archbishopric should henceforth lose their venom. This was a special temptation to Moses Charas. He was strong on vipers. He had made medicine of many of them, he had written a book about them, and he knew all there was to know about them. He knew something about archbishops too, which ought to have prevented him from publicly demonstrating the vanity of the proclamation. But he must needs show to some influential friends a local viper he had caught and make it bite two chickens, both of which died promptly. This demonstration got talked about, and Charas was prosecuted on a charge of attempting to overthrow an established belief. He was imprisoned by the Inquisition, but after four months he abjured Protestantism, and was set free. It must be remembered that he was 72 years of age. On his return to France Louis XIV received him kindly, and had him elected to the Academy of Sciences. Charas's chief work was a Pharmacopœia, which was in great vogue, and was translated into all the principal modern languages, even into Chinese.

Nicolas Lemery (born at Rouen, 1645, died 1715), a self-taught chemist and pharmacist, exercised an enormous influence in science and medicine. He opened a pharmacy in the Rue Galande, Paris, and there taught chemistry orally and practically. His course was an immense success. Fashionable people thronged to his lectures, and students came from all countries to get the advantage of his teaching. He, too, was a Protestant, and was struck by the storm of religious animosity. Charles II had the opportunity of showing him hospitality in London, and seems to have manifested towards him much friendliness. The University of Berlin likewise made him tempting proposals, but Lemery could only feel at home in France. Things seemed quieter and he returned, only to find in a short time that the condition was worse for Protestants than ever. The Revocation of the Edict of Nantes prevented him from following either of his professions, pharmacy or medicine; and for their sake he adopted the Catholic faith. His "Universal Pharmacopœia" and his "Dictionary of Simple Drugs" were published after these troubles, and they are the works by which he won his lasting reputation.

Gilles François Boulduc (1675–1742) was for many years first apothecary to Louis XIV, and an authority on pharmaceutical matters in his time. By his essays he helped to popularise Epsom, Glauber's, and Seignette's salts in France.

Antoine Baumé (born at Senlis, 1728, died 1804), the son of an innkeeper, after an imperfect education in the provinces, got into the famous establishment of Geoffrey at Paris and made such good use of his opportunities that he became Professor of Chemistry at the College of France when he was 25. A practical and extraordinarily industrious chemist, he wrote much, invented the areometer which bears his name, founded a factory of sal ammoniac, and bleaching works for silk by a process which he devised. Baumé did good service, too, in dispelling many of the traditional superstitions of pharmacy, such as the complicated formulas and disgusting ingredients which were so common in his time. He was never content to accept any views on trust.

The three medallions which follow are those of Lavoisier, Berthollet, and Chaptal; great chemists whose right to be represented cannot be challenged, but whose works were not specially associated with pharmacy. These three all lived at the time of the Revolution. Lavoisier was one of its most distinguished victims, Berthollet became the companion and adviser of Napoleon in Egypt, and Chaptal was the chemist commissioned by the Convention to provide gunpowder for its ragged troops. He became one of Napoleon's Ministers under the Consulate.

André Laugier (1770–1832), who comes next, was a relative and pupil of Fourcroy, and became an Army pharmacist, serving through Bonaparte's Egyptian campaign. His works were mostly on mineralogical subjects.

Georges Simon Serullas (1774–1832) was another military pharmacist who served in the Napoleonic wars. He was, later, chief pharmacist at the military hospital of Val de Grace, where he devoted much study to many medicinal chemicals, such as cyanic acid, iodides, bromides, and chlorides of cyanogen, hydrobromic ether, etc.

Thénard (1777–1857), the eminent chemist, follows. He was very poor when he asked Vauquelin to receive him as a pupil without pay. He only secured the benefit he asked for because the chemist's sister happened to want a boy at the time to help her in the kitchen. He became a peer of France in 1832. To him we owe peroxide of hydrogen.

Nicolas J. B. Guibourt (1790–1867), Professor of Materia Medica at the School of Pharmacy, was author of a well-known "History of Simple Drugs," and other works. He is often quoted in "Pharmacographia."

Achille Valenciennes (1794–1865) was noted as a naturalist, and especially as a zoologist. He was Cuvier's most trusted assistant in the preparation of certain of his works. For many years Valenciennes was Professor of Zoology at the School of Pharmacy, Paris.

Baron Liebig (1803–1873), was placed in a pharmacy at Heppenheim as a youth, but remained there only ten months. His chemical works are well known.

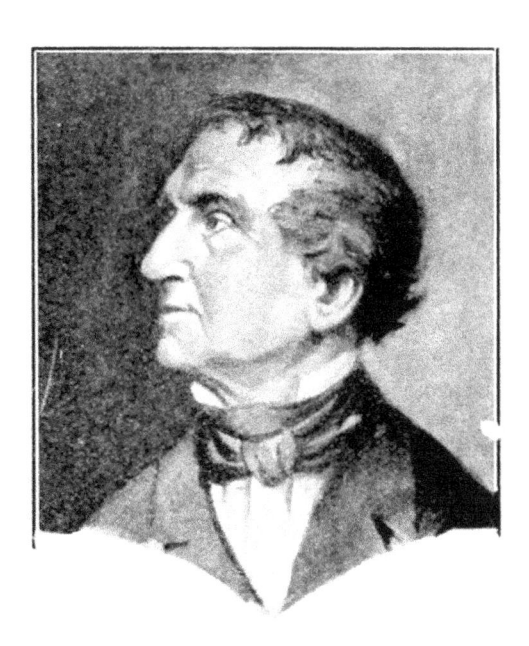

Baron Liebig.

Charles Frederick Gerhardt (1816–1856), born at Strasburg (then a French city), one of Liebig's most brilliant pupils, was for some years Professor of Chemistry at Montpellier in succession to Balard. Later, he founded a laboratory at Paris, and finally accepted the Chair of Chemistry at Strasburg. He was one of the founders of modern organic chemistry, and the originator of the type theory.

Theophile Jules Pelouze (1807–1867) held a position in the pharmaceutical service of the Salpêtrière Hospital at Paris, when, one day in the country, he was overtaken by a torrential storm. A carriage passing, the pedestrian appealed to the driver to take him inside. No notice was taken of his request, so the indignant young pharmacist ran after the vehicle and seized the reins. Having stopped the horse, he delivered a severe lecture to the driver on his lack of courtesy and humanity. The passenger in the carriage invited him to enter and share the shelter. This gentleman was M. Gay-Lussac, the most eminent chemist in Paris at the time. The acquaintance thus curiously commenced resulted in Pelouze becoming Gay-Lussac's laboratory assistant. He ultimately succeeded his employer at the Polytechnic School and, later still, was promoted to the Chair which Thénard had occupied at the College of France. Pelouze was a voluminous writer, and did useful work on the production of native sugar. In conjunction with Liebig he discovered œnanthic ether.

Sir Humphry Davy served an apprenticeship with a Mr. Borlase, an apothecary of Penzance, but afterwards exchanged physic for science. He died at Geneva in 1829 at the age of 51, after a life crowded with scientific triumphs.

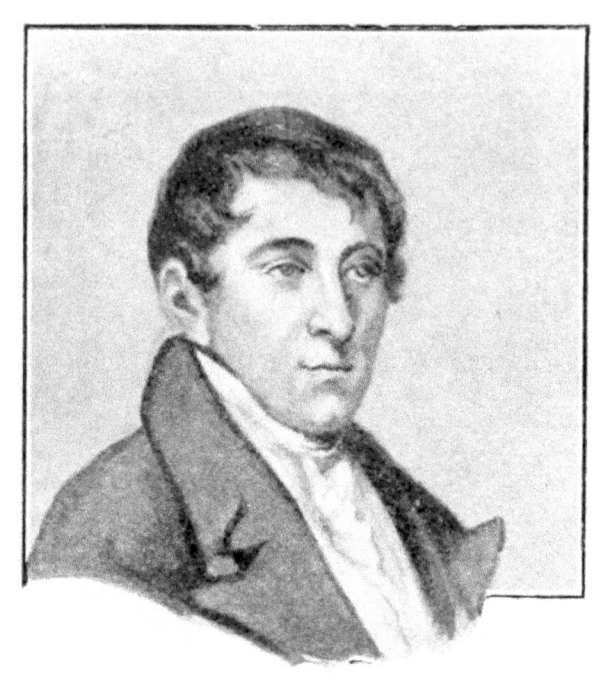

Sir Humphry Davy.

Antoine Jussieu was the eldest of the three sons of Laurent Jussieu, a master in pharmacy at Lyons. Antoine was born in 1686, and began to collect plants from his childhood. His two brothers, Bernard and Joseph, followed in his steps, and they, and Bernard's son, Antoine Laurent, constitute the famous Jussieu dynasty, from whom we have received the natural system of botanical classification. The story is a long and interesting one, but it is outside the scope of these notes. It must be remarked, however, that to Antoine Jussieu is due the credit of the introduction of the coffee plant into the western hemisphere. The island of Martinique was where the first coffee shrub was planted.

Fourcroy, another chemist of the Revolutionary period, comes next and is followed by

Nicolas Houel (1520–1584), who was the founder of the School of Pharmacy of Paris. He was an apothecary, and out of the ample fortune which he had made from his profession, endowed a "House of Christian Charity." He stipulated that it was to be a school for young orphans born of legal marriages, there to be instructed to serve and honour God, to acquire good literary instruction, and to learn the art of the apothecary. He also provided that the establishment should furnish medicines to the sick poor, who did not wish to go to the hospital, gratuitously. The institution consisted of a chapel, a school, a complete pharmacy, a garden of simples, and a hospital. The charity was duly authorised by Henri III and Queen Loise of Lorraine, but this did not prevent Henri IV taking possession of it in 1596, and using it as a home for his wounded soldiers. That was the origin of the Hotel des Invalides. Louis XIII transferred the Invalides to the Château of Bicêtre, and gave the school to the Sisters of St. Lazare. In 1622, however, the Parliament of Paris took the matter in hand and restored the property to the corporation of Apothecaries on condition that they would carry out the bequest of Houel. In 1777 Louis XVI made it the College of Pharmacy, and after the Convention the Directory declared it to be the Free School of Pharmacy. When pharmacy was reorganised in France during Napoleon's consulate, the institution became the Paris School of Pharmacy.

Jan Swammerdam, a famous Dutch anatomist (1637–1680), comes next, and after him, Claude Bernard, the physiologist (1813–1878), who began his career in a poor little pharmacy at Lyons. Jean Baptiste Dumas, born 1800, and living when the medallion was placed, also commenced his career in a small pharmacy at Alais (Gard), his native town. Dumas was one of the greatest chemists of the century. The doctrine of substitution of radicles in chemical compounds was suggested by him. He died April 11, 1884, at Cannes.

XII
ROYAL AND NOBLE PHARMACISTS.

> We know what Heaven or Hell may bring,
>
> But no man knoweth the mind of a King.
>
> RUDYARD KIPLING—"Ballad of the King's Jest."

In the "Myths of Pharmacy" it has been shown that some of the most honoured of the deities of the ancient world interested themselves in pharmacy. To a greater or less extent many important personages in the world's history since have occupied some of their leisure in the endeavour to extract or compound some new and effective remedies.

CLASSICAL LEGENDS.

Chin-Nong, Emperor of China, who died 2699 B.C., is reckoned to have been the founder of pharmacy in the Far East. He studied plants and composed a Herbal used to this day. It is related of him that he discovered seventy poisonous plants and an equal number of antidotes to them. He describes how to make extracts and decoctions, what they are good for, and had some notions of analysis. Chin-Nong was the second of the nine sovereigns who preceded the establishment of the Chinese dynasties. To him is also attributed the invention of the plough.

The Emperor Adrian, whose curiosity and literary tastes led him to the study of astrology, magic, and medicine, composed an antidote which was known as Adrianum, and which consisted of more than forty ingredients, of which opium, henbane, and euphorbium were the principal.

Attalus III, the last king of Pergamos in Asia Minor, who died about 134 B.C., bequeathing his kingdom to the Romans who already controlled it, was a worthless and cruel prince, but of some reputation in pharmacy. Having poisoned his uncle, the reigning king, Attalus soon wearied of public affairs, and devoted his time to gardening, and especially to the cultivation of poisonous and medicinal plants. Plutarch expressly mentions henbane, hellebore, hemlock, and lotus as among the herbs which he studied, and Justin reports that he amused himself by sending to his friends presents of fruits, mixing poisonous ones with the others. He is credited with the invention of our white lead ointment and Celsus and Galen mention a plaster and an antidote as among his achievements. Marcellus has preserved a prescription which he says Attalus devised for diseases of the liver and spleen, for dropsy, and for improving a lurid complexion. It consisted of saffron, Indian nard, cassia, cinnamon, myrrh, schœnanthus, and costus, made into an electuary with honey, and kept in a silver box.

Gentius, King of Illyria, discovered the medicinal value of the gentian and introduced it into medical practice. The plant is supposed to have acquired its name from this king. Gentius was induced by Perseus, King of Macedon, to declare war against the Romans, Perseus promising to support him with money and other aid. This he failed to do and Gentius was defeated and taken prisoner by Anicius after a war which lasted only thirty days.

MITHRIDATIUM.

Mithridates VI, commonly called "the Great," King of Pontus in Asia Minor, was born 134 B.C., and succeeded his father on the throne at the age of twelve. Next to Hannibal he was the most troublesome foe the Roman Republic had to deal with. His several wars with that power occupied twenty-six years of his life. Sylla, Lucullus, and Pompey, in succession, led Roman armies against him, and gained battles again and again, but he was only at last completely conquered by the last-named general after long and costly efforts.

Mithridates was a valiant soldier and a skilful general, but a monster of cruelty. He was apparently a learned man, or at least one who took interest in learning. The fable of his medicinal secrets took possession of the imagination of the Romans. They were especially attracted by the stories of his famous antidote. According to some he invented this himself; others say the secret was communicated to him by a Persian physician named Zopyrus. Celsus states that a physician of this name gave a similar secret to one of the Egyptian Ptolemies. This may have been the same Zopyrus, for Mithridates lived in the time of the Ptolemies. The Egyptian antidote was handed down to us under the name of Ambrosia.

When Pompey had finally defeated Mithridates he took possession of a quantity of the tyrant's papers at Nicopolis, and it was reported that among these were his medicinal formulas. Mithridates meanwhile was seeking help to prosecute the war. But his allies, his own son, and his soldiers were all tired of him. In his despair he poisoned his wife and daughters, and then took poison himself. But according to the legend, propagated perhaps by some clever advertising quacks in Rome, he had so successfully immunised his body to the effects of all poisons that they would now take no effect. Consequently he had to call in the assistance of a Gallic soldier, who despatched his chief with a spear. The story of his defeat and death are historic; the poison story is legend which, however it was originated, was no doubt good value in the drug stores of Rome, where the confection of Mithridates was soon sold. As will be stated immediately there is abundant reason to believe that the alleged formula which Pompey was said to have discovered and to have had translated was devised at home.

In 1745 when a new London Pharmacopœia was nearly ready for issue, a scholarly exposure of the absurdity of the compound which still occupied space in that and in all other official formularies, along with its equally egregious companion, Theriaca, was published by Dr. William Heberden, a leading physician of the day, and though it was too late to cause the deletion of the formulas in the edition of 1746, that was the last time they appeared in the Pharmacopœia, though they had been given in all the issues of that work from 1618 onwards. No better completion of the history of this preparation can be given than that which Dr. Heberden wrote 165 years ago. The King of Pontus, he assumed, like many other ancient royalties, was pleased to affect special skill in the production of medicines, and it is not surprising that his courtiers should have flattered him on this accomplishment. Thus the opinion prevailed among his enemies as well as in his own kingdom that his achievements in pharmacy approached the miraculous. His conqueror, Pompey, apparently shared the popular belief, and took uncommon care in the ransack of his effects, after Mithridates had been compelled to fly from the field, to secure for himself his medical writings. According to Quintus Serenus Samonicus, however, the Roman general was amused at his own credulity when, instead of a vast and precious arcana he found himself in possession of only a few trifling and worthless receipts.

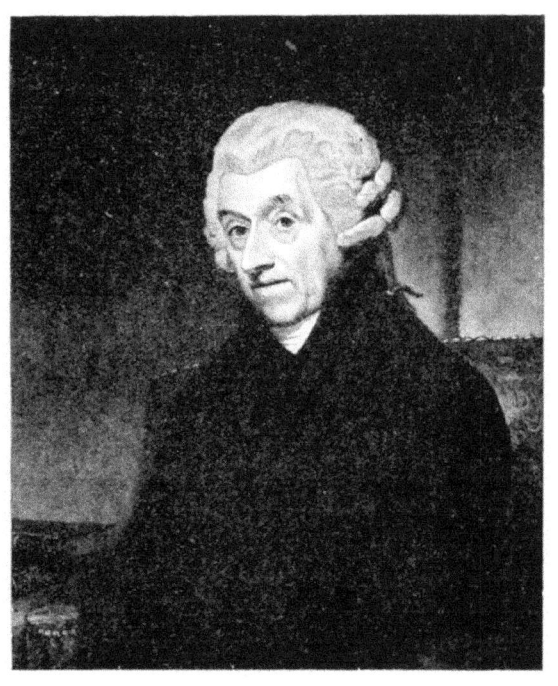

Dr. William Heberden. 1710–1801.

(From a mezzotint in the British Museum.)

The anticipation of some marvellous secrets was so universal, and the Roman publishers so well disposed to cater for this, that it is not to be wondered at that a confection of Mithridates and stories of its miraculous power soon found their way into literature. A pompous formula, which it was professed had been discovered among the papers of Mithridates captured by Pompey came to be known under the title of Antidotum Mithridatium. It is noteworthy that Plutarch, who in his life of Pompey mentions that certain love letters and documents helping to interpret dreams were among these papers, makes no allusion to the medical recipe; while Samonicus states explicitly that, notwithstanding the many formulæ which had got into circulation pretending to be that of the genuine confection, the only one found in the cabinet of Mithridates was a trivial one for a compound of 20 leaves of rue, 1 grain of salt, 2 nuts, and 2 dried figs. So that, Dr. Heberden remarks, the King of Pontus may have been as much a stranger to the medicine to which his name was attached as many eminent physicians of this day are to medicines associated with their names.

The compound, made from the probably spurious formula, however, acquired an immense fame. Some of the Roman emperors are declared to have compounded it with their own hands. Galen says that whoever took a proper dose in the morning was ensured against poison throughout that day. Great physicians studied it with a view of making it, if possible, more perfect. The most important modification of the formula was made by Andromachus, Nero's physician, who omitted the scink, added vipers, and increased the proportion of opium. He changed the name to Galene, but this was not retained, and in Trajan's time the name of Theriaca was the accepted designation, a title which has lasted throughout the subsequent centuries.

Dr. Heberden's criticism of the composition is as effective now as when he wrote, but it should be remembered that in his day there was a Theriacal party in medicine; to us the comments seem obvious. He points out that in the formula as it then appeared in the Pharmacopœia no regard was had to the known virtues of the simples, nor to the rules of artful composition. There was no foundation for the wonderful stories told concerning it, and the utmost that could then be said of it was that it was a diaphoretic, "which is commonly the virtue of a medicine which has none."

But even if undesigning chance did happen to hit upon a mixture which possessed such marvellous virtues, what foundation was there, he asked, for believing that any other fortuitous concourse of ingredients would be similarly successful? This preparation had scarcely continued the same for a hundred years at a time. According to Celsus, who first described it, it consisted of thirty-eight simples. Before the time of Nero five of these had been struck out and twenty new ones added. Andromachus omitted six and added twenty-eight; leaving seventy-five net. Aetius in the fifth century, and

Myrepsus in the twelfth gave very different accounts of it, and since then the formulas had been constantly fluctuating. Some of the original ingredients were, Dr. Heberden said, utterly unknown in his time; others could only be guessed at. About a century previously a dispute about Balm of Gilead, which was one of the constituents, had been referred to the Pope, who, however, prudently declined to exercise his infallibility on this subject.

Authorities were not agreed whether it was better old or new. Galen said the virtue of the opium was mitigated by keeping; Juncker said it fermented, and by fermentation the power of the opium was exalted three or fourfold.

A Pharmaceutical Pope.

Peter of Spain, a native of Lisbon, was a physician who became Pope under the title of John XXI. He died in 1277. He wrote a treatise on medicine, or rather made a collection of formulas, including most of the absurd ones then current and adding a few of his own. One was to carry about a parchment on which were written the names of Gaspard, Balthasar, and Melchior, the three wise men of the East, as a sure preservative from epilepsy. Another was a method of curing a diarrhœa by filling a human bone with the excrements of a patient, and throwing it into a river. The diarrhœa would cease when the bone was emptied of its contents.

Henry VIII (of England)

was fond of dabbling with medicine. In Brewer's history of his reign, referring to the years 1516–18, we are told:—

"The amusements of court were diversified by hunting and out-door sports in the morning; in the afternoon by Memo's music, by the consecration and distribution of cramp rings, or the invention of plasters and compounding of medicines, an occupation in which the King took unusual pleasure."

In the British Museum among the Sloane MSS. there is one numbered 1047, entitled Dr. Butt's Diary, which records many of these pharmaceutical achievements of the monarch. Dr. Butt was the King's physician and was no doubt his guide in these experiments. Dr. Butt, or Butts, is referred to in Strype's "Life of Cranmer" and in Shakespeare's "Henry VIII." Many of the liniments and cataplasms formulated are for excoriations or ulcers in the legs, a disease, as Dr. Brewer notes, "common in those days, and from which the King himself suffered."

Among the contents of the Diary are "The King's Majesty's own Plaster." It is described as a plaster devised by the king to heal ulcers without pain. It was a compound of pearls and guaiacum wood. There are in the manuscript formulas for other plasters "devised by the King at Greenwich and made at Westminster" to heal excoriations, to heal swellings in the ankles, one for my lady Anne of Cleves "to mollify and resolve, comfort and cease pain of cold and windy causes"; and an ointment to cool and "let" (prevent) inflammations, and take away itch.

Other formulas by Dr. Butt himself, and by other contemporary doctors, are comprised in this Diary.

Sir H. Halford, in an article "On the Deaths of Some Eminent Persons," printed in 1835, says of Henry VIII, who died of dropsy at the age of 56, that he was "a great dabbler in physic, and offered medical advice on all occasions which presented themselves, and also made up the medicines."

QUEEN ELIZABETH OF ENGLAND

appears to have been an amateur prescriber. Etmuller states that she sent a formula for a "cephalica-cardiac medicine" to the Holy Roman Emperor, Rudolf II, himself a dabbler in various scientific quackeries. It consisted of amber, musk, and civet, dissolved in spirit of roses. It is further on record that the English queen selected doctors and pharmacists for Ivan the Terrible of Russia. In Wadd's Memorabilia, one of her Majesty's quarter's bills from her apothecary, Hugo Morgan, is quoted. It amounted to £83 7s. 8d., and included the following items:—A confection made like manus Christi with bezoar stone and unicorn's horn, 11s.; a royal sweetmeat with incised rhubarb, 1s. 4d.; rose water for the king of Navarre's ambassador, 1s.; a conserve of barberries with preserved damascene plums, and other things for Mr. Ralegh, 6s.; sweet scent to be used at the christening of Sir Richard Knightley's son, 2s.

THE QUEEN OF HUNGARY'S WATER.

Rosemary has at times enjoyed a high reputation among medicinal herbs. Arnold of Villa Nova affirms that he had often seen cancers, gangrenes, and fistulas, which would yield to no other medicine, dry up and become perfectly cured by frequently bathing them with a spirituous infusion of rosemary. His disciple, Raymond Lully, extracted the essential oil by distillation.

The name probably assisted the fame of the plant. In the middle ages it was believed to be associated with the Virgin. It was in fact derived from Ros and Maris, meaning Dew of the Sea; probably because it grew near the shores of the Mediterranean.

"Here's rosemary for you; that's for remembrance." So says Ophelia in Hamlet; and many other poets and chroniclers relate how the plant was used at funerals and weddings as a symbol of constancy. It is supposed that this signification arose from the medicinal employment of rosemary to improve the memory. It may easily have happened, however, that the medicinal use followed the emblematical idea.

Old books and some modern ones tell the legend of the Queen of Hungary and her rosemary remedy. It is alleged in pharmaceutical treatises published in the nineteenth century that a document is preserved in the Imperial Library at Vienna, dated 1235, and written by Queen Elisabeth of Hungary, thus expressed:—

> "I, Elisabeth, Queen of Hungary, being very infirm and much troubled with gout, in the seventy-second year of my age, used for a year this recipe given to me by an ancient hermit, whom I never saw before nor since; and was not only cured but recovered my strength, and appeared to all so remarkably beautiful that the King of Poland asked me in marriage, he being a widower and I a widow. I, however, refused him for the love of my Lord Jesus Christ, from one of whose angels I believe I received the remedy."

> The royal formula is as follows:—"Take aqua vitae, four times distilled, 3 parts; the tops and flowers of rosemary, 2 parts; put these together in a closed vessel, let them stand in a gentle heat fifty hours, and then distil them. Take one teaspoonful of this in the morning once every week, and let your face and diseased limb be washed with it every morning."

Beckmann investigated this story and came to the conclusion that the name "Eau de La Reine d'Hongrie" had been adopted by some vendors of a spirit of rosemary "in order to give greater consequence and credit to their commodity"; in other words, he suggests that the interesting narrative was only a clever advertisement.

The only Queen Elisabeth of Hungary was the wife of King Charles Robert, and daughter of Ladislaus, King of Poland. She died in 1380, and for more than ten years before that date either her brother, Casimir II, or her son Louis, was the reigning sovereign in Poland, and neither of these can be supposed to have been her suitor. The alleged date of the document quoted would better suit St. Elisabeth of Hungary, and some old writers attribute the formula and the story to her. But she was never queen of Hungary, and moreover she died in 1231 at the age of 25. Beckmann also denies the statement that the document pretended to be in Queen Elisabeth's writing is preserved in the Imperial Library at Vienna. The whole narrative is traced to a German named Hoyer, in 1716, and he apparently copied it from a French medical writer named Prevot, who published it in 1659. Prevot attributes the story to "St. Elisabeth, Queen of Hungary," and says he copied both the history and the formula from an old breviary in the possession of his friend, Francis Podacather, a Cyprus nobleman, who had inherited it from his ancestors. This is the one little possibility of truth in the record, for it appears that Queen Elisabeth of Hungary did mention two breviaries in her will, and it may have been that one of these was the one which the Cyprus nobleman possessed.

THE ROYAL TOUCH.—THE KING'S EVIL.

There are several instances in ancient history illustrating the healing virtue residing or alleged to reside in the person of a king. Pyrrhus, King of Epirus, according to Plutarch, cured colics and affections of the spleen by laying patients on their backs and passing his great toe over their bodies. Suelin relates that when the Emperor Vespasian was at Alexandria a poor blind man came to him saying that the god Serapis had revealed to him that if he, the Emperor, would touch his eyes with his spittle, his sight would be restored. Vespasian was angry and would have driven the man away, but some of those around him urged him to exercise his power, and at last he consented and cured the poor man of his blindness and some others of lameness. Cœlius Spartianus declares that the Emperor Adrian cured dropsy by touching patients with the tips of his fingers. The Eddas tell how King Olaf healed the wounds of Egill, the Icelandic hero, by laying on of hands and singing proverbs. A legend of the counts of Hapsburg declares that at one time they could cure a sick person by kissing him.

The superstition crystallised itself in the practice of the English and French kings of touching for the cure of scrofula, or king's evil as the disease consequently came to be named. The term scrofula is itself one of the curiosities of etymology. Scrofula is the diminutive of scrota, a sow, and means a little pig. It is conjectured that the name was adopted from the idea of pigs burrowing under the surface of straw and likening to that the pig's back sort of shape of the ulcers characteristic of the disease.

The first English king who undertook this treatment, so far as is known, was Edward the Confessor, who reigned from 1042 to 1066. But there is evidence that the French kings had practised it earlier. Robert the Pious (970–1031), son of Hughes Capet, is said to have exercised the miraculous power, and Church legend goes back five hundred years before this, attributing the origin of the gift to the date of the conversion of Clovis, A.D. 496. On that occasion the holy oil for the coronation of the Conqueror was brought direct from heaven in a phial carried by a dove, and the healing faculty was conferred at the same time. Most of the French kings down to Louis XV continued to touch, and it was even suggested that the practice should be resumed by Louis XVIII after the Restoration in 1815, but that monarch's advisers prudently resolved that it would not do to risk the ridicule of modern France.

The records of Edward the Confessor's miraculous feats of healing are obtained from William of Malmesbury, who wrote his Chronicles in the first half of the 12th century, about a hundred years after the Confessor's reign. The earliest printed edition of the Chronicles appeared in 1577, and Shakespeare undoubtedly drew from it the description of the ceremony which is given in Macbeth (Act iv, Sc. 3). Malcolm and Macduff are represented as being in England "in a room of the King's palace" (Edward the Confessor's). The doctor tells them

> There are a crew of wretched souls
>
> That stay his cure: their malady convinces
>
> The great assay of art; but at his touch—
>
> Such sanctity hath heaven given his hand—
>
> They presently amend.

Asked about the nature of the disease the doctor says "'Tis called the evil," and he adds

> How he solicits Heaven
>
> Himself best knows: but strangely visited people,
>
> All swoln and ulcerous, pitiful to the eye,
>
> The mere despair of surgery, he cures,
>
> Hanging a golden stamp about their necks,
>
> Put on with holy prayers: and 'tis spoken,
>
> To the succeeding royalty he leaves
>
> The healing benediction.

There is no evidence that any of the Norman kings performed the rite, but it is on record that Henry II performed cures by touching, and allusions to the practice by Edward II, Edward III, Richard II, and Henry IV have been found in old manuscripts. It is probable, too, that the other kings preceding the Tudors followed the fashion when the interval between their wars gave them the necessary leisure. From Henry VII to Queen Anne all our rulers except Cromwell "touched." Oliver, not being able to claim the virtue by reason of his descent, would certainly not have been trusted, and Dutch William had no sympathy with the superstition. It is recorded of him that once he yielded to importunity and went through the form of touching. "God gave thee better health and more sense" was the unsentimental benediction he pronounced. Queen Anne, as is well known, "touched" Dr. Johnson in his childhood, but it is recorded that in this case no cure was effected.

Boswell says that Johnson's mother in taking the child (who was then between two and three years old) to London for the ceremony was acting on the advice of Sir John Floyer, who was at that time a noted physician at Lichfield. The "touch-piece" presented by Queen Anne to Dr. Johnson is preserved in the British Museum. The Pretender, Charles Edward, touched someone at Holyrood House, Edinburgh, and his partisans said a cure was effected in three weeks. Which proved his right to the throne of England.

The story told by William of Malmesbury about Edward the Confessor is that "a young woman that had a husband about the same age as herself, but no child, was afflicted with overflowing of humours in her neck, which broke out in great nobbs, was commanded in a dream to apply to the King to wash it. To court she goes, and the King being at his Devotions all alone dip'd his fingers in water and dabbel'd the woman's neck, and he had no sooner taken away his hand than she found herself better." William goes on to tell that within a week she was well, and that within a year she was brought to bed of twins.

Modern doctors have forgotten and despised the strange story of this royal touch, but two and three centuries ago they very seriously discussed it. Reports of marvellous and numerous cures were confidently related, and the writers who had no faith in the virtue of the performance admitted the genuineness of many of the cases. Sergeant-Surgeon Dickens, Queen Anne's surgeon, narrated the most curious instance. At the request of one young woman he brought her to the Queen to be touched. After the performance he impressed upon her the importance of never parting with the gold medal which was given to all patients; for it appears that he had reason to expect that she was likely to sell it. She promised always to retain it, and in due course she was cured. In time, thinking all risk had passed, she disposed of the touch-piece; the disease returned; she confessed her fault penitently to Dr. Dickens, and by his aid was touched again, and once more cured. Surgeon Wiseman, chief surgeon in Charles I's army, and afterwards Sergeant-Surgeon in Charles II's household, described the cures effected by that monarch. He had been an eye-witness of hundreds of cures, he says. Many other testimonies of the same kind might be quoted, but it is as well to remark that a habit grew up of describing the touching itself as a cure.

Careful and intelligent inquiries into the alleged success of the practice by investigators who were by no means believers in any actual royal virtue, but who yet admitted unhesitatingly the reality of many of the claimed cures, are on record. Among treatises of this character may be mentioned "A Free and Impartial Inquiry into the Antiquity and Efficacy of Touching for the King's Evil," by William Beckett, F.R.S., a well known surgeon, 1722, and "Criterion, or Miracles Examined," by Dr. Douglas, Bishop of Salisbury, 1754. Both of these writers admit that cures did result from the King's touch;

the Bishop says that he personally knew a man who had been healed. Mr. Beckett deals with these cures with much judgment. He points out how likely it was that the excitement of the visit to the court, both in anticipation and in realisation, and the impressive ceremony there conducted, would in many instances so affect the constitution, causing the blood to course through the veins more quickly, as to effect a cure.

Mr. Beckett also gives extremely good reasons for doubting whether Edward the Confessor ever did "touch" for scrofula. The gift is not mentioned in the Bull of Pope Alexander III by which the Confessor was canonised, nor by several earlier writers than William of Malmesbury, monks only too eager to glorify their benefactor.

Henry VII was the first to surround the ceremony of touching with an imposing religious service, and to give a touch-piece to the patient. Henry VIII does not seem to have followed the practice of his father to any great extent, and there was some disturbance about it in the next few reigns. The Catholics denied that Queen Elizabeth could possess the healing virtue, and when actual cures were cited to them one of their bishops declared that these were due, not to the royal virtue, but to the virtue of the sign of the cross. All the Stuart kings, Charles II particularly, exercised their hereditary powers most diligently. Macaulay states that Charles II touched nearly one hundred thousand persons during his reign. In his record year, 1682, he performed the rite eight thousand five hundred times.

Evelyn gives the following account of the performance, which, as will be seen, was no light duty. He describes it thus:

"Sitting under his state in the Banqueting House, the chirurgeons cause the sick to be brought or led up to the throne, where, they kneeling, ye King strokes their faces and cheeks with both his hands at once, at which instant a chaplaine in his formalities says:—'He put his hands upon them and healed them.' This he said to every one in particular. When they have been all touched, they come up again in the same order; and the other chaplaine kneeling, and having an angel of gold strung on white ribbon on his arms delivers them one by one to His Majestie, who puts them about the necks of the touched as they passe, while the first chaplaine repeats 'That is ye true light which came into ye world.' Then follows an epistle (as at first a gospel) with the liturgy, prayers for the sick, with some alteration, and then the Lord Chamberlain and the Comptroller of the Household bring a basin, ewer, and towel, for his Majesty to wash."

In 1684 Thomas Rosewell, evidently an unrepentant Puritan, was tried before Judge Jeffries on a charge of high treason, the indictment alleging that he had said "the people made a flocking to the king upon pretence of being healed of the king's evil, which he could not do." Rosewell had further declared that he and others, being priests and prophets, could do as much as the king. And Rosewell had told how Jeroboam's hand had dried up when he would have seized the man of God who had prophesied against him, and how the king's hand had been restored on the prayer of the prophet. In his defence Rosewell had sneered at the Latin of the indictment, which spoke of the "Morbus Regni Anglici," which, as he said, would mean the disease of the English kingdom, not the king's evil. Jeffries, having taunted the prisoner and his witnesses with being "snivelling saints," insisted on a verdict of guilty, and would no doubt have had the mocker's ears cut off; but it is satisfactory to know that Charles II, who probably had not more faith in his healing power than the accused, ordered him to be pardoned.

The English prayer-book contained a form of service for this ceremony up to the year 1719.

Queen Anne was the last ruler in England to touch. There is no record of any of the Georges attempting the miracle, but the young Pretender, Charles Edward, when claiming to be Prince of Wales, touched a female child at Holyrood House in 1745, and is said to have effected a cure, and after his death in 1780 his brother, Cardinal York, still touched at Rome.

Louis XV was the last King of France who touched. Louis XIV fulfilled the duty on a larger scale, and doubtless with the utmost confidence in his royal virtue. The formula used by the kings of France when they had touched a patient was "Le roi te touche, Dieu te guerisse" ("The king touches thee; may God heal thee"). It is said that Henri of Navarre, when in the thick of the fight at Ivry (1590), as he laid about him with his sword right and left, gaily shouted this familiar expression.

CRAMP RINGS.

Faith in "cramp rings" corresponds in many respects with the reverential confidence in the royal touch as a cure for scrofula. The former, however, appears to have been of entirely English origin. Legend attributes the first cramp ring to Edward the Confessor.

St. Edward on his death-bed is alleged to have given a ring from his finger to the Abbot of Westminster with the explanation that it had been brought to him not long before by a pilgrim from Jerusalem to whom it had been given by a mysterious stranger, presumably a visitant from the world of spirits, who had bidden him give the ring to the king with the message that his end was near. The ring was preserved as a relic at Westminster for some time, and was found to possess miraculous efficacy for the cure of epilepsy and cramp. It was next heard of at Havering in Essex, the very name of which place, according to Camden, furnished evidence of the accuracy of the tradition. Havering was obviously a contraction of "have the ring." So at least thought the old etymologists.

When the relic disappeared is not recorded; but the Tudor kings were in the habit of contributing a certain amount of gold and silver as an offering to the Cross every Good Friday, and the metal being made into rings was consecrated by them, in accordance with a form of service which was included in old English prayer books (see Burnett's History of the Reformation, Part 2, Book 2, No. 25). This was actually used until the reign of Queen Anne. Andrew Boorde, in his "Breviary of Health," 1557, says: "The kynges of England doth halow every yere cramp rynges ye which rynges worn on one's finger doth helpe them whyche hath ye cramp." They seem to have been regarded especially as a protection against epilepsy, and courtiers were much importuned to obtain some for persons afflicted.

The process of hallowing the rings is described in Brand's "Popular Antiquities." A crucifix was laid on a cushion in the royal chapel, and a piece of carpet was spread in front of it. The king entered in state, and when he came to the carpet crept on it to the crucifix. There the rings were brought to him in a silver dish, and he blessed them.

In the Harleian Manuscripts (295 f119) a letter is preserved dated the xxi. daie of June, 1518, from Lord Berners (the translator of Froissart), then ambassador to the Emperor Charles V. He writes from Saragoza "to my Lord Cardinall's grace" (Wolsey), "If your grace remember me with some crampe rynges ye shall doo a thing muche looked for; and I trust to bestowe thaym well with Goddes grace, who evermor preserve and encrease your most reverent astate."

It does not appear certain that the royal consecration of these rings was continued after the reign of Queen Mary; but cramp rings continued in esteem almost until our own time in some parts of the country. In Brand's book, and in several numbers of *Notes and Queries* references to superstitions in connection with these, their production and the wearing of them particularly against epilepsy, are recorded. Sometimes, to be effective, the rings must have been made from coffin handles, or coffin nails, the coffins from which they have been taken having been buried; or rings of silver or gold, manufactured while the story of the Passion of the Saviour was being read, would possess curative power. So would a ring made from silver collected at a Communion service, preferably on Easter Sunday. In Berkshire, a ring made from five sixpences collected from five bachelors, none of whom must know the purpose of the collection, and formed by a bachelor smith into a ring was believed in; and in Suffolk, not very long since, nine bachelors contributed a crooked sixpence each to make a ring for a young woman in the village to wear for the cure of epileptic fits to which she was subject.

THE EARL OF WARWICK'S POWDER.

The Earl of Warwick's Powder is named in many old English, and more frequently still in foreign dispensatories and pharmacopœias, appearing generally under the title of "Pulvis Comitis de Warwick, or Pulvis Warwiciensis," sometimes also as "Pulvis Cornacchini." It is the original of our Pulv. Scammon Co, and was given in the P.L. 1721 in its pristine form, thus:—

- Scammony, prepared with the fumes of sulphur, 2 ounces.
- Diaphoretic antimony, 1 ounce.
- Cream of tartar, ½ ounce.

In the P.L. 1746 the pulvis e scammonio compositus, made from four parts of scammony and three parts of burnt hartshorn, was substituted for the above, but neither this nor the modern compound scammony powder, consisting of scammony, jalap, and ginger, can be regarded as representing the original Earl of Warwick's powder.

The Earl of Warwick from whom the powder acquired its name was Robert Dudley, son of the famous Earl of Leicester, Queen Elizabeth's favourite, and of Kenilworth notoriety. His mother was the widow of Lord Sheffield, and there was much dispute about the legitimacy of the child, but the evidence goes to show that Leicester married her two days before the birth of the boy. He afterwards abandoned her, but he left his estates to the boy. Young Robert Dudley grew up a singularly handsome and popular youth. He led an adventurous life, voyaging, exploring, and fighting Spanish ships. He failed to establish his claims to his titles and estates in England, and ultimately settled at Florence, where he became a Catholic, and distinguished himself as an engineer and architect. He won the favour of Ferdinand II, Emperor of Austria, who created him Earl of Warwick and Duke of Northumberland, and the Pope recognised his nobility. He died in Italy in 1649. The chroniclers of the time refer to a book he is said to have written under the title of *Catholicon*, which was "in good esteem among physicians." If it existed it was probably a collection of medical formulæ, but it is not unlikely that this supposed book has been confused with one written by a Dr. Cornacchini, of Pisa, and dedicated to Dudley. In that work, which is known, the powder is described, and its invention is attributed to the Earl. It is alleged to have possessed marvellous medicinal virtues.

Duke of Portland's Gout Powder.

Under this title a powder had a great reputation about the middle of the eighteenth century, and well on into the nineteenth century. The powder was composed of aristolochia rotunda (birthwort root), gentian root, and the tops and leaves of germander, ground pine, and centaury, of each equal parts. One drachm was to be taken every morning, fasting, for three months, and then ½ drachm for the rest of the year. Particular directions in regard to diet were given with the formula.

The compound was evidently only a slight modification of several to be found in the works of the later Latin authors, Aetius, Alexander of Trailles, and Paul of Egineta. These were entitled Tetrapharmacum, Antidotus Podagrica ex duobus centauriae generibus, Diatesseron, and other names. The "duobus" remedy was an electuary prescribed by Aetius, and a piece the size of a hazel nut had to be taken every morning for a year. Hence it was called medicamentum ad annum. This, or something very like it, was in use in Italy for centuries under the name of Pulvis Principis Mirandolæ, and spread from there to the neighbouring countries. An Englishman long resident in Switzerland had compiled a manuscript collection of medical formulæ, and his son, who became acquainted with the Duke of Portland of the period, persuaded him to give this gout remedy a trial. The result was so satisfactory that the Duke had the formula and the diet directions printed on leaflets, and these were given to anyone who asked for them.

Sir Walter Raleigh's Great Cordial.

During his twelve years' imprisonment in the Tower in the earlier part of the reign of James I, Sir Walter Raleigh was allowed a room in which he fitted up a laboratory, and divided his time between chemical experiments and literary labours. It was believed that Raleigh had brought with him from Guiana some wonderful curative balsam, and this opinion, combined with the knowledge that he dabbled largely with retorts and alembics in the Tower, ensured a lively public interest in his "Great Cordial" when it was available.

The Queen, Anne of Denmark, and Prince Henry, were both warm partisans of Raleigh, and did their best to get him released. The Queen was convinced that the "Great Cordial" had saved her life in a serious illness, and Prince Henry took a particular interest in Raleigh's experiments. When the Prince was on his death-bed Raleigh sent him some of the cordial, declaring, it was reported, that it would certainly cure him provided he had not been poisoned. This unwise suggestion coming to James's ears greatly incensed him, and darkened Raleigh's prospects of life and freedom considerably.

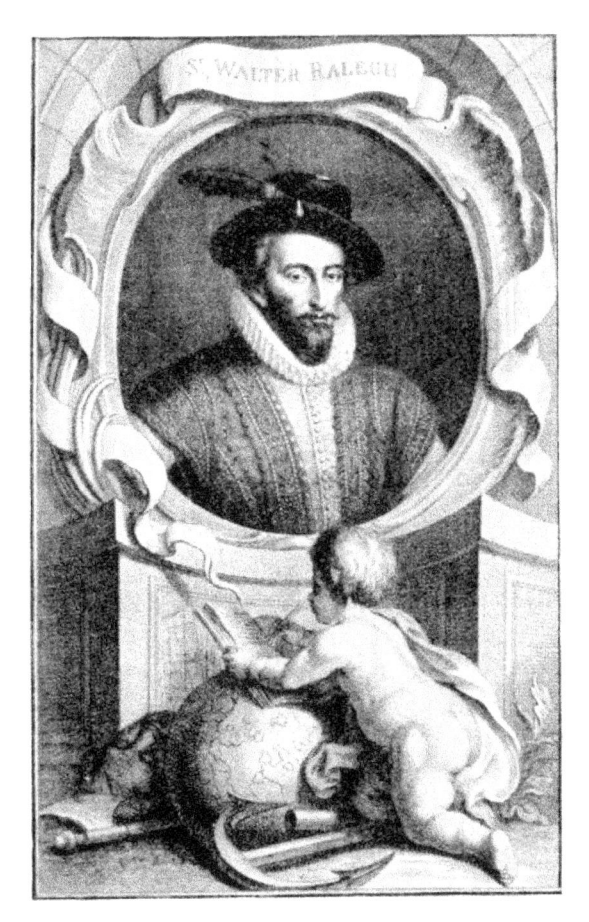

Sir Walter Raleigh.

(From a mezzotint in the British Museum.)

No known authentic formula of the cordial exists, but Charles II was curious about it, and his French apothecary, Le Febre, on the king's command, prepared some of the compound from data then available, and wrote a treatise on it which was afterwards translated into English by Peter Lebon. Evelyn records in his diary the demonstration of the composition given by Le Febre to the Court on September 20, 1662.

The cordial then consisted of forty roots, seeds, herbs, etc., macerated in spirit of wine, and distilled. With the distillate were combined bezoar stones, pearls, coral, deer's horn, amber, musk, antimony, various earths, sugar, and much besides. Vipers' flesh, with the heart and liver, and "mineral unicorn" were added later on the suggestion of Sir Kenelm Digby. The official history of this strange concoction is appended.

Confectio Raleighana was first official in the London Pharmacopœia of 1721. The formula was—

> Rasurae C. Cervi lb. i.
>
> Carnis viperarum c. cordibus et hepatibus, 6 oz.
>
> Flor. Borag., rosmar., calendulae, roris solis, rosarum rub., sambuci, ana lb. ss.
>
> Herb. scordii, cardui benedicti, melissæ, dictamni cretici, menthæ, majoranæ, betonicæ, ana manipules duodecim.
>
> Succi Kermis, Sem. card. maj., cubebarum, Bacc. junip., macis, nuc. mosch., caryoph., croci, ana 2 oz.
>
> Cinnam. opt., cort. lign. sassaf., cort. flav. malorum citriorum, aurantiorum, ana 3 oz.
>
> Lign. aloes, sassafras, ana 6 oz.
>
> Rad. angelic., valerian, sylvest., fraxinell, seu dictamni alb., serpentar. Virginianæ, Zedoariæ, tormentillæ bistort, Aristoloch. long., Aristoloch. rotund., gentianæ, imperatoriæ, ana 1½ oz.

These were to be cut up or crushed, and a tincture made from them with rectified spirit. The tincture was to be evaporated in a sand-bath, the expressed magma was then to be burned, and the ashes, lixiviated in water, were to be added to the extract.

Then the following powders were to be added to this liquid to form a confection:—Bezoar stone, Eastern and western, of each 1½ oz.; Eastern pearls, 2 oz.; red coral, 3 oz.; Eastern Bole, Terra Sigillata, calcined hartshorn, ambergris, of each 1 oz.; musk, 1½ drachms; powdered sugar, 2 lb.

In the P.L. 1746 Confectio Raleighana appears as Confectio Cardiaca. It is expressly stated that this new name is substituted for the old one. The formula is simplified, but the resemblance to the original can be traced. It runs thus:—Summitatum Rorismar, recent., Bacc, Junip., ana lb. i; Sem. card., min. decort., Zedoariæ, Croci. ana lb. ss. Make a tincture with these with about 1½ gallons of diluted spirit, and afterwards reduce it to 2½ lb. by evaporating at a gentle heat; then add the following, all in the finest powder:—Compound powder of crabs' shells, 16 oz. This was prepared powder of crab shells, 1 lb.; pearls and red coral, of each 3 oz.; cinnamon and nutmegs, of each 2 oz.; cloves, 1 oz.; sugar, 2 lb. To make a confection.

In the P.L. 1788 the compound is still further simplified, and acquires the name of Confectio Aromatica. The index of that work gives "Confectio

Aromatica vice Confectio Cardiaca." The formula now runs thus:—
Zedoaria, coarsely powdered, saffron, of each, ½ lb.; water, 3 lb. Macerate
for 24 hours, express and strain. Evaporate the strained liquor to 1½ lb., and
add the following, all in fine powder:—compound powder of crabs' shells,
16 oz.; cinnamon, nutmeg, of each 2 oz.; cloves, 8 oz.; cardamom seeds, ½
oz.; sugar, 2 lb. Make a confection.

In the 1809 P.L. the zedoary is abandoned, the quantity of saffron is reduced
to 2 ounces, the pulv. chelis cancrorum co. is described as testarum præp.,
and there is no maceration of any of the ingredients. The powders are simply
mixed, and the water added little by little until the proper consistence is
attained.

This formula is retained in the Pharmacopœias of 1824 and 1836, but in that
of 1851 the powdered shells became prepared chalk. In the Edinburgh
Pharmacopœia of 1841, and in that of Dublin of 1850, the confection was
made from aromatic powders of similar composition, made into confections
in P.E. with syrup of orange peel, and in P.D. with simple syrup and clarified
honey. All that remains of this historic remedy is Pulvis Cretæ Aromaticus
B.P., and from this the saffron has been entirely removed.

Raleigh's Cordial occasionally turns up in histories. In Aubrey's "Brief
Lives," it is stated that "Sir Walter Raleigh was a great chymist, and amongst
some MSS. receipts I have seen some secrets from him. He made an excellent
cordiall, good in feavers. Mr. Robert Boyle has the recipe and does great
cures by it."

In Strickland's "Lives of the Queens of England" (Vol. VIII, p. 122) we are
told that, according to the newspapers of the day, William III, in his last
illness was kept alive all through his last night by the use of Sir Walter
Raleigh's Cordial.

In Lord John Hervey's "Memoirs of the Reign of George II" (Vol. III, p.
294), the details of the last illness of Queen Caroline, who died in 1737, are
narrated. Snake root and Sir Walter Raleigh's Cordial were prescribed for her.
As the latter took some time to prepare, Ransby, house surgeon to the King,
said one cordial was as good as another, and gave her Usquebaugh. She,
however, took the other mixture when it came. Afterwards Daffy's Elixir and
mint water were administered.

Tar Water as a Panacea.

George Berkeley was born in 1685 in Kilkenny county, Ireland, but claimed
to be of English extraction. He graduated at Trinity College, Dublin, and
became a Fellow of that College. His metaphysical speculations made him

famous. He was the originator of the view that the actual existence of matter was not capable of proof. Having been appointed Dean of Derry he was well provided for, but just then he became enthusiastically desirous to convert and civilise the North American Indians. With this object in view he proposed to establish a University at Bermuda to train students for the work. He got some college friends to join him, collected about £5,000 from wealthy supporters, and after long negotiations persuaded the House of Commons to recommend George I. to grant him a contribution of £20,000 which never came. It was during that time that he learned of the medicinal efficacy of tar water from some of the Indian tribes whom he visited. Some time after his return he was made Bishop of Cloyne, and worked indefatigably in his diocese. A terrible winter in 1739–40 caused great distress and was followed by an epidemic of small-pox. It was then that the Bishop remembered his American experiences. He gave tar water as a remedy and tar water as a prophylactic, with the result, as he reported, that those who took the disease had it very mildly if they had taken tar water. Convinced of its value he gave it in other illnesses with such success that with characteristic enthusiasm he came to believe that he had discovered a panacea. Some reports of this treatment had been published in certain magazines, but in the spring of 1744 a little book by the Bishop appeared giving a full account of his experiences. It was entitled "A Chain of Philosophical Reflections and Enquiries concerning the virtues of Tar Water, and divers other subjects connected together and arising one from another." The treatise was eagerly read and discussed both in Ireland and England. A second edition was required in a few weeks, and to this the author gave the short title "Siris" (Greek for chain).

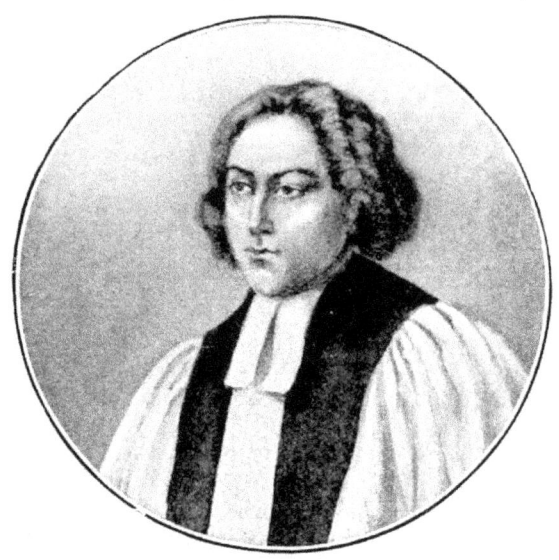

Berkeley.

(From the British Museum.)

The Bishop's theory was an attractive one. The pine trees he argued, had accumulated from the sunlight and the air a large proportion of the vital element of the universe, and condensed it in the tar which they yielded. The vital element could be drawn off by water and conveyed to the human organism.

It is not necessary here to follow out his chain of reasoning from the vital element in tar up to the Supreme Mind from which that vital principle emanated. On the way the author quoted freely and effectively from Plato and Pythagoras, from Theophrastus and Pliny, from Boerhaave and Boyle, and from many other authorities. He showed how the balsams and resins of the ancient world were of the same nature as tar. Van Helmont said, "Whoever can make myrrh soluble by the human body has the secret of prolonging his days," and Boerhaave had recognised that there was truth in this remark on account of the anti-putrefactive power of the myrrh. This was the power which tar possessed in so large a degree. Homberg had made gold by introducing the vital element in the form of light into the pores of mercury. The process was too expensive to make the production of gold by this means profitable, but the fact showed an analogy with the concentration of the same element in the tar.

Berkeley's process for making the tar water was simply to pour 1 gallon of cold water on a quart of tar; stir it with a wooden ladle for five or six minutes, and then set the vessel aside for three days and nights to let the tar subside. The water was then to be drawn off and kept in well-stoppered bottles. Ordinarily half a pint might be taken fasting morning and night, but to cure disease much larger doses might be given. It had proved of extraordinary value not only in small-pox, but also in eruptions and ulcers, ulceration of the bowels and of the lungs, consumptive cough, pleurisy, dropsy, and gravel. It greatly aided digestion, and consequently prevented gout. It was a remedy in all inflammatory disorders and fevers. It was a cordial which cheered, warmed, and comforted, with no injurious effects.

The nation went wild over this discovery. "The Bishop of Cloyne has made tar water as fashionable as Vauxhall or Ranelagh," wrote Duncombe.

The Bishop's book was translated into most of the European languages, and tar water attained some degree of popularity on the Continent. It owed no little of its success in this country to the opposition it met with from medical writers. The public at once concluded that they were very anxious about their "kitchen prospects," to use the symbolism of Paracelsus. Every attack on tar water called forth several replies. Berkeley himself responded to some of the criticisms by very poor verses, which he got a friend to send to the journals with strict injunctions to keep his name secret.

Paris in "Pharmacologia" refers to the tar water mania, asking "What but the spell of authority could have inspired a general belief that the sooty washings of rosin would act as a universal remedy?" It need hardly be pointed out that the general belief was rather a revolt against authority than an acceptance of it.

Dr. Young, the author of "Night Thoughts," wrote: "They who have experienced the wonderful effects of tar water reveal its excellences to others. I say reveal, because they are beyond what any can conceive by reason or natural light. But others disbelieve them though the revelation is attested past all scruple, because to them such excellences are incomprehensible. Now give me leave to say that this infidelity may possibly be as fatal to morbid bodies as other infidelity is to morbid souls. I say this in honest zeal for your welfare. I am confident if you persist you'll be greatly benefited by it. In old obstinate, chronical complaints, it probably will not show its virtue under three months; though secretly it is doing good all the time."

KINGS BUY SECRET REMEDIES.

In past times it was not unusual for monarchs to purchase from the inventors of panaceas the secrets of their composition for publication for the benefit of their subjects. Several instances are mentioned in other chapters of this book. Among these may be noted Goddard's Drops, bought by Charles II., Glauber's Kermes Mineral or Poudre des Chartres, Talbor's Tincture of Bark, and Helvetius's Ipecacuanha, the secrets of which were obtained by Louis XIV for fancy prices. In Louis XIV's reign the French Government purchased from the Prieur de Cabrier an arcanum to cure rupture without bandages or operations. The recipe, which was made public, was that a few drops of spirit of salt were to be taken in red wine frequently during the day. Mr. Stephens's Cure for the Stone was transferred to the public by a payment authorised by Act of Parliament.

The Emperor Joseph II of Austria paid 1,500 florins somewhere about the year 1785 for the formula for a secret febrifuge which was at that time enjoying extreme popularity. It proved to be simply an alcoholic tincture of box bark (*Buxus sempervirens*). The remedy lost its prestige as soon as the secret was gone.

Nouffer's Tapeworm Cure.

Louis XVI gave 18,000 livres (about £700) to a Madame Nouffer or Nuffer for a noted cure for tapeworm, which she had inherited from her deceased husband. As the result of the king's purchase, a little book was published in 1775 explaining fully the treatment.

Nouffer was a surgeon living at Morat, in Switzerland. He had practised his special worm cure treatment for many years, and by it he had acquired a considerable local fame. After his death his widow, who knew all about the secret, continued to receive patients. Among those who came to her was a Russian, Prince Baryantinski, who was staying in the neighbourhood and had heard of the cure. He had been troubled for years with tapeworm, and Madame Nouffer's remedy cured him. The Prince reported the facts to his regular physician at Paris, and consequently cases were sent from that city to the Swiss lady. She was so successful that the king was induced to give her the sum named for the revelation of her method, which was briefly as follows:—

For a day or two the patient was fed on buttered toast only. Meanwhile enemas of mallow and marshmallow with a little salt and olive oil were administered. Then, early in the morning, 3 drachms of powder of male fern in a teacupful of water was taken. Candied lemon was chewed after the dose to relieve the nauseousness, and the mouth was washed out with an aromatic water. If the patient vomited the medicine another dose was given. Two hours after the male fern a bolus containing 12 grains each of calomel and resin of scammony, with 5 grains of gamboge, and with confection of hyacinth as the excipient, had to be taken. A cup of warm tea was recommended shortly after the bolus. The doses quoted were regarded as average ones. They might be modified according to the strength of the patient. Generally the treatment narrated sufficed to expel the worm. If it did not, the whole proceeding was repeated.

Male fern was a remedy mentioned by Dioscorides and other ancient writers, but it had been forgotten for centuries until Madame Nouffer's system brought it to the recollection of medical practitioners. It again fell out of use, but a French physician named Jobert revived its popularity in 1869. He was assisted in the preparation of the remedy by Mr. Hepp, pharmacien of the Civil Hospital of Strasburg.

Bestucheff's Tincture and La Mothe's Golden Drops.

Alexis Petrovitch Bestoujeff-Rumine, commonly called Count von Bestoujeff or Bestucheff, was in the service of the Elector George of Hanover when that Prince was called to reign over Great Britain. He thereupon became George's ambassador at St. Petersburg. On the death of Peter the Great Bestucheff withdrew from the British diplomatic service, and commenced a varied and stormy political career, under the three Empresses Anna, Elizabeth, and Catherine II, who, with brief intervals, succeeded each other on the Russian throne. He was Foreign Minister under the first, Grand Chancellor and then a disgraced exile under the second, recalled and highly honoured by Catherine. During his banishment he interested himself in a remedy which became enormously popular at that epoch, known in France as the Golden Drops of General La Mothe, and in Germany and Russia as Bestucheff's Tincture. La Mothe had been in the service of Leopold Ragotzky, Prince of Transylvania, but retiring from the Army he went to live at Paris and took these golden drops with him. They were a tincture of perchloride of iron with spirit of ether, but the public believed them to be a solution of gold. They were recommended as a marvellous restorative medicine, and sold (in Paris) at 25 livres (nearly £1) for the half-ounce bottle. So famous were they that Louis XV sent 200 bottles to the Pope as a particularly precious gift. Subsequently Louis gave La Mothe a pension of 4,000 livres a year for the right of making the drops for his Hotel des Invalides, La Mothe and his widow after him retaining the right to sell to the public.

Bestucheff sold his recipe to the Empress Catherine for 3,000 roubles, and by her orders it was passed on to the College of Medicine of St. Petersburg, which published it under the title of the Tinctura Tonica Nervina Bestucheffi. The formula at first published was chemically absurd, but Klaproth corrected it, and the prestige of the quack medicine was destroyed. But an ethereal tincture of perchloride of iron was adopted in most of the Continental pharmacopœias.

It is not clear whether Bestucheff and La Mothe were in association at any time, but their preparations were similar if not identical.

Under the rule of Napoleon I the French Government bought several formulas of secret remedies for about £100 each. None of them either had or has since acquired any popular reputation. The formulas were published in the medical and pharmaceutical journals of the time.

XIII
CHEMICAL CONTRIBUTIONS TO PHARMACY

> Chymistry. "An art whereby sensible bodies contained in vessels, or capable of being contained therein, are so changed by means of certain instruments, and principally fire, that their several powers and virtues are thereby discovered, with a view to philosophy or medicine."—BOERHAAVE. Quoted as a definition in Johnson's Dictionary, 1755.

ACIDS, ALKALIES, AND SALTS.

Under the above title almost the entire history of chemistry might be easily comprehended. The gradual growth of definite meanings attached to these terms has been coincident with the attainment of accurate notions concerning the composition of bodies. To the ancient philosophers sour wine, acetum vinæ, or acetum as it is still called, was the only acid definitely known. When the alchemists became busy trying to extract the virtue out of all substances they produced several acids by distillation. These they called, for example, spirit of vitriol, spirit of nitre, spirit of salt, meaning our sulphuric, nitric, and hydrochloric acids respectively. They regarded everything obtained by distillation as a spirit. When the theorists came forward, Becher, Stahl, and their followers, they treated these acids as original constituents of the substances from which they were obtained. Thus, when sulphur was burned phlogiston was set free, and acid remained. Lavoisier believed that the acidifying principle had been discovered in oxygen, and it was on this theory that he gave that element its name. But this idea broke down when Davy proved that there was no oxygen in the so-called muriatic, or oxy-muriatic acid. It was the subsequent recognition of the law of substitution which made it clear that the acids are, in fact, salts of hydrogen or of some metal substituted for the hydrogen.

The history of alkalies is as varied as is that of acids. The distinction between caustic alkalies and mild alkalies was a problem as far back as Dioscorides. By burning limestone caustic lime is produced. It was not an unreasonable presumption that the fire had created this causticity, and this theory was held with regard to all the alkalies until it was proved by Joseph Black, in 1756, that the caustic alkali was the result of a gas, fixed air, he named it, being driven off from the mild alkali.

The ancient Jews prepared what they called Borith (translated "soap" in Jeremiah, ii, 22, and Malachi, iii, 2) by filtering water through vegetable ashes. Borith was therefore an impure carbonate of potash. It is probable that the salt-wort was generally employed for this purpose, and some of the old versions of the Old Testament give the herb "Borith" as the proper sense of the passages referred to above. In any case the alkaline solution produced from vegetable ashes was used for bleaching and cleansing purposes. The Roman "lixivium" was similarly prepared, and the process is still followed in some countries where there are dense forests. The Arabic word "al-kali" was apparently applied to the product from the word "qaly," which meant "to roast." The earliest known use of the term is, however, found in the works of Albertus Magnus, early in the thirteenth century. A process of making caustic potash by filtering water through vegetable ashes with quicklime is described in the works attributed to Geber, but this is in a treatise now known to have been written in the thirteenth or fourteenth century. It was only in 1736 that the three alkalies, soda, potash, and ammonia, were definitely distinguished by Duhamel as mineral, vegetable, and animal or volatile alkalies.

A formula for a solution of caustic potash was given in the P.L., 1746, under the title of Lixivium Saponarium. Equal parts of Russian potashes and quicklime were mixed, wetted until the lime was slaked, water afterwards added freely, and after agitation the solution poured off. This was ten years before Black's classic investigation already referred to. Before Black, and for some time afterwards, there were several theories in explanation of the action of the lime on the potashes. The lime had been tamed, but the potash had become more virulent. One popular suggestion was that the lime had withdrawn a kind of mucilage from the potashes; another that it had the effect of developing the power of the potashes by a mechanical process of comminution. A German chemist named Meyer, who vigorously opposed Black's conclusions, maintained that the lime contained a certain Acidum Causticum or Acidum Pingue, which potashes extracted from it.

In the P.L., 1788, the process was altered by increasing the proportion of the lime, and the product was described as Aqua Kali Puri. Subsequently the proportion of the lime employed was reduced.

The word "salt" is traced back to the Greek "hals," the sea, from which was formed the adjective "salos," fluctuating (like the waves), and subsequently the Latin "sal." Marine salt was therefore the original salt, and salts in chemistry were substances more or less resembling sea-salt. Generally, the term was limited to solids which had a taste and were soluble in water, but the notion was developed that salt was a constituent of everything, and this salt was extracted, and was liable to get a new name each time. Salt of wormwood, for instance, is one of the names which has survived as a synonym for salt of tartar, or carbonate of potash. Paracelsus insisted that all the metals were composed of salt, sulphur, and mercury, but these substances were idealised in his jargon and corresponded with the body, soul, and spirit, respectively.

Lavoisier was the first chemist who sought to define salts scientifically. He regarded them as a combination of an acid with a basic oxide. But when the true nature of chlorine was discovered it was found that this definition would exclude salt itself. This led to the adoption of the terms "haloid" and "amphide" salts, the former being compounds of two elements (now the combination of chlorine, bromine, iodine, cyanogen, or fluorine with a metal), and the latter being compounds of two oxides. The names were invented by Berzelius. Since then salts have been the subjects of various modern theories, electric and other, but they are always substances in which hydrogen or a metal substituted for it is combined with a radical. In a wide sense the acids are also salts.

ALCOHOL.

Al-koh'l was an Arabic word indicating the sulphide of antimony so generally used by Eastern women to darken their eyebrows, eyelashes, and the eyes themselves. Similar words are found in other ancient languages. Cohal in Chaldee is related to the Hebrew kakhal used in Ezekiel, xxiii, 40, in the sense of to paint or stain. The primary meaning of alcohol therefore is a stain. Being used especially in reference to the finely levigated sulphide of antimony, the meaning was gradually extended to other impalpable powders, and in alchemical writings the alcohol of Mars, a reduced iron, the alcohol of sulphur, flowers of brimstone, and similar expressions are common. As late as 1773 Baumé, in his "Chymie Experimentale," gives "powders of the finest tenuity" as the first definition, and "spirit of wine rectified to the utmost degree" as the second explanation of the term alcohol. As certain of the finest powders were obtained by sublimation the transfer of the word to a fluid produced by a similar method is intelligible, and thus came the alcohol of wine, which has supplanted all the other alcohols.

Distillation is a very ancient process. Evidence exists of its use by the Chinese in the most remote period of their history, and possibly they distilled wine. But so far as can be traced spirit was not produced from wine previous to the thirteenth century. Berthelot investigated some alleged early references to it and came to the conclusion indicated. Aristotle alludes to the possibility of rendering sea water potable by vaporising it, and he also notes elsewhere that wine gives off an exhalation which emits a flame. Theophrastus mentions that wine poured on a fire as in libations can produce a flame. Pliny indicates a particular locality which produced a wine of Falerno, which was the only wine that could be inflamed by contact with fire. At Alexandria, in the first century of the Christian era, condensing apparatus was invented, and descriptions of the apparatus used are known, but no allusion to the distillation of wine occurs in any existing reference to the chemistry of that period. Rhazes, who died in A.D. 925, is alleged to have mentioned a spirit distilled from wine, but Berthelot shows that this is a misunderstanding of a passage relating to false or artificial wines.

Water distilled from roses is mentioned by Nicander, about 140 B.C., and the same author employs the term ambix for the pot or apparatus from which this water was obtained. The Arabs adopted this word, and prefixing to it their article, al, made it into alembic. This in English appeared for some centuries in the abbreviated form of limbeck. The Greek ambix was a cup-shaped vessel which was set on or in a fire, as a crucible was used.

Pissaeleum was a peculiar form of distillation practised by the Romans. It was an oil of pitch made by hanging a fleece of wool over a vessel in which pitch was being boiled. The vapour which collected was pressed out and used.

Distilled waters from roses and aromatic herbs figured prominently in the pharmacy of the Arabs, and Geber, perhaps in the eighth century, describes the process, and may have used it for other than pharmaceutical purposes. Avicenna likens the body of man to a still, the stomach being the kettle, the head the cap, and the nostrils the cooling tube from which the distillate drips.

M. Berthelot gives the following from the Book of Fires of Marcus Grecas, which he says could not be earlier than 1300, as the first definite indication of a method of producing what was called aqua ardens. "Take a black wine, thick and old. To ¼ lb. of this add 2 scruples of sulphur vivum in very fine powder, and 2 scruples of common salt in coarse fragments, and 1 or 2 lbs. of tartar extracted from a good white wine. Place all in a copper alembic and distil off the aqua ardens." The addition of the salt and sulphur, M. Berthelot explains, was to counteract the supposed humidity.

Albucasis, a Spanish Arab of the eleventh century, is supposed from some obscure expressions in his writings to have known how to make a spirit from wine; but Arnold of Villa Nova, who wrote in the latter part of the thirteenth century, is the first explicitly to refer to it. He does not intimate that he had discovered it himself, but he appears to treat it as something comparatively new. Aqua vini is what he calls it, but some name it, he says, aqua vitæ, or water which preserves itself always, and golden water. It is well called water of life, he says, because it strengthens the body and prolongs life. He distilled herbs with it such as rosemary and sage, and highly commended the medicinal virtue of these tinctures.

It is worth remarking that when Henry II invaded and conquered Ireland in the twelfth century the inhabitants were making and drinking a product which they termed uisge-beatha, now abbreviated into whisky, the exact meaning of the name being water of life.

Raymond Lully, who acquired much of his chemical lore from Arnold of Villa Nova, was even more enthusiastic in praise of the aqua vitæ than his teacher. "The taste of it exceedeth all other tastes, and the smell all other smells," he wrote. Elsewhere he describes it as "of marveylous use and commoditie a little before the joyning of battle to styre and encourage the soldiers' minds." He believed it to be the panacea so long sought, and regarded its discovery as evidence that the end of the world was near. The process for making the aqua vitæ as described by Lully was to digest limpid and well-flavoured red or white wine for twenty days in a closed vessel in fermenting horse-dung. It was then to be distilled drop by drop from a gentle fire in a sand-bath.

The chemical constitution of alcohol was speculated upon rather wildly by the chemists who experimented on it before Lavoisier. It was held to be a combination of phlogiston with water, but the phlogiston-philosophers disagreed on the question whether it contained an oil. Stahl, however, later supported by Macquer, found that an oil was actually separated from it if mixed with water and allowed to evaporate slowly in the open air, after treating it with an acid. Lavoisier, in 1781, carefully analysed spirit of wine and found that 1 lb. yielded 4 oz. 4 drms. 37½ grains of carbon, 1 oz. 2 drms. 5½ grains of inflammable gas (hydrogen), and 10 oz. 1 drm. 29 grains of water. It was de Saussure who later, following Lavoisier's methods of investigation, but with an absolute alcohol which had been recently produced by Lowitz, a Russian chemist, showed that oxygen was a constituent of alcohol. Berthelot succeeded in making alcohol synthetically in 1854. His process was to shake olefiant gas (C_2H_4) vigorously with sulphuric acid, dilute the mixture with eight to ten parts of water, and distil. Meldola, however ("The Chemical Synthesis of Vital Products," 1904), insists that an English chemist, Henry Hennell, anticipated Berthelot in this discovery.

ALUM.

Alum is a substance which considerably mystified the ancient chemists, who knew the salt but did not understand its composition. Ancient writers like Pliny and Dioscorides were acquainted with a product which the former called alumen and which is evidently the same as had been described by Dioscorides under the name of Stypteria. Pliny says there were several varieties of this mineral used in dyeing, and it is clear from his account that his alumen was sometimes sulphate of iron and sometimes a mixture of sulphate of iron with an aluminous earth. It is the fact that where the various vitriols are found they are generally associated with aluminous earth.

Alum as we know it was first prepared in the East and used for dyeing purposes. Alum works were in existence some time subsequent to the twelfth century at a place named Rocca in Syria, which may have been a town of that name on the Euphrates, or more probably was Edessa, which was originally known as Roccha. It has been supposed that it was the manufacture of alum at this place which bequeathed to us the name of Rock or Rocha alum, but the Historical English Dictionary says this derivation is "evidently unfounded."

The alchemists were familiar with alum and knew it to be a combination of sulphuric acid with an unknown earth. Van Helmont was the first to employ alum as a styptic in uterine hæmorrhage, and Helvetius made a great reputation for a styptic he recommended for similar cases. His pills were composed of alum 10 parts, dragon's blood 3 parts, honey of roses q.s., made into 4 grain pills, of which six were to be taken daily. Alum and nutmeg equal parts were given in agues. Paris says the addition of nutmeg to alum corrects its tendency to disturb the bowels. It has also been advocated in cancer and typhoid, but these internal uses have been generally abandoned. Spirit of Alum is occasionally met with in alchemical writings. It was water charged with sulphuric acid obtained by the distillation of alum over a naked fire.

Until the fifteenth century the only alum factories from which Europe was supplied were at Constantinople, Smyrna, and Trebizonde. Beckman relates that an alum factory was founded in the Isle of Ischia, on the coast of Tuscany, by a Genoese merchant named Bartholomew Perdix, who had learnt the art at Rocca. Very soon afterwards John de Castro, a Paduan who had been engaged in cloth dyeing at Constantinople but had lost all his property when that city was captured by Mahomet II in 1453, was appointed to an office in the Treasury of the Apostolic Chamber, and in the course of his duties found what he believed to be an aluminous rock at Tolfa, near Civita Vecchia. He asked the Pope, Pius II, to allow him to experiment, but it was some years before the necessary permission was granted. When at last the truth of Castro's surmise was established the Pope was greatly interested. He looked upon the discovery as a great Christian victory over the Turks, and handsomely rewarded de Castro, to whom, besides, a monument was erected in Padua inscribed "Joanni de Castro, Aluminis inventor." The factory brought in a splendid revenue to the Apostolic exchequer, and the Pope did his utmost to retain the monopoly, for when in consequence of the extravagant prices to which the Tolfa alum was raised merchants began again to buy the Eastern product his Holiness issued a decree prohibiting Christians from purchasing from the infidels under pain of excommunication. Later, when, in Charles I's reign, Sir Thomas Challoner discovered an aluminous deposit near his home at Guisborough in Yorkshire, and persuaded some of the Pope's workmen to come there to work the schist, he and those whom he had tempted away were solemnly and most vigorously "cursed."

Meanwhile the nature of the earth with which the sulphuric acid was combined remained unknown to chemists. Stahl worked at the problem and came to the conclusion that it was lime. The younger Geoffroy, a famous pharmacist of Paris, ascertained (1728) that the earth of alum was identical with that of argillaceous earth and Alumina was for some time called Argile. Marggraf observed that he could not get alum crystals from a combination of argile and sulphuric acid, but noting that in the old factories it had been the custom to add putrid urine to the solution, for which carbonate of potash was subsequently substituted, went so far as to make the salt, but did not appreciate that it was actually a double salt. The name alumina which the earth now bears was given to it by Morveau. It was Vauquelin (another pharmacist) who clearly proved the composition of alum, and Lavoisier first suggested that alumina was the oxide of a metal. Sir Humphry Davy agreed with this view but failed to isolate the metal. Oersted was the first to actually extract aluminium from the oxide, but his process was an impracticable one, but in 1828 Woehler, and in 1858 Deville, found means of producing the metal in sufficient abundance to make it a valuable article of industry.

AMMONIA.

The chemical history of ammonia commences in Egypt with Sal Ammoniac. This is mentioned by Pliny under the name of Hammoniacus sal. Dioscorides also alludes to it; but in neither case does the description given fit in satisfactorily with the product known to us. Dioscorides, for instance, states that sal ammoniac is particularly prized if it can lie easily split up into rectangular fragments. It has been conjectured that what was called sal ammoniac by the ancient writers was, at least sometimes, rock salt.

The name is generally supposed to have been derived from that of the Egyptian deity, Amn or Amen, or Ammon as the Greeks called him, and in the belief that he was the same god as Jupiter he is referred to in classical literature as Zeus-Ammon or Jupiter-Ammon. The principal temple of this god was situated in an oasis of the Libyan desert which was then known as Ammonia (now Siwah), and if, as is supposed, the salt was found or produced in that locality its name is thus accounted for. Gum ammoniacum was likewise so called in the belief that it was obtained in that district, though the gum with which we are familiar and which comes from India and Persia, is quite a different article from the African gum the name of which it has usurped. Pliny derives the name of the salt from the Greek "ammos," sand, as it was found in the sand of the desert; an explanation which overlooks the fact that the stuff was called by a similar name in a country where the sand was not called ammos. In old Latin, French, and English writings "armoniac" is often met with. This was not inaccurate spelling; it was suggested by the opinion that the word was connected with Greek, armonia, a fastening or joining, from the use of sal ammoniac in soldering metals.

That Pliny did sometimes meet with the genuine sal ammoniac is conjectured by his allusion to the "vehement odour" arising when lime was mixed with natrum. Probably this natrum was sal ammoniac. Among the Arabs the term sal ammoniac often means rock salt; but in the writings attributed to Geber, some of which may be as late as the twelfth or thirteenth century, our sal ammoniac is distinctly described. It is also exactly described by Albertus Magnus in the thirteenth century, who mentions an artificial as well as a natural product, but does not indicate how the former was made. From this time sal ammoniac became a common and much-prized substance in alchemical investigations, as from it chlorides were obtained. The "volatile spirit of sal ammoniac" was made by distilling a solution of sal ammoniac with quicklime, and of course the same product was obtained in other ways, especially by distilling harts' horns, and this was always regarded as having peculiarly valuable properties. A "sal ammoniacum fixum" was known to the alchemists of the fifteenth century. It was obtained as a residue after sal ammoniac and quicklime had been sublimed. It was simply chloride of calcium.

The so-called natural sal ammoniac was for centuries brought from Egypt, and was supposed to have been mined in the earth or sand of that country. In 1716 the younger Geoffroy came to the conclusion that it must be a product of sublimation, and he read a paper to the French Academy giving his reasons for this opinion. Homberg and Lemery opposed this view with so much bitterness, however, that the paper was not printed. In 1719 M. Lemaire, French Consul at Cairo, sent to the Academy an account of the method by which sal ammoniac was produced in Egypt, and this report definitely confirmed the opinion which Geoffroy had formed. It was, said M. Lemaire, simply a salt sublimed from soot. The fuel used in Egypt was exclusively the dung of camels and other animals which had been dried by the sun. It consisted largely of sal ammoniac, and this was retained in the soot. For a long time an artificial sal ammoniac had been manufactured at Venice, and a commoner sort also came from Holland. These were reputed to be made from human or animal urine. The manufacture of sal ammoniac was commenced in London early in the eighteenth century by a Mr. Goodwin.

A formula for Sal Ammoniacum Factitium in Quincy's Dispensatory (1724) is as follows:—Take of Urine lb. x.; of Sea-salt lb. ii.; of Wood soot lb. i.; boil these together in a mass, then put them in a subliming pot with a proper head, and there will rise up what forms these cakes. Dr. James (1764) states that at Newcastle one gallon of the bittern or liquor which drains from common salt whilst making, was mixed with 3 gallons of urine. The mixture was set aside for 48 hours to effervesce and subside. Afterwards the clear liquor was drawn off and evaporated in leaden vessels to crystallisation. The crystals were sublimed. A sal ammoniacum volatile was made by subliming sal ammoniac and salt of tartar (or lime or chalk) together. Sometimes some spices were put into the retort. This salt was used for smelling-bottles. Aqua regia was made by distilling sal ammoniac and saltpetre together.

Sal Volatile Oleosum was introduced by Sylvius (de la Boe) about the year 1650. It became a medicated stimulant of the utmost popularity, and there were many formulas for it. One of the most famous was Goddard's Drop. (See page 319).

Ammonia in gaseous form was first obtained by Priestley in 1774. He called it alkaline air. Scheele soon after established that it contained nitrogen and Berthollet proved its chemical composition in 1785.

SPIRITUS AMMONIÆ AROMATICUS

was first inserted in the P.L. 1721, under the title of "Spiritus Salis Volatilis Oleosus." Cinnamon, mace, cloves, citron, sal ammoniac, and salts of tartar were distilled with spirit of wine. In 1746 the process was altered, sal ammoniac and fixed alkali being first distilled with proof spirit to yield "spiritus salis anmioniaci dulcis," to which essential oils of lemon, nutmeg, and cloves were added, and the mixture was then re-distilled. In 1788 the spirit became spiritus ammoniæ compositus, and the redistillation when the oils had been added was omitted. The name spiritus ammoniæ aromaticus was first adopted in the P.L. 1809, and has been retained ever since, though the process of making it has been frequently varied. That title was first given to it in the Dublin Pharmacopœia of 1807. Spiritus Salinus Aromaticus was the first title adopted in the Edinburgh Pharmacopœia. It was a preparation similar to that of the P.L., but angelica, marjoram, galangal, anthos flowers, orange, and lemon were additional flavours.

Quincy (1724) credits Sylvius with the invention of this spirit, which he refers to as "mightily now in use," and as "a most noble cephalic and cordial." It had "almost excluded the use of spirit of hartshorn." This preparation, invented by Sylvius, was called the Carminative Spirit of Sylvius.

Mindererus's Spirit, made from distilled vinegar and the volatile spirit of hartshorn, is believed by many competent authorities to have possessed virtues which are not contained in the modern liquor ammonii acetati. The late Professor Redwood was one of these. He believed that the old preparation contained a trace of cyanic ether. The new liquor, he said, made from strong caustic solution of ammonia and strong acetic acid, "is but the ghost of the old preparation. It is as unlike the true Mindererus's Spirit as a glass of vapid distilled water is unlike the sparkling crystal water as it springs from a gushing fountain" (*Pharm. Jnl.*, Vol. V., N.S. p. 408). Mindererus was a physician of Augsburg who died in 1621. It was Boerhaave in 1732 who advocated the use of Mindererus's Spirit and made it popular.

Eau de Luce, which was official in the P.L. 1824, under the title of Spiritus Ammoniæ Succinatus, was an ammonia compound which became popular in France, and, in some degree all over Europe, about the middle of the eighteenth century, and was apparently first sold for removing grease from cloth and other fabrics. It is said that one of the pupils of Bernard Jussieu, having been bitten by a viper, applied some of the preparation, and was cured by it. It thence acquired a medical fame, which it still retains. The P.L. formula ordered 3 drachms of mastic, 4 minims of oil of amber, and 14 minims of oil of lavender to be dissolved in 9 fluid drachms of rectified spirit, and mixed with 10 fluid ounces of solution of ammonia. In some of the Continental pharmacopœias a much larger proportion of oil of amber is prescribed, and sometimes only that and spirit of ammonia. In some soap is ordered. In the P.L., 1851, the oil of amber was omitted. It has been recommended for external application in rheumatism and paralysis.

It has been generally asserted that this preparation was devised by a pharmacist of Lille (some say of Amsterdam), of the name of Luce. It is also asserted that a Paris pharmacist named Dubalen originated it, and that he and his successor Juliot made it popular; that Luce of Lille imitated it, but that not being able to get it purely white added some copper and gave it a blue tint which came to be a mark of its genuineness. Among the names applied to it have been Aqua Luccana, Aqua Sancti Luciæ, Aqua Lucii, and Eau de Lusse.

BROMINE.

Bromine, isolated by Balard in 1826, was named by the discoverer Muride, from Muria, brine. Its actual name was suggested by Gay Lussac from Bromos, a stench.

Schultzenberger relates, on the authority of Stas, that some years before the discovery of bromine by Balard, a bottle of nearly pure bromine was sent to Liebig by a German company of manufacturers of salt, with the request that he would examine it. Somewhat carelessly the great chemist tested the product and assumed that it was chloride of iodine. But he put away the bottle, probably with the intention of investigating it more closely when he had more leisure. When he heard of Balard's discovery he turned to this bottle and realised what he had missed. Schultzenberger says he kept it in a special cupboard labelled "Cupboard of Mistakes," and would sometimes show it to his friends as an example of the danger of coming to a conclusion too promptly.

COLLODION.

Pyroxylin was discovered by Schönbein in 1847, and the next year an American medical student at Boston, Massachussets, described in the American Journal of the Medical Sciences his experiments showing the use that could be made of this substance in surgery when dissolved in ether and alcohol. By painting it on a band of leather one inch wide and attaching this to the hand, he caused the band to adhere so firmly that it could not be detached by a weight of twenty pounds.

EPSOM SALTS.

The medicinal value of the Epsom springs was discovered, it is believed, towards the end of the sixteenth century, in the reign of Queen Elizabeth. According to a local tradition the particular spring which became so famous was not used for any purpose until one very dry summer, when the farmer on whose land it existed bethought him to dig the ground round about the spring, so as to make a pond for his cattle to drink from. Having done this he found that the animals would not touch the water, and on tasting it himself he appreciated their objection to it. The peculiar merits of the water becoming known, certain London physicians sent patients to Epsom to drink it, and it proved especially useful in the cases of some who suffered with old ulcers. Apparently the sores were washed with it. The name of the farmer who contributed this important item to medical history was Henry Wicker or Wickes.

In 1621 the owner of the estate where the spring had been found walled in the well, and erected a shed for the convenience of the sick visitors, who were then resorting to Epsom in increasing numbers. By 1640 the Epsom Spa had become famous. The third Lord North, who published a book called the Forest of Varieties in 1645, claimed to have been the first to have made known the virtues of both the Epsom and the Tonbridge waters to the King's sick subjects, "the journey to the German Spa being too expensive and inconvenient to sick persons, and great sums of money being thereby carried out of the kingdom."

After the Restoration Epsom became a fashionable watering-place. Before 1700 a ball-room had been built, and a promenade laid out; a number of new inns and boarding-houses had been opened; sedan-chairs and hackney coaches crowded the streets; and sports and play of all kinds were provided. Pepys mentions visits to Epsom more than once in his Diary, and Charles II and some of his favourites were there occasionally. The town reached its zenith of gaiety in the reign of Queen Anne, who with her husband, Prince

George of Denmark, frequently drove from Windsor to Epsom to drink the waters.

An apothecary living at Epsom in those times, and who had prospered abundantly from the influx of visitors, is alleged to have done much to check the hopeful prospects of the Surrey village. Much wanted more, and Mr. Levingstern, the practitioner referred to, thought he saw his way to a large fortune. He found another spring about half a mile from the Old Wells, bought the land on which it was situated, built on it a large assembly room for music, dancing, and gambling, and provided a multitude of attractions, including games, fashion shops, and other luxuries. At first he drew the crowds away from the Old Wells. But his Epsom water did not give satisfaction. For some reason it brought the remedial fame of the springs generally into disrepute. Then Levingstern bought the lease of the Old Wells, and, unwisely it may be thought, shut them up altogether. The glory of Epsom had departed, and though several efforts were made subsequently to tempt society back to it, they were invariably unsuccessful. The building at the Old Wells was pulled down in 1802, and a private house built on the site. This house is called The Wells, and the original well is still to be seen in the garden. The very site of Mr. Levingstern's "New Wells" is now doubtful. He died in 1827.

In 1695 Nehemiah Grew, physician, and secretary of the Royal Society, wrote a treatise "On the Bitter Cathartic Salt in the Epsom Water." Dr. Grew names 1620 as about the date when the medicinal spring was discovered at Epsom by a countryman, and he says that for about ten years the countrypeople only used it to wash external ulcers. He relates that it was Lord Dudley North, who apparently lived near by, who first began to take it as a medicine. He had been in the habit of visiting the German spas, as he "laboured under a melancholy disposition." He used it, we are told, with abundant success, and regarded it as a medicine sent from heaven. Among those whom he induced to take the Epsom waters were Maria de Medicis, the mother of the wife of Charles I, Lord Goring, the Earl of Norwich, and many other persons of quality. These having shown the way, the physicians of London began to recommend the waters, and then, Dr. Grew tells us, the place got crowded, as many as 2,000 persons having taken the water in a single day.

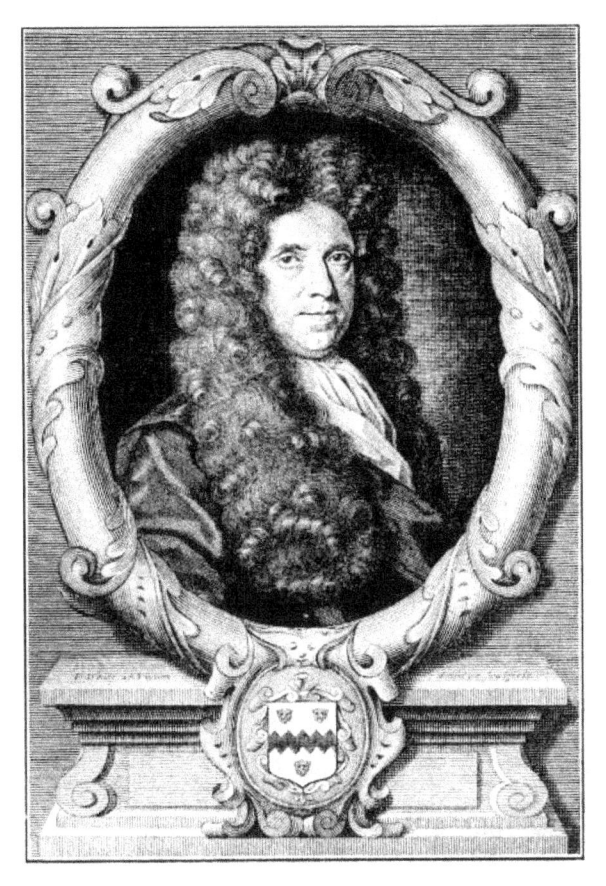

Dr. Nehemiah Grew.

Born, 1628; died, 1711.

(From an engraving by R. White, from life.)

>Dr. Grew was for many years secretary of the Royal Society and editor of the *Philosophical Transactions*. He was one of the pioneers of the science of structural botany and author of *The Anatomy of Plants*.

It was Dr. Grew who first extracted the salt from the Epsom water, and his treatise deals principally with that. He describes the effect of adding all sorts of chemicals, oil of vitriol, salt of tartar, nitre, galls, syrup of violets, and other substances to the solution; explains how it differs from the sal mirabilis (sulphate of soda); and writes of its delicate bitter taste as if he were commenting on a new wine. It most resembles the crystals of silver, he says, in the similitude of taste.

As to the medicinal value of this salt Dr. Grew says it is free from the malignant quality of most cathartics, never violently agitates the humours, nor causes sickness, faintings, or pains in the bowels. He recommends it for digestive disorders, heartburn, loss of appetite, and colic; in hypochondriacal distemper, in stone, diabetes, jaundice, vertigo, and (to quote the English translation) "in wandering gout, vulgarly but erroneously called the rheumatism." It will exterminate worms in children in doses of 1½ to 2 drachms, if given after 1, 2, or 3 grains of mercurius dulcis, according to age. Epsom salts were not to be given in dropsy, intermittent fevers, chlorosis, blood-spitting, to paralytics, or to women with child.

"I generally prescribe," writes the doctor, "one, two, or three pints of water, aromatised with a little mace, to which I add ½ oz. or 1 oz., or a greater dose of the salt." He gives a specimen prescription which orders 1 oz. or 10 drachms of the salt in 2 quarts of spring water, with 1 drachm of mace. This dose (2 quarts, remember) was to be taken in the morning in the course of two hours, generally warm, and taking a little exercise meanwhile. This was what was called an apozem. You might add to the apozem, if thought desirable, 3 drachms of senna and 1½ oz. or 2 oz. of flaky manna.

Mr. Francis Moult, Chymist, at the sign of the Glauber's Head, Watling Street, London, translated Dr. Grew's treatise into English, and gave a copy to buyers of the Bitter Purging Salts. Probably he was the "furnace philosopher" referred to by Quincy (see below), though it is difficult to see what there was to object to in his action.

George and Francis Moult (the latter was, no doubt, the chymist who kept the shop in Watling Street) in about the year 1700 found a more abundant supply of the popular salt in a spring at Shooter's Hill, where it is recorded they boiled down as much as 200 barrels of the water in a week, obtaining some 2 cwt. of salt from these. Some time after, a Dr. Hoy discovered a new method of producing an artificial salt which corresponded in all respects with the cathartic salts obtained from Epsom water, and which by reason of the price soon drove the latter out of the market, and caused the Shooter's Hill works to be closed. It was known that Hoy's salt was made from sea water, and at first it was alleged to be the sal mirabilis of Glauber, sulphate of soda. But this was disproved, and experiments were carried on at the salt works belonging to Lady Carrington at Portsmouth, and later at Lymington, where the manufacture settled for many years, the source being the residue after salt had been made, called the bittern—salts of magnesium, in fact. This was the principal source of supply, though it was made in many places and under various patents until in 1816 Dr. Henry, of Manchester, took out a patent for the production of sulphate of magnesia from dolomite.

It should be mentioned that it was by the examination of Epsom salts that Black was led to his epoch-making discovery of the distinction between the alkaline earths, and also of fixed air, in 1754.

In Quincy's "Dispensatory" (1724), medicinal waters like those of Epsom are described as Aquæ Aluminosæ. It is stated that there are many in England, scarce a county without them. The principal ones about London are at Epsom, Acton, Dulwich, and North-hall. They all "abound with a salt of an aluminous and nitrous nature," and "greatly deterge the stomach and bowels." But it is easy to take them too frequently, so that "the salts will too much get into the blood, which by their grossness will gradually be collected in the capillaries and glands to obstruct them and occasion fevers." After some more advice Quincy adds—

> "It is difficult to pass this article without setting a mark upon that abominable cheat which is now sold by the name of Epsom waters. Dr. Grew, who was a most worthy physician and an industrious experimenter, made trial how much salt these waters would leave upon evaporation, and found that a gallon left about two drams, or near, according to my best remembrance, for I have not his writings by me. He likewise found the salt thus procured answered the virtues of the water in its cathartic qualities. Of this an account was given before the Royal Society in a Latin dissertation. But the avaricious craft of a certain furnace-philosopher could not let this useful discovery in natural knowledge rest under the improvement and proper use of persons of integrity; but he pretended to make a great quantity for sale; and to recommend his salt translated the Doctor's Lecture into English to give away as a quack-bill."

Quincy proceeds to tell us how other competitors came in, and how the price was so reduced that what was first sold at one shilling an ounce, and could not honestly be made under (Quincy apparently refers to the salt made by evaporation), came down in a short time to thirty shillings per hundredweight.

ETHER.

The action of sulphuric acid on spirit of wine is alluded to in the works of Raymond Lully in the thirteenth century, and in those attributed to Basil Valentine, by whom the product is described as "an agreeable essence and of good odour." Valerius Cordus, in 1517, described a liquor which he called Oleum Vitrioli Dulce in his "Chemical Pharmacopœia." This was intended to represent the Spiritus Vitrioli Antepilepticus Paracelsi. It was prepared by distilling a mixture of equal parts of sulphuric acid and spirit of wine, after this mixture had been digested in hot ashes for two months. Probably the product obtained by Cordus was what came to be called later the sweet oil of wine, and not what we know as sulphuric ether.

The first ether made for medicinal purposes was manufactured in the laboratory directed by Robert Boyle, and it is said that he and Sir Isaac Newton made some experiments with it at the time. A paper describing his ether investigations was published by Newton in the "Philosophical Transactions" for May, 1700. In 1700 a paper on ether was published by Dr. Frobenius in the "Philosophical Transactions," and in the same publication in 1741 a further paper appeared giving the process by which Frobenius had prepared his "Spiritus Vini Ethereus." Equal parts of oil of vitriol and highly rectified spirit of wine by weight were distilled until a dense liquid began to pass; the retort was then cooled, half the original weight of spirit was added, and the distillation again renewed. This process was repeated as long as ether was produced. Frobenius had been associated with Ambrose Godfrey in Boyle's laboratory, and Godfrey had been supplying ether for some years, but he does not seem to have published his process. It was in Frobenius's first paper, published in 1730, that the name of ether was first proposed for the product, which had been previously known as Aqua Lulliana, Aqua Temperata, Oleum Dulce Paracelsi, and such-like fancy titles. Frobenius, it was understood, was a *nom de plume*. Ambrose Godfrey Hanckwitz, Boyle's chemist, sharply criticised Frobenius's article, said it was a rhapsody in the style of the alchemists, and that the experiments indicated had been already described by Boyle. Godfrey was, in fact, at that time making and selling this interesting substance. In France, the Duke of Orleans, a clever chemist, who was suspected to have had some association with the famous poisonings of his time, and whose laboratory was at the Abbaye Ste. Genevieve, was the first to produce ether in quantities of a pint at a time.

Hoffmann's "Mineral Anodyne Liquor," the original of our Spiritus Ætheris Co., was a semi-secret preparation much prescribed by the famous inventor. He said it was composed of the dulcified spirit of vitriol and the aromatic oil which came over after it. But he did not state in what proportion he mixed these, nor the exact process he followed.

The chemical nature of sulphuric ether was long in doubt. Macquer, who considered that ether was alcohol deprived of its aqueous principle, was the most accurate of the early investigators. Scheele held that ether was dephlogisticated alcohol. Pelletier described it as alcohol oxygenised at the expense of the sulphuric acid. De Saussure, Gay-Lussac, and Liebig studied the substance, but it was Dumas and Boullay in 1837, and Williamson in 1854, who cleared up the chemistry of ethers.

Ether is alcohol, two molecules deprived of H_2O [alcohol, C_2H_5O HO; ether, $(C_2H_5)_2O$]. Distilling spirit of wine and sulphuric acid together, it seemed obvious that the sulphuric acid should possess itself of the H_2O, and leave the ether. But on this theory it was not possible to explain the invariable formation of sulphovinic acid (a sulphate of ethyl) in the process, nor the simultaneous distillation of water with the ether. Williamson proved that the acid first combined with the alcohol molecule, setting the water free, and that then an excess of alcohol decomposed the sulphovinic acid thus formed into free sulphuric acid and ether, this circuit proceeding continuously.

SPIRIT OF NITROUS ETHER.

This popular medicine has been traced back to Raymond Lully in the thirteenth century, and to Basil Valentine. But the doctor who brought it into general use was Sylvius (de la Boe) of Leyden, for whom it was sold as a lithontryptic at a very high price. It first appeared in the P.L., 1746, as Spiritus Nitri dulcis. In English this was for a long time called "dulcified spirit of nitre," and in the form of sweet spirit of nitre still remains on our labels. In the P.L., 1788, the title was changed to Spiritus Ætheris nitrosi, and in that of 1809 to Spiritus Ætheris nitrici. The process ordered in the first official formula was to distil 6 oz. (apoth. weight) of nitric acid of $1·5$ specific gravity, with 32 fluid oz. of rectified spirit. Successive reductions were made in the proportion and strength of the acid in the pharmacopœias of 1809, 1824, and 1851, to 3½ fluid ounces of nitric acid, sp. gr. $1·42$, with 40 fluid ounces of rectified spirit, and a product of 28 fluid ounces. The object of these several modifications was to avoid the violent reaction which affected the nature of the product.

ETHIOPS.

Æthiops or Ethiops originally meant a negro or something black. The word is alleged to have been derived from aithein, to burn, and ops, the face, but this etymology was probably devised to fit the facts. There is no historical evidence in its favour. Most likely the word was a native African one of unknown meaning. It became a popular pharmaceutical term two or three hundred years ago, but is now almost obsolete, at least in this country. In France several mercurial preparations are still known by the name of Ethiops. There are, for instance, the Ethiops magnesium, the Ethiops saccharine, and the Ethiops gommeux; combinations of mercury with magnesia, sugar, and gum acacia respectively. These designations echo the mysteries of alchemy.

Ethiops alone meant Ethiops Mineral. This was a combination of mercury and sulphur, generally equal parts, rubbed together until all the mercury was killed. It was a very uncertain preparation, but was believed to be specially good for worms. "Infallible against the itch," says Quincy, 1724. Its chemical composition varied from a mere mixture of the two substances to a mixture of sulphur and bisulphide of mercury, according to the conditions in which it was kept. It was formerly known as the hypnotic powder of Jacobi.

Ethiops Martial was the black oxide of iron. It was a mixture of protoxide and sesquioxide of iron. Lemery's process was the one usually recommended, but perhaps not always followed. It was to keep iron filings always covered with water and frequently stirred for several months until the oxide was a smooth black powder. Lemery's Crocus Martis was a similar preparation but contained more of the sesquioxide. The Edinburgh and Dublin Pharmacopœias of 1826 ordered simply scales of iron collected from a blacksmith's anvil, purified by applying a magnet, and reduced to a fine powder. This was a favourite preparation of iron with Sydenham. Made into pills with extract of wormwood, the Ethiops Martial constituted the pilula ferri of Swediaur.

Ethiopic pills were similar to Plummer's pills (pil. calomel. co.). Guy's ethiopic powder was once a well-known remedy for worms. It was composed of equal parts of pure rasped tin, mercury, and sulphur. Vegetable ethiops was the ashes of fucus vesiculosus which were given in scrofulous complaints and in goitre before iodine was discovered. The ashes contain a small proportion of iodine. Dr. Runel ("Dissertation on the Use of Sea Water," 1759) says it far exceeds burnt sponge in virtue.

Huxham recommended an Aethiops Antimoniale, composed of two parts of sulphide of antimony and one part of flowers of sulphur. The older Aethiops Antimoniale was a combination of antimony chloride with mercury, and was given in venereal and scrofulous complaints. Mercury with chalk was sometimes called absorbent ethiops, or alkalised ethiops.

IODINE

was discovered by Bernard Courtois in 1811. Courtois, who was born at Dijon in 1777, was apprenticed to a pharmacist at Auxerre named Fremy, grandfather of the noted chemist of that name, and was afterwards associated as assistant with Seguin, Thénard, and Fourcroy. He had worked with the first-named of these in the isolation of the active principle of opium, whereby Seguin so nearly secured the glory of the discovery of the alkaloids. In 1811 Courtois was manufacturing artificial nitre, and experimenting on the extraction of alkali from seaweed. He had crystallised soda from some of the mother liquor until it would yield no more crystals, and then he warmed the liquor in a vessel to which a little sulphuric acid had been accidentally added. He was surprised to see beautiful violet vapours disengaged, and from these scales of a grayish-black colour and of metallic lustre were deposited.

Courtois was too busy at the time to follow up his discovery, but he brought it to the notice of a chemist friend named Clement. The latter presented a report of his experiments to the Academy of Sciences on November 20th, 1813, two years after Courtois's first observation. No suggestion was made by Courtois or Clement of the new substance being an element.

This deduction became the occasion of an acrimonious dispute between Gay-Lussac and Humphry Davy. The English chemist happened to be in Paris (by special favour of Napoleon) at the time when Clement read his paper. He immediately commenced experimenting, and was apparently the first to suspect the elementary nature of iodine. His claim was confirmed by a communication he made to Cuvier. But Gay-Lussac forestalled his announcement in a paper he read at the Academy on December 6th, 1813. Davy complained of the trick Gay-Lussac played him, and Hofer, who investigated the circumstances, came to the conclusion that Davy was certainly the first to recognise iodine as a simple *body*, and to give it its name from the Greek, Ion, violet. Ion was originally Fion, but had lost its initial. The Latin viola was derived from the original word.

Jean Francois Coindet, of Geneva (an Edinburgh graduate), suspected that iodine was the active constituent of burnt sponge, which had long been empirically employed in goitre and scrofula, and having proved that this was the case, was the first physician to use iodine as a remedy. The pharmaceutical forms and the medical uses of iodine have been very numerous during the century which has almost elapsed since its introduction, but it would be impossible even to detail them here.

Iodoform was first prepared by Serullas about 1828, and its chemical composition was elucidated by Dumas soon after. It was first used in medicine by Bouchardat in 1836, and then dropped out of practice for about twenty years, when it again appeared in French treatises, and its use soon became general as an antiseptic application.

Bernard Courtois was awarded 6,000 francs by the Academy of Sciences in 1832, but he died in Paris in 1838 in poverty. He had been ruined in 1815 by the competition of East Indian saltpetre with the artificial nitre which he was manufacturing. In that year the prohibitive duty on the native product was removed. When the Academy awarded 6,000 francs to Courtois it also voted 3,000 francs to Coindet, who had so promptly made medical use of Courtois' discovery.

LITHIUM.

Lithium, the oxide of which was discovered in 1807 by Arfwedson, was first suggested as a remedy for gout by Dr. Ure in 1843. He based his proposal on an observation by Lipowitz of the singular power of lithium in dissolving uric acid. Dr. Garrod popularised the employment of the carbonate of lithium in medicine. Most of the natural mineral waters which had acquired a reputation in gouty affections have been found to contain lithium.

Magnesia.

The first use of carbonate of magnesia medicinally was in the form of a secret medicine which must have acquired much popularity in the beginning of the eighteenth century. It was prepared, says Bergmann, by a regular canon at Rome, sold under the title of the powder of the Count of Palma, and credited with almost universal virtues. The method of preparation was rigidly concealed, but it evidently attracted the attention of chemists and physicians, for it appears that in 1707 Valentini published a process by which a similar product could be obtained from the mother liquor of "nitre" (soda) by calcination. In 1709 Slevogt obtained a powder exactly resembling it by precipitating magnesia from a solution of the sulphate by potash. Lancisi reported on it in 1717, and in 1722 Hoffmann went near to explaining the distinction between the several earthy salts, which in his time were all regarded as calcareous.

Hoffmann's process to obtain the powder was to add a solution of carbonate of potash to the mother liquor from which rough nitre had been obtained (solution of chloride of magnesium), and collect the precipitate. This being yielded by two clear solutions gave to the carbonate of magnesia precipitated the name of Miraculum Chemicum.

Magnesia was the name of a district in Thessaly, and of two cities in Asia Minor. The Greek "magnesia lithos," magnesian stone, has been frequently applied to the lodestone, but this can hardly have been correct, as the magnesian stone was described as white and shining like silver. Liddell and Scott think talc was more probably the substance. The alchemists sometimes mention a magnesia, but the name seems to have been a very elastic one with them. The Historical English Dictionary quotes the following reference to the word from "Norton Ord. Alch.," 1477:—"Another stone you must have ... a stone glittering with perspicuitie ... the price of an ounce conveniently is Twenty Shillings. Her name is Magnetia. Few people her knows."

Paracelsus uses the term in the sense of an amalgam. He writes of the Magnesia of Gold. In Pomet's "History of Drugs," 1712, magnesia meant manganese. Hoffmann, 1722, first applied the name to oxide of magnesia, adapting it from the medical Latin term, magnes carneus, flesh magnet, because it adheres so strongly to the lips, the fancy being that it attracts the flesh as the lodestone attracts iron.

Hoffmann's observations on magnesia and its salts, which were published in the first quarter of the eighteenth century, were very intelligent, and undoubtedly it was he who first distinguished magnesia from chalk. He says "A number of springs, among which I may mention Eger, Elster, Schwalbach, and Wilding, contain a neutral salt which has not yet received a name, and which is almost unknown. I have also found it in the waters of Hornhausen which owe to this salt their aperient and diuretic properties. Authors commonly call it nitre; but it has nothing in common with nitre. It is not inflammable, its crystallising form is entirely different, and it does not yield aqua fortis. It is a neutral salt similar to the arcanum duplicatum (sulphate of potash), bitter in taste, and producing on the tongue a sensation of cold." He further states that the salt in question appears to proceed from the combination of sulphuric acid with a calcareous earth of alkaline nature. The combination "is effected in the bosom of the earth." In another of his works Hoffmann distinguishes the magnesian salt from one of lime, showing particularly that the latter was but slightly soluble and had scarcely any taste. Crabs' eyes and egg shells he notes combine with sulphuric acid and form salts with no taste. The sulphate of this earth (Epsom salt) he found had a strong bitter taste.

The true character of magnesia and its salts was not clearly understood until Joseph Black unravelled the complications of the alkaline salts by his historic investigation, which became one of the most noted epochs of chemistry by its incidental revelation of the combination of the caustic alkalies with what Black termed "fixed air," subsequently named carbonic acid gas by Lavoisier in 1784. When Black was studying medicine at Edinburgh a lively controversy was in progress in medical circles on the mode of action of the lithontriptic medicines which had lately been introduced. Drs. Whytt and Aston, both university professors, were the leaders in this dispute. Whytt held that lime water made from oyster shells was more effective for dissolving calculi in the bladder than lime water prepared from ordinary calcareous stone. Alston insisted that the latter was preferable. Black was interested, and his experiments convinced him of the scientific importance of his discoveries. He postponed taking his degree for some time in order to be sure of his facts. His graduation thesis, which was dated June 11, 1754, was entitled "De humore acide cibis orto et magnesia alba." His full treatise, "Experiments upon magnesia alba, quicklime, and some other alkaline substances," was published in 1756. It had been previously believed that the process of calcining certain alkaline salts whereby caustic alkalies were produced was explained by the combination with the salt of an acrid principle derived from the fire. Now it was shown that something was lost in the process; that the calcined alkali weighed less than the salt experimented with. The something expelled Black proved was an air, and an air different from that of the atmosphere, which was generally supposed to be the one air of the universe. He identified it with the "gas sylvestre" of Van Helmont, and named it "fixed air." Magnesia alba first appeared in the London Pharmacopœia of 1787 under that name.

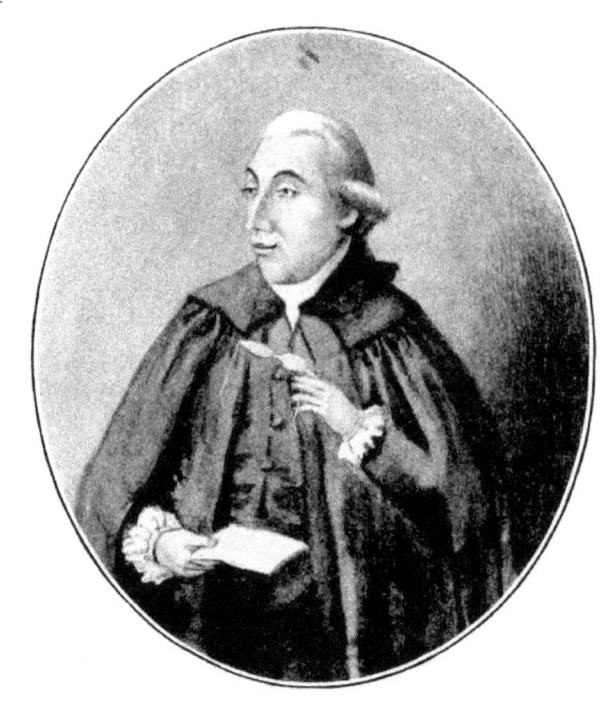

Joseph Black Lecturing (after John Ray)

(From a print in the British Museum.)

The oxide of magnesia was believed to be an elementary substance until Sir Humphry Davy separated the metal from the earth by his electrolytic method in the presence of mercury. By this means he obtained an amalgam, and by oxidising this he reproduced magnesia and left the mercury free, thus proving that the earth was an oxide of a metal. In 1830 Bussy isolated the magnesium by heating in a glass tube some potassium covered with fragments of chloride of magnesium, and washing away the chloride of potassium formed. Magnesium in small globules was left in the tube. The metal is now prepared on an industrial scale either by electrolysis, or by fusing fluor-spar with sodium. At present the uses of magnesium and of its derivatives are infinitesimal in comparison with the vast quantities available in deposits, as in dolomite, and in the sea.

NITRE

among the ancient Greeks and Romans generally meant carbonate of soda, sometimes carbonate of potash. The Arab chemists, however, clearly described nitrate of potash. In the works attributed to Geber and Marcus

Græcus, especially, its characters are represented. Raymond Lully, in the thirteenth century, mentions sal nitri, and evidently alludes to saltpetre, and Roger Bacon always meant nitrate of potash when he wrote of nitre. It was not, however, until the seventeenth century that the term acquired the definite meaning which we attach to it.

At the beginning of that century there was much discussion as to the formation of nitre, as it had been held that the acid which combined with the alkali was ready formed in the atmosphere. Glauber was the first to argue that vegetables formed saltpetre from the soil. Stahl taught that the acid constituent of nitre was vitriolic acid combined with phlogiston emanating from putrefying vegetable matter.

After gunpowder had become a prime necessity of life, saltpetre bounded upwards in the estimation of kings and statesmen. In France in 1540 an Edict was issued commissioning officials called "salpêtriers" in all districts who were authorised to seek for saltpetre in cellars, stables, dovecotes, and other places where it was formed naturally. No one was permitted to pull down a building of any sort without first giving due notice to the salpêtriers. The "Salpêtrière" Asylum in Paris recalls one of the national factories of nitre. During the French Revolution citizens were "invited" to lixiviate the soil and ceilings of their cellars, stables, etc., and to supply the Republic with saltpetre for gunpowder. The Government paid 24 sous, 1s., a pound for the nitre thus procured, though, as this was no doubt paid in assignats, it was cheap enough. It was estimated that 16,000,000 lbs. a year were thus provided.

PETROLEUM.

Under the name of naphtha and other designations petroleum has been known and used from the earliest times. The Persians were the first, as far as is known, to employ it for lighting, and also for cooking. They likewise made use of it as a liniment for rheumatism. So in this country, a kind of petroleum was sold as a liniment under the name of British oil; and in America, long before the great oil industry had been thought of, petroleum was popular as a liniment for rheumatism under the name of Seneca Oil.

Asphalt, or Bitumen of Judæa, was used by the Egyptians for embalming. Probably they reduced its solidity by naphtha. Naphtha was employed by Medea to render the robe which she presented to her rival Glauca inflammable, and this legend is given to account for the name of Oil of Medea, by which petroleum was anciently known. It was no doubt the principal ingredient in the Greek Fire of the middle ages.

Petroleum has been called by many other names. Oil of Peter or Petre was a common one, meaning, like petroleum, simply rock oil. Myrepsus, in the thirteenth century, refers to it as Allicola. The monks called it sometimes oil of St. Barbarus, and oil of St. Catherine.

Dioscorides said naphtha was useful as an application in dimness of sight. Two centuries ago it was occasionally given in doses of a few drops for worms, and was frequently applied in toothache. Petroleum Barbadense, Barbadoes tar, had some reputation in pectoral complaints in the seventeenth and eighteenth centuries, and was admitted into the P.L. as the menstruum for sulphur in the balsamum sulphuris Barbadense.

PHOSPHORUS.

Phosphorus, or its Latin equivalent, Lucifer, was the name given by the ancient astronomers to the planet Venus when it appeared as a morning star. When it shone as an evening star they called it Hesperus. Do we invent such seductive names now, or do they only seem attractive to us because they are ancient or foreign?

The phosphorescent properties of certain earths had been occasionally noticed by naturalists, but no observation of the kind has been traced in ancient writings. The earliest allusion to a "fire-stone" known occurs in the work of a gossipy French historian named De Thou. In a history of his own times this writer relates that in 1550, when Henri II made his state entry into Boulogne on the occasion of its restoration to France by the English, a stranger in foreign costume presented the king with a fire-stone which, he said, had been brought from India. De Thou narrates that this wonderful stone glowed with inconceivable splendour, was so hot that it could not be touched without danger, and that if confined in a close space it would spring with force into the air.

Sometime early in the seventeenth century, a shoemaker of Bologna, one Vincent Cascariolo, who, in addition to his ordinary business dabbled in alchemy, discovered a stone in the neighbourhood of his city which was luminous in the dark. The stone, which is now known to have been a sulphate of barium, and which the shoemaker calcined, ground, and formed into little round discs about the size of a shilling, and sold for a fancy price, was called the sun-stone. The discs, exposed to a strong light for a few minutes and then withdrawn into a dark room, gave out the incandescent light which we know so well. The discovery excited keen interest among scientific men all over Europe.

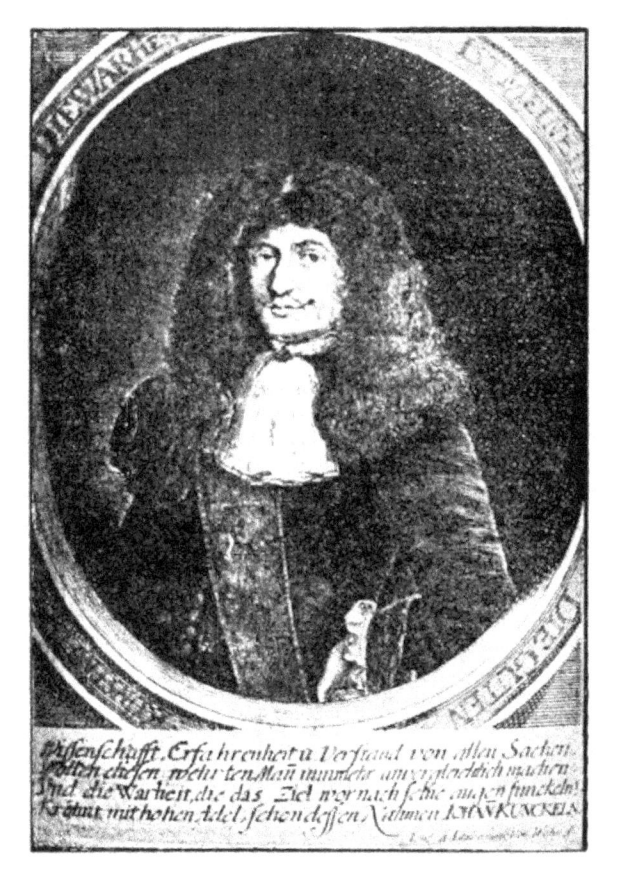

Johann Kunckel.

(From the Collection of Etchings in the Royal Gallery at Berlin.)

About 1668 two alchemists named Bauduin and Frueben, who lived at Grossenhayn in Saxony, conceived the idea of extracting by chemical processes the spirit of the world (Spiritus Mundi). Their notion was to combine earth, air, fire, and water in their alembic, and to obtain the essences of all of these in one distillate. They dissolved lime in nitric acid, evaporated to dryness, exposed the residue to the air, and let it absorb humidity. They then distilled this substance and obtained the humidity in a pure form. History does not tell us what questions they put to their spirit of the world when they had thus caught it. It appears, however, that the stuff attained a great sale. It was supplied at 12 groschen the loth, equal to about 1s. 6d. per ounce, and lords and peasants came after it eagerly. Rain-water would have been just as good, Kunckel, who tells the story, remarks. But one day Bauduin broke one of the vessels in which was contained some of the calcined nitrate of lime, and he observed that this, like the Bologna stone, was luminous in the dark after exposure to sunlight. Bauduin appreciated the importance of his discovery, and, taking some of his earth to Dresden, talked about it there. Kunckel, who was then the Elector's pharmacist, and keenly interested in new discoveries, heard about this curious substance, and was very curious to find out all he could. He visited Bauduin and tried to draw from him the details of his process. But Bauduin was very shy of Kunckel, and the latter has left an amusing account of an evening he spent with his quarry. Kunckel tried to talk chemistry, but Bauduin would only take interest in music. At last, however, Kunckel induced Bauduin to go out of the room to fetch a concave mirror to see if with that the precious phosphorus (for Bauduin had already appropriated this name to the stuff) would absorb the light. While Bauduin was gone Kunckel managed to nip a morsel with his finger-nail. With this, aided by the fragments of information he had been able to steal from Bauduin's conversation, he commenced to experiment by treating chalk with nitric acid, and ultimately succeeded in producing the coveted luminous earth. He sent a little lump of it to Bauduin as an acknowledgment of the pleasant musical evening the latter had given him.

It was now 1669. Kunckel was visiting Hamburg, and there he showed to a scientific friend a piece of his "phosphorus." To his surprise the friend was not at all astonished at it, but told Kunckel that an old doctor in Hamburg had produced something much more wonderful. Brandt was the name of the local alchemist. He had been in business, had failed, and was now practising medicine enough to keep him, but was devoting his heart and soul and all his spare time to the discovery of the philosopher's stone. The two friends visited Brandt, who showed them the real "phosphor" which he had produced, to which, of course, the other substances compared as dip candles might to the electric light, but nothing would induce the old gentleman to disclose any details of his process. Kunckel wrote to a scientific friend happily named Krafft at Dresden about the new "phosphor." Honour seems to have been cheap among scientific friends at that time, for Krafft posted off to Hamburg, without saying anything to Kunckel about his intention, caught Brandt in a different humour, or perhaps specially hard-up, and bought his secret for 200 thalers.

According to another story, the German chemist Homberg also succeeded in securing Brandt's secret by taking to him as a present one of those weather prognosticators in which a figure of a man and another of a woman come out of doors or go in when it is going to be wet or fine, as the case may be; a toy which had just then been invented.

Stimulated perhaps by Brandt's obstinacy and Krafft's treachery, Kunckel set to work and in time succeeded in manufacturing phosphorus. It may be taken as certain that he had picked old Brandt's brains a little, and his own skill and shrewdness enabled him to fill up the gaps in his knowledge. However he acquired the art, he soon became the first practical manufacturer of phosphorus.

Brandt discovered phosphorus because he had arrived at the conviction that the philosopher's stone was to be got from urine. In the course of his experiments with that liquid, phosphorus came out unexpectedly from the process of distilling urine with sand and lime.

The new substance excited great curiosity in scientific circles all over Europe, but the German chemists who knew anything about it kept their information secret, and only misleading stories of its origin were published. Robert Boyle, however, who was travelling on the Continent when the interest in the discovery was keenest, got a hint of the method of manufacture, and on his return to England proceeded to experiment. His operator and assistant in these investigations was Ambrose Godfrey Hanckwitz, who became the founder of a London pharmaceutical business which still exists. Ultimately Boyle and Hanckwitz were completely successful, and for many years the "English phosphorus" supplied by Hanckwitz from his laboratory in Southampton Street, Strand, monopolised the European market. According to a pamphlet published by him, entitled "Historia Phosphori et Fama," the continental phosphorus was an "unctuous, dawbing oyliness," while his was the "right glacial" kind.

In 1680 Boyle deposited with the Royal Society, of which he was then president, a sealed packet containing an account of his experiments and of his process for the production of the "Icy Noctiluca," as he called his phosphorus.

It is related in the Memoirs of the Academy of Sciences of Paris for 1737 that in that year a stranger appeared in Paris and offered for a stipulated reward to communicate the process of making phosphorus to the French Government. A committee of the Academy, with Hellot as its president, was appointed to witness the stranger's manipulation. According to the report of this committee, the experiment was completely successful.

It only remains to add, to complete the history, that in 1769, Gahn, a Swedish mine owner, discovered phosphorus in bones, and that working from this observation Scheele in 1775 devised the process for the manufacture of phosphorus which is still followed.

Such a remarkable substance as phosphorus, extracted as it had been from the human body, was evidently marked out for medical uses. Experiments were soon commenced with it. Kunckel's "luminous pills" were the first in the field, so far as is known. His report was published in the "Chemische Anmerkungen" in 1721. He gave it in three-grain doses, and reported that it had a calmative effect! Subsequently it was tried in various diseases by continental practitioners. Mentz commended it in colic, Langensalz in asthenic fevers, Bonneken in tetanus, Wetkard in apoplexy, and Trampel in gout.

In 1769 Alphonse Leroy, of Paris, reported a curious experience. He was sent for to a patient apparently on the point of death from phthisis. Seeing that the case was hopeless, he prepared and administered a placebo of sugared water. Calling the next day, Leroy found his patient somewhat revived, and on examining the sugar which he had used for his solution, he found that some phosphorus had been kept in it for a long time. The patient was much too far gone to recover, but she survived for fifteen days, and Leroy attributed this amelioration to the phosphorised water which he had accidentally given her.

Gahn discovered phosphorus in the bones in 1768, and in 1779 another German chemist named Hensing ascertained its presence in a fatty matter which he extracted from the brain. Medical theories were naturally based on these observations. Couerbe, a French chemist quoted by Dr. Churchill, wrote thus in 1830:

> "The want of phosphorus in the brain would reduce man to the sad condition of the brute; an excess of this element irritates the nervous system, excites the individual, and throws him into that terrible state of disturbance called madness, or mental alienation; a moderate proportion gives rise to the sublimest ideas, and produces that admirable harmony which spiritualists call the soul."

British practitioners took but very little notice of phosphorus as a remedy in the first century of its career, although it remained for a large part of that period an English product.

It is rather curious, too, that neither in this country nor on the Continent did it get into the hands of the empirics, as mercury, antimony, and other dangerous drugs did. It may be supposed that it was not so much the danger that checked them as the pharmaceutical difficulties in the way of preparing suitable medicines. The earliest preparations of phosphorus, such as Kunckel's pills, were a combination of it in a free state with conserve of roses. This method was gradually abandoned on account of the difficulty of subdividing the phosphorus so perfectly that the dose could be measured accurately. But as Dr. Ashburton Thompson remarks,[3] "although it is not so specifically mentioned, the uncertainty of action which imperfectly divided phosphorus exhibits" had something to do with the rejection of the old formulas. That is putting it very gently. The three-grain doses must have killed more people than they cured. The author just quoted says that in the early days "the dose employed seldom fell below 3 grains, while it occasionally rose as high as 12 grains." Even Leroy, he adds, instituted his experiments by taking a bolus of 3 grains, and he did not seriously suffer from it. The recommended dose has been regularly declining. In 1855 Dr. Hughes Bennett gave it at one-fortieth to one-eighth of a grain. The Pharmacopœia now prescribes one-hundredth to one-twentieth of a grain.

THE HYPOPHOSPHITES.

The hypophosphites in the form of syrup were introduced by Dr. J. F. Churchill, of Paris, as specifics in consumptive diseases about 1857. His preference of these salts over the phosphates was based on the theory that the deficiency in the system in a phthisical condition was not of phosphates, which had been completely oxidised, but of a phosphide in an oxidisable condition, and this requirement was fulfilled by the hypophosphites. The latter he compared to wood or coal, the phosphates to ashes, so far as active energy was concerned. Dr. Churchill's interest in a special manufacture of the hypophosphite syrups prejudiced the medical profession against his theories, and it is not certain that he got a fair hearing in consequence. The general verdict was that his results were not obtained by other experimenters, but for a good many years past syrups of the hypophosphites have been among the most popular of our general tonics.

Phosphorus is soluble in alcohol, ether, chloroform, bisulphide of carbon, and to a very small extent in water.

Phosphor paste as a vermin killer was ordered by the Prussian Government to be substituted for arsenical compounds in 1843, and it is probable that to some degree the alteration has been successful, though in France it was found that phosphorus in this form became a popular agent for suicide and criminal poisoning.

SAL PRUNELLA

was at one time in high esteem, as it was believed that by the process adopted for making it the nitre was specially purified. Purified nitre was melted in an iron pot and a little flowers of sulphur (1 oz. to 2 lb.) was sprinkled on it, a little at a time. The sulphur deflagrating was supposed to exercise the purifying influence on the nitre. The actual effect was to convert a small part of the nitrate of potash into sulphate. It was first called Sal Prunella in Germany from the belief that it was a specific against a certain plum-coloured quinsy of an epidemic character. Boerhaave advised the omission of the sulphur, but believed that melting the pure nitre and moulding it was of medicinal value by evaporating aqueous moisture.

Nitre and flowers of sulphur were deflagrated together before the Sal Prunella theory was invented, equal quantities being employed. The resulting combination, which was of course sulphate of potash, was known as Sal Polychrestum, the Salt of Many Virtues.

SAL GEMMÆ.

Sal Gemmæ or Sal Fossile was the name given to rock salt, particularly to the transparent and the tinted varieties. It was believed to be more penetrating than the salt derived from sea water, and this property Lemery ascribed to the circumstance that it had never been dissolved in water, and therefore retained all its native keenness.

SPIRIT OF SALT.

Spiritus Salis Marini Glauberi was one of the products discovered by Glauber, to whom we owe the name of spirit of salt. He was a keen observer and remarked on the suffocating vapour yielded as soon as oil of vitriol was poured on sea-salt. It is astonishing to his biographers that he just missed discovering chlorine. The spirit of salt was highly recommended for many medicinal uses; for exciting the appetite, correcting the bile, curing gangrene, and dissolving stone. Its remarkable property of assisting nitric acid to dissolve gold was soon observed and was attributed to its penetrating power.

TARTAR.

Tartarus was the mythological hell where the gods imprisoned and punished those who had offended them. Virgil represents it as surrounded by three walls and the river Phlegethon, whose waters were sulphur and pitch. Its entrance was protected by a tower wrapped in a cloud three times as black as the darkest night, a gate which the gods themselves could not break, and guarded by Cerberus.

There is nothing to associate this dismal place with the tartar of chemistry, except that in old books it is said that Paracelsus so named the product because it "produces oil, water, tincture, and salt, which burn the patient as Tartarus does." Paracelsus did not invent the name of tartar; it is found in many alchemical books long before his time. The earliest found use of it is in an alchemical work by Hortulcuus, an English alchemist of the eleventh century.

Paracelsus was writing about "tartarous diseases" ("De Morbis Tartareis"), those, that is, which resulted from the deposit of concretions. Stone, gravel, and gout were among these diseases of tartar, and evidently it was this morbid tartar which he associated with the legendary Tartarus. The word tartar, applied to the deposit from wine, is sometimes supposed to have descended from an Egyptian term, dardarot, meaning an eternal habitation, and etymologists generally prefer it as the origin of the name. If it was, the sense development of the term as applied to the chemical is not clear. The Greek word *tartarizein*, meaning to shiver with cold, does not help much in tracing the history of the word. Another frequently advocated derivation is the Arab, *durd*, dregs, sediment, which it is said was actually applied to the tartar of wine. It appears, too, that the Arabs used this term also as we do to represent the deposit on teeth; they also had a word, *dirad*, to mean a shedding of teeth, and by *darda* they signified a toothless old woman. Some etymologists consider, however, that the transition from durd to tartar would be most unlikely.

When the alchemists began to experiment with tartar their first process would be to distil it. The residue left in their retorts they called the salt of tartar. They knew this substance under other names, salt of wormwood, for instance, but they did not recognise the identity. By treating tartar with vinegar they produced acetate of potash, which they called regenerated tartar. Oswald Crollius, the compiler of the first European pharmacopœia, gave the name of vitriolated tartar to what we now know as sulphate of potash.

The iatro-chemists of the next century, who obtained it by various methods, gave to sulphate of potash distinct names which show in what esteem it was held. Among other designations it appears as Specificum purgans, Arcanum duplicatum, Nitrum fixum, Panacea holsatica, and Sel de duobus. Glaser, who produced it from sulphur, saltpetre, and urine distilled together, sold it as Sal Polychrest of Glaser.

Cream of tartar was known to the ancients under the name of Fæx Vini, which is the designation for it used by Dioscorides.

The tartar of wine was found to be only soluble in water with difficulty; but if boiled in water a turbid liquor was yielded which in the boiled condition continually threw up a sort of skin or scum. This was taken off with a skimmer and dried; it was naturally called Cream of Tartar.

Paracelsus and other chemists distilled this cream and got an oil from it which they called oil or spirit of tartar. It was chiefly a pyro-tartaric acid with some empyreumatic constituents. It was a thin, light yellow, bitter tasting but rather tart, and pleasant smelling oil, and was credited with remarkable penetrating powers. It was used in disorders of the ligaments, membranes, and tendons. Particularly surprising to them was the fact that the residue of a distinctly acid substance was a strong alkali. This "salt of tartar" was found to yield another oil called oleum tartari per deliquium, or lixivium tartari, which was the name by which it was called in the Pharmacopœia. Salt of tartar and cream of tartar together yielded the tartarum tartarisatus. It was when making this that Seignette produced by accident his double tartrate of potash and soda, now familiarly known as Rochelle salt.

Vitriol.

Visitando Interiora Terræ Rectificando Invenies Occultum Lapidem Veram Medicinam. (Visiting the interior of the earth you may find, by rectifying the occult stone, the true medicine.) This acrostic is first found in the works attributed to Basil Valentine.

The vitriols enjoyed an enormous reputation in medicine, at least until their chemical composition was definitely explained by Geoffrey in 1728. It was certainly known that the green vitriols contained iron, and they were sometimes named vitriol of Mars; that the blue vitriols contained copper, which obtained for them the designation of vitriol of Venus; and the white was understood to be associated with calamine, though by some it was supposed to be only green vitriol which had been calcined.

The name of vitriol cannot be traced further back than to Albertus Magnus in the thirteenth century. He expressly applies the term to atramentum viride, the Latin name for sulphate of iron. Presumably it was given to the salt on account of its glassy appearance. The alchemists, on distilling these vitriols found that they always yielded a spirit or oil, to which they naturally gave the name of spirit or oil of vitriol.

In Greek the vitriols were called chalcanthon, as they were extracted from brass; the common name in Latin was atramentum sutorium, because they were employed for making leather black. Dioscorides states that this substance is a valuable emetic, should be taken after eating poisonous fungi, and will expel worms. Pliny recommends it for the cure of ulcers, and Galen used it as a collyrium. There was a good deal of confusion between the vitriols and the alums, and the Greek stypteria and the Latin alumens were often an aluminous earth combined with some vitriol. Pliny gives a test for the purity of what he calls alum, which consists in dropping on it some pomegranate juice, when, he says, it should turn black if it is pure. Evidently his alum contained sulphate of iron.

Paracelsus declared that, with proper chemical management, vitriol was capable of furnishing the fourth part of all necessary medicine. It contained in itself the power of curing jaundice, gravel, stone, fevers, worms, and epilepsy.

Mayerne was another strong advocate of the medicinal virtues of vitriol. According to him it possessed the most diverse properties. It was hot and cold, attenuative and incressant, aperitive and astringent, coagulative and dissolvant, corroborative, purgative, and sudorific.

A multitude of medicines were made from the vitriols. A vitriolum camphoratum was included in the P.L. of 1721 by distilling spirit of camphor from calcined vitriol; but Quincy remarks:—"Its intention I am not acquainted with, nor have ever met with it in prescription." In Dr. Walter Harris's "Pharmacopœia Anti-Empirica," 1683, allusion is made to a remedy made by one Bovius, which consisted of spirit of vitriol, and was designed to lie a universal remedy. Added to an infusion of balm, marjoram, and bugloss, it would cure headache and vertigo; with rose water, fevers; with fumitory water, itch; with fennel water it would restore decayed memory; with plantain water it was a remedy against diarrhœa; and with lettuce water it became a narcotic. "A rare fellow," quaintly comments the doctor. Homberg's narcotic salt of vitriol was a combination of green vitriol and borax made after a very complicated process. The Gilla Vitrioli was a purified white vitriol used as an emetic. Spiritus Vitrioli dulcis was an imitation of Hoffmann's Anodyne. This distilled with hartshorn made the Diaphoretic Vitriol.

One of the precious secrets of the alchemists, occasionally sold to kings and wealthy amateurs, was that of converting iron into copper by means of blue vitriol. A strong solution of the salt was prepared, and an iron blade, or any iron instrument, was immersed in it for a certain time. When taken out it appeared to be a blade or instrument of copper. Kunckel was the first chemist to explain the fallacy.

Elixir of Vitriol was devised by Adrian Mynsicht, a famous German physician, in the early part of the seventeenth century. He published an Armamentarium Medico-Chymicum which became very popular. His Elixir (under the name of Elixir Vitrioli Mynsichti) was first given in the P.L. of 1721 as follows:—cinnamon, ginger, cloves, of each 3 drachms: calamus aromaticus, 1 oz.; galangal root, 1½ oz.; sage, mint, of each ½ oz.; cubebs, nutmegs, of each 2 oz.; lign. aloes, lemon peel, of each 1 drachm; candied sugar, 3 oz. Digest in spirit of wine, 1½ lb., and oil of vitriol 1 lb. for twenty days. Then filter.

In the P.L. 1746 the formula was simplified by mixing 4 oz. of oil of vitriol with 1 lb. of Aromatic Tincture, and the title was changed to Elixir Vitrioli Acidum. In the P.L. 1778 there was no Elixir of Vitriol, dilute sulphuric acid taking its place. This was then called Acidum Vitriolicum Dilutum. Under the name of Acidum Sulphuricum Aromaticum, however, an acidulated tincture, flavoured with ginger and cinnamon, was retained, and this, with the synonym of Elixir of Vitriol, is still in the B.P.

Quincy (1724) states that this medicine had lately come greatly in practice, and deservedly. "It mightily strengthens the stomach," he says, "and does good service in relaxations from debauches and overfeeding."

The alga "nostoch," so-called by Paracelsus, who also described it as flos cœlorum, acquired the name of vegetable vitriol, and sometimes spittle of the stars, because it appeared after rains in places where it had not been seen before.

XIV
MEDICINES FROM THE METALS

> Metals are all identical in their essence; they only differ by their form. The form depends on accidental causes which the artist must seek to discover. The accidents interfere with the regular combinations of sulphur and mercury; for every metal is a combination of these two substances. When pure sulphur meets pure mercury, gold results sooner or later by the action of nature. Species are immutable and cannot be transformed from one into the other; but lead, copper, iron, silver, &c., are not species. They only appear to be from their diverse forms.
>
> ALBERTUS MAGNUS:—"De Alchemia." (About 1250.)

ANTIMONY.

Some of the old writers insisted that antimony (the native sulphide) was used as a medicine by Hippocrates who called it Tetragonon, which simply meant four-cornered, and of which we also know that it was made up with the milk of a woman. The reason which the iatro-chemists gave for believing that this compound was made from antimony was worthy of the age when it was the practice to apply enigmatic names to medicinal substances, a practice, however, quite foreign to Hippocrates. They understood the term to imply four natures or virtues, and they said antimony had four virtues, namely, sudorific, emetic, purgative, and cordial; therefore tetragonon meant antimony.

THE ETYMOLOGY OF ANTIMONY.

The name of this metal is one of the curiosities of philology. The old legend was that Basil Valentine, testing his medicine on some of his brother monks, killed a few of them. "Those who have ears for etymological sounds," says Paris in "Pharmacologia," "will instantly recognise the origin of the word antimonachos, or monks-bane." Another version of the monk story is to the effect that after Basil Valentine had been experimenting with antimony in his laboratory he threw some of his compounds out of the window, and pigs came and ate them. He noticed that after the purgative action had passed off the pigs fattened. On this hint he administered the same antimonial preparation to certain monks who were emaciated by long fasts, and they died through the violence of the remedy.

These stories were probably the invention of some French punster, who worked them into shape out of the French name of the substance, antimoine, which, without the change of a letter, might mean bad for the monk. Littré entirely demolished any possibility of their truth by discovering the name in the writings of the Salernitan physician, Constantine, the African, who lived at the end of the eleventh century, three or four hundred years before the earliest dates suggested for Basil Valentine.

Other suggested derivations have been anti-monos, for the reason that the sulphide was never found alone; anti-menein, in reference to its tonic properties; and anti-minium, because it was used as an eye paint in the place of red lead. These are all guesses unsupported by evidence.

The modern philological theory is that the early Latin stibium and the late Latin antimonium have the same etymological origin. Stibium was the Latinised form of the Greek stimmi. Stimmi declined as stimmid—and this may have found its way into the Arabic through a conjectural isthimmid to the known Arabic name uthmud, which via athmud and athmoud became Latinised again into antimonium.

AL-KOHOL.

The antimony known to the ancients as stibium or stimuli was the native sulphide which Eastern women used for darkening their eyelashes. Probably it was used by Jezebel when, expecting Jehu at Samaria, "she painted her eyes and tired her head." The Hebrew expression is "she put her eyes in paint," and the Hebrew word for the paint is Phuph; (2 Kings, c. 9, v. 30). In Ezekiel, c. 23, v. 40, a debauched woman is described who painted her eyes, and in this case the Hebrew word employed is Kohol. The Septuagint translated both Phuph and Kohol by stimmi. The method is still used by Arabic women. They have a little silver or ivory rod which they damp and dip into a finely levigated powder called ismed, and draw this between the eyelids. Karrenhappuch, one of Job's daughters, meant a vessel of antimony. The writer of the Book of Enoch says that the angel Azazel taught the practice to women before the Flood. He "taught men to make swords, and knives, and shields, and coats of mail, and made known to them metals, and the art of working them; bracelets, and ornaments, and the use of antimony, and the beautifying of the eyebrows, and the most costly and choicest stones, and all colouring tinctures, so that the world was changed." Some of the early Christian fathers condemned the vanity. "Inunge oculos non stibio diaboli, sed collyrio Christi," writes Tertullian.

ALCHEMICAL HOPES OF ANTIMONY.

The alchemists and the early chemical physicians had great hopes of antimony. "They tormented it in every possible manner," says Fourcroy, "in the hope of getting from it a universal remedy." With it, too, they were convinced that they were coming near to the transmutation of other metals into gold. Noticing how readily it formed alloys with other metals they named it Lupus Metallorum, the Wolf of Metals. Their process for getting the Powder of Projection, as well as can be gathered from their mystic jargon was to first fuse the crude antimony, the sulphide, with iron which withdrew the sulphur from the antimony. The metal thus obtained they called the Martial Regulus of Antimony. Regulus, or little king, implied an impure gold. Combining this with corrosive sublimate and silver, and subliming the mixture they got the lunar butter of antimony. The sublimation had to be repeated eight or ten times, the residue, or fæces, being added to the sublimate every time. At last the sublimed butter of antimony was transferred to an oval glass vessel capable of containing twelve times its quantity, and hermetically sealed. The Philosophic Egg, as the vessel with its contents was called, was then placed in a sand-bath and kept at a moderate heat for several months. When it had become converted into a red powder, the operation was finished. This powder was the Powder of Projection. It was sprinkled on other metals in a state of fusion, mercury being an ingredient of the fused mass, and yellow gold was produced.

Antimonial Compounds.

By other processes the early experimenters obtained various other products. By simply heating crude antimony in a crucible they would sometimes get a vitreous substance in consequence of some of the silica of the crucible combining with the antimony. That was their glass of antimony, which was generally an oxide with some sulphide. In other cases the so-called liver of antimony resulted, a compound containing a larger proportion of the sulphide. This they also called crocus metallorum or saffron of the metals, and one or other of these products was originally the basis of antimonial wine.

It was digested with Rhine wine, and the tartar of the wine formed a tartrate of antimony, but, as may be supposed, the composition of the wine was very variable. Emetic tartar was subsequently substituted for the liver.

The crystalline protoxide of antimony obtained by inflaming, volatilising, and condensing the regulus was known as argentine flowers of antimony. The regulus heated with nitric acid yielded a compound of metal with antimonious acid, and was called mineral bezoar; a compound, really a suboxide, got by fusing sulphide of antimony and nitre was called diaphoretic antimony; the chloride, first made by distilling crude antimony (the native sulphide) with corrosive sublimate, yielded the thick soft butter of antimony; the addition of water to this chemical caused the precipitation of a white oxychloride which was long known as Algaroth's powder, or mercury of life. It contained no mercury, but was the most popular emetic before the introduction of the tartrate. Victor Algarotti, who introduced it, was a physician, of Verona, who died in 1603. It was alleged that he was poisoned by his local rivals in consequence of the success of his remedy. He was also the inventor of a quintessence of gold.

The regulus of antimony in alloy with some tin was used to make the antimony cups from which antimonial wine originated. It was also made into the pilulæ perpetuæ, or everlasting pills, which, passing through the body almost unchanged, were kept as a family remedy and taken again and again. It is probable that the surface of these pills became slightly oxidised, and consequently acquired a medicinal effect.

Kermes Mineral.

One of the most famous of the antimony compounds was the kermes mineral, which it is understood was invented by Glauber about 1651. He made it by treating a solution of the oxide of antimony with cream of tartar, and then passing a current of sulphuretted hydrogen through the solution. An orange-red powder was obtained, and famous cures were effected by it. Glauber kept his process secret, but a Dr. de Chastenay learnt it after Glauber's death from one of his pupils and confided it to a surgeon named La Ligerie, who in his turn communicated it to Brother Simon, a Carthusian monk, who at once commenced successfully to treat his brother monks with it, and soon after the Poudre des Chartres was one of the most popular remedies in France for many serious diseases, small-pox, ague, dropsy, syphilis, and many others. In 1720 Louis XIV bought the formula for its preparation for a considerable sum from La Ligerie. It has been agreed by chemists, Berzelius and others, who have studied Kermes Mineral, that it is a mixture of about 40 per cent. or less of oxide of antimony with a hydrated sulphide of the metal, and a small proportion of sulphide of sodium or potassium (according to the method of preparation). It is still official in the Pharmacopœias of the United States and of many Continental countries.

From the solution from which the Kermes had been deposited a further precipitate was obtained by the addition of hydrochloric acid. This, too, was a mixture, consisting of protosulphide and persulphide of antimony with some sulphur. It was the golden sulphuret which in association with calomel became so noted in the form of Plummer's powder and Plummer's pills. The powder was at first known as Plummer's Æthiops Medicinalis.

It would be tedious to go through the multitude of antimonial compounds which have become official, and it would be impossible in any reasonable space even to enumerate the quack medicines with an antimonial base which were so recklessly sold in this and other countries, especially in the earlier half of the seventeenth century. The most important of all the antimonial compounds, or, at least, the one which has maintained the favour of the medical profession in all countries, is, of course, the tartrate of antimony and potassium, emetic tartar.

EMETIC TARTAR.

Adrian Mynsicht, physician to the Duke of Mecklenburg in the early part of the seventeenth century, is generally credited with the invention of emetic tartar. Certainly the earliest known description of it is found in his "Thesaurus Medico-Chymicum," published in 1631. But Hofer has pointed out that the mixture known as the Earl of Warwick's Powder, which consisted of scammony, diaphoretic antimony (a binantimoniate of potash) and cream of tartar, which Cornachinus of Pisa described in 1620, was really its forerunner, and he considers that the salt was recognised in medicine before Mynsicht published his description.

Glauber, in 1648, described the process of making Mynsicht's emetic tartar from cream of tartar and argentine flowers of antimony.

ANTIMONY CONTROVERSY.

No medicine has been more violently attacked or so enthusiastically praised as antimony. The virulent antagonism to it manifested by the Faculty of Physicians of Paris was unquestionably the exciting cause of much of the fame to which it attained. It is generally stated that on the instigation of the Faculty the Parliament of Paris decreed that it should not be employed in medicines at all. This, however, has been proved to be incorrect. Certainly the Faculty in 1566 did, in fact, forbid its own licentiates to use it, and actually expelled one of their most able associates, Turquet de Mayerne, because he had disobeyed their injunction. But M. Teallier has shown by documentary evidence that the decree of the Parliament did not go beyond requiring that antimony should not be supplied for medicinal use except on the order of a qualified physician. The action of the Faculty, although approved for a time, was later almost disregarded, and when the court physicians cured the young king, Louis XIV, in 1657, by the administration of antimony, the defeat of the anti-antimonists was completed. The repeal of the decree against antimonials was dated 1666, just a century after its promulgation.

Louis XIV was taken dangerously ill at Calais, in 1657, when he was 19 years of age. A physician (Voltaire says a quack) of Abbeville had the audacity to treat him by the administration of emetic tartar, and the King himself and his Court were convinced that he owed his life to this remedy. The opponents of antimony were silenced, though they did not yield in their opinion. Gui Patin, who had termed the new medicine "tartre stygiè" (its usual French name was tartre stibié), protested against the attempt to canonise this poison, and asserted that the cure of the king was due to his own excellent constitution.

To illustrate the earnestness, not to say the ferocity, of medical controversy at the beginning of the seventeenth century, the record of the expulsion of Turquet de Mayerne from the College of Physicians of Paris, in 1603, quoted from the minutes of the College and translated by Nedham, may be given. It should be remembered that Turquet was the favourite physician of Henri IV, and, nominally, his offence was that he had published a defence of his friend, Quercetanus, who had prescribed mercurial and antimonial medicines. The minute is in the following terms:—

> The College of Physicians in the University of Paris, being lawfully congregated, having heard the Report made by the Censor to whom the business of examining the Apology published under the name of Turquet de Mayerne, was committed, do with unanimous consent condemn the same as an infamous libel, stuffed with lying reproaches and impudent calumnies, which could not have proceeded from any but an unlearned, impudent, drunken, mad fellow: And do judge the said Turquet to be unworthy to practise physick in any place because of his rashness, impudence, and ignorance of true physick: But do exhort all physicians which practise Physick in any nations or places whatsoever that they will drive the said Turquet and such like monsters of men and opinions out of their company and coasts; and that they will constantly continue in the doctrine of Hippocrates and Galen. Moreover, they forbid all men that are of the Society of the Physicians of Paris, that they do not admit a consultation with Turquet or such like person. Whosoever shall presume to act contrary shall be deprived of all honours, emoluments, and privileges of the University and be expunged out of the regent Physicians.
>
> Dated December 5, 1603.

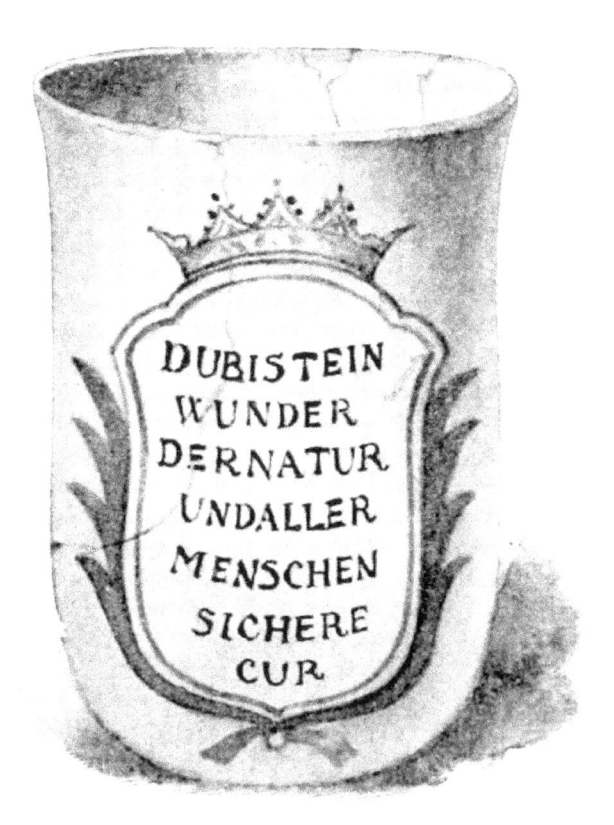

Antimony Cup.

(From an illustration to a note by Professor Redwood in the *Pharmaceutical Journal*, July 1, 1858.)

ANTIMONY CUPS (POCULA EMETICA)

were in use in the sixteenth and seventeenth centuries, more perhaps in Germany than in this country. The one illustrated is in the Museum of Practical Geology, Jermyn Street. It was bought for a shilling at a sale at Christies' in 1858, and was described in the catalogue as "An old metal cup, with German inscription and coronet, gilt, in woodcase." The cups are said to have been made of an alloy of tin and antimony, and wine standing for a time in one of them would become slightly impregnated with emetic tartar, the tartar of the wine acting on the film of oxide of antimony which would form on the inner surface of the cup. How far these cups were used in families does not appear, but it is said they were common in monasteries, and that monks who took too much wine were punished by having to drink some more which had been standing in the poculum emeticum. Dr. Walter Harris, in "Pharmacopœia Anti-Empirica" (1683) refers to the cups, and says, "their day is pretty well over. It is rare to meet with one now."

It was supposed by the early chemical physicians that antimony imparted emetic properties to wine without any loss of weight. Angelo Sala tells of a German who attained some fame in his time by letting out a piece of glass of antimony on hire. The patient was instructed to immerse this in a cup of wine for three, four, or five hours (according to the strength of the person prescribed for), and then to drink the wine. The practitioner charged a fee of a dozen fresh eggs for the use of his stone, and, as he had hundreds of clients, patients had to wait their turn for their emetic.

BISMUTH.

Bismuth, the metal, was not known to the ancients nor to the Arabs. It was first mentioned under that name by Agricola, in 1546, in "De Natura Fossilium," and was not then regarded as a distinct body. Agricola considered it to be a form of lead, and other mining chemists believed that it gradually changed into silver. The Magistery (trisnitrate or oxynitrate) was the secret blanc de fard which Lemery sold in large quantities as a cosmetic. He bought the secret from an unknown chemist and made a large fortune out of it. His process was to dissolve one ounce of the metal in two ounces of nitric acid and to pour on the solution five or six pints of water in which one ounce of sea-salt had been dissolved. The sea-salt would yield a proportion of bismuth oxychloride in the precipitate. Lemery made a pomatum, ʒi to the ounce, and a lotion, ʒi to ʒiv of lily water.

Until the latter part of the eighteenth century bismuth salts were regarded as poisonous and were scarcely used in medicine by way of internal administration. Even Odier, of Geneva, to whom we owe the introduction of this medicine in dyspepsia and diarrhœa, prescribed it in 1 grain doses with 10 grains each of magnesia and sugar.

Lemery says the bismuth of his time was a compound made in England from the gross and impure tin found in the English mines. "The workmen mix this tin with equal parts of tartar and saltpetre. This mixture they throw by degrees into crucibles made red hot in a large fire. When this is melted they pour it into greased iron mortars and let it cool. Afterwards they separate the regulus at the bottom from the scoriæ and wash it well. This is the tin-glass, which may be called the regulus of tin." Pomet says much the same about the composition. He adds, "It is so true that tin-glass is artificial that I have made it myself, and am ready to show it to those who won't believe me."

Those writers belonged to the first quarter of the eighteenth century. A quarter of a century later Quincy is telling us that the metal called Bismuth "is composed of tin, tartar, and arsenic, made in the northern parts of Germany, and from thence brought to England."

Meanwhile Stahl and Dufay had been studying bismuth and had established its character and elementary nature.

Liquor Bismuthi et Ammonii Citratis was introduced into the B.P. 1867, as an imitation of the proprietary Liquor Bismuthi, which Mr. G. F. Schacht, pharmaceutical chemist, of Clifton, had invented a few years previously. It was found that the official preparation differed from the proprietary one in taste and action principally because no attempt had been made to free it from the nitric acid used to dissolve the bismuth. This was corrected in 1885 by a liquor prepared from citrate of bismuth dissolved by solution of ammonia. This method has been further elaborated. Continental physicians have not favoured a solution of bismuth. They consider that the remedial value of bismuth depends on its insolubility; this view now obtains in England also.

Trochisci Bismuthi Compositi of the B.P. 1864, were believed to be intended to imitate the "Heartburn Tablets," made by Dr. Burt, an eminent medical practitioner of Edinburgh in the early part of the nineteenth century, and sold for him at a guinea a pound. Notwithstanding the price, perhaps because of it, these tablets attained to considerable popularity. It was said that Dr. Burt and his apprentices made all he supplied in his kitchen. Some said that his tablets contained no bismuth, the antacid properties being due entirely to chalk. In 1867 rose-flavour was substituted for cinnamon in the official lozenges, and in 1898 the oxynitrate of bismuth gave place to oxycarbonate.

GOLD.

> For gold in physick is a cordiall,
>
> Therefore he loved gold in special.
>
> Chaucer's *Doctour of Phisike*.

The employment of gold as a remedy is but rarely mentioned in ancient medical literature. Gold leaf was probably used by the Egyptians to cover abrasions of the skin. Pieces of it have been found on mummies apparently so applied. Some of the Arab alchemists, Geber among them, are believed to have made some kind of elixir of life from gold, but their writings are too enigmatical to be trusted. Avicenna mentions gold among blood purifiers, and the gilding of pills originated with the Eastern pharmacists. Probably it was believed that the gold added to the efficacy of the pills. It was not, however, until the period of chemical medicine in Europe that gold attained its special fame.

Arnold of Villa Nova, and Raymond Lully were among the advocates of the medicinal virtues of gold; but in the century before Paracelsus appeared, Brassavolus, Fallopius, and other writers questioned its virtues. With

Paracelsus, Quercetanus, Libavius, Crollius, and others of that age, however, gold entered fully into its kingdom. They could hardly exalt it too highly. But it is difficult to ascertain from the writings of this period what the chemical physicians understood by gold.

Paracelsus says it needs much preparation before it can be administered. To make their aurum potabile some of the alchemists professed to separate the salt from the fixed sulphur, which they held was the real principle of gold, its seed, as some of them called it, and to obtain this in such a form that it could be taken in any liquor. The seed of gold was with many of them the universal medicine which would cure all diseases, and prolong life indefinitely. It was the sulphur of the sun with which that body revivifies nature.

Paracelsus prescribed gold for purifying blood, and intimates that it is useful as an antidote in cases of poisoning, and will prevent miscarriages in women. He considered it not so cordial as emeralds, but more so than silver. He also states that if put into the mouth of a newly-born babe it will prevent the devil from acquiring power over the child.

The Archidoxa Medicinæ of Paracelsus, his famous Elixir of Long Life, is believed to have been a compound of gold and corrosive sublimate. He recommended gold especially in diseases connected with the heart, the organ which the sun was supposed to rule. Among the earlier Paracelsians Angelo Sala wrote a treatise on gold, entitled "Chrysologia, seu Examen Auri Chymicum," Hamburg, 1622. Sachsens prepared a Tinctura Solis secundem secretiorem Paracelsi Mentem preparata. But Thurneyssen, who carried on his quackeries on the largest scale, did the most to push the gold business. His Magistery of the Sun attained to great popularity in Germany, and these and his other preparations, together with the astrological almanacks and talismans which he sold, enabled him to live in great splendour at Frankfort, where he is said to have employed 200 persons in his laboratory. His fame departed, however, and he died in poverty at Cologne, in 1595.

Aurum Potabile.

Roger Bacon is said to have held that potable gold was the true elixir of life. He told Pope Nicholas IV that an old man in Sicily, ploughing, found one day a golden phial containing a yellow liquid. He thought it was dew, drank in off, and was immediately transformed into a hale, robust, handsome, and highly accomplished youth. He entered into the service of the King of Sicily, and remained at court for the next eighty years.

Francis Anthony was a famous quack in the reigns of Queen Elizabeth and James I. The College of Physicians took proceedings against him several times, fined him and imprisoned him, but aristocratic influences were exerted on his behalf and ultimately the College found it prudent to let him alone. His panacea "Aurum potabile" professed to be a solution of gold, and the wealthy classes of the period had unbounded belief in its wonderful remedial virtues. Some years after the death of Anthony the famous Honourable Robert Boyle (the "Father of philosophy and brother of the Earl of Cork") in the "Sceptical Chymist" wrote that though he was prejudiced against all such compositions, he had known (and he describes) some such wonderful cures resulting from this aurum potabile that he was compelled to bear testimony to its efficacy. Boyle also states that he had seen in part the preparation of this nostrum. He rather enigmatically reports that there was but a single ingredient associated with the gold, that this came from above, and was reputed to be one of the simplest substances in nature.

Anthony claimed that his product would cure most diseases; vomitings, fluxes, stoppages, fevers, plague, and palsies were included among the evils which it overcame. Several of the well-known physicians of the time wrote angry pamphlets denouncing Anthony's pretensions. Dr. Matthew Gwynne's "Aurum non aurum," and Dr. Cotta's "Cotta contra Antonium" were two of the most noted. Of course these gave Anthony opportunities of reply, and largely promoted the business. In one of his later publications Anthony boldly offered to exhibit his process to a committee of proper and unbiassed witnesses with the object of proving that the compound was truly a solution of gold. The challenge appears to have been accepted, and the Master of the Mint, Baron Thomas Knivet, and other experts were present when the test was made. According to Gwynne the result was failure, but I do not find any unprejudiced report of the experiment.

The writer of the life of Anthony in the old "Biographia Britannica," who is his warm partisan, gives what he declares to have been the genuine formula for the aurum potabile. It had long been in the possession of Anthony's descendants, he says, and was given to him (the author of the biography) by an eminent chemist. If this is true it is evident that a solution of gold would not have resulted from the process.

This is what the alleged Anthony's manuscript prescribes:—The object, Anthony says, is to so far open the gold that its sulphur may become active. To open it a liquor and a salt are required, these together forming the menstruum. The liquor was 3 pints of red wine vinegar distilled from a gallon; the salt was block tin burnt to ashes in an iron pan; these to be mixed and distilled again and again. Take one ounce of filed gold, and heat it in a crucible with white salt; take it out and grind the mixture; heat again; wash with water until no taste of salt is left; mix this with the menstruum, one ounce to the pint, digest, and evaporate to the consistence of honey. The Aurum Potabile was made by dissolving this in spirit of wine.

Whatever may have been the opinion of the experts who watched Anthony make his Aurum Potabile, the sale of the panacea was not destroyed, perhaps not injured by the result. Anthony made a handsome fortune out of it and continued to sell it largely until his death in 1623, and according to the authority already quoted, his son John Anthony, who qualified as an M.D. and held the licence of the College, derived a considerable income from the sale of the remedy. Dr. Munk, however, in the "Roll of the College of Physicians" intimates that this gentleman was free from the hereditary stain. "He succeeded to the more reputable part of his father's practice," is the pleasant way in which Dr. Munk describes John Anthony, M.D. John, however, wrote the following epitaph on his father:

> Though poisonous Envy ever sought to blame
>
> Or hide the fruits of thy Intention;
>
> Yet shall all they commend that high design
>
> Of purest gold to make a Medicine
>
> That feel thy Help by that thy rare Invention.

Glauber (1650) expounds "the true method of making Aurum Potabile," knowledge of which, he says, was bestowed on him from the highest. "Haply there will be some," he remarks at the beginning of his treatise on this subject, who will deny "that gold is the Son of the Sun, or a metallic body, fixed and perfect, proceeding from the rays of the Sun; asking how the Solary immaterial rays can be made material and corporeal?" But this only shows how ignorant they are of the generation of metals and minerals. Disposing of such incredulity by a few comments, and referring the sceptics to his treatise De Generatione Metallorum, he deals with several other irrelevant matters, and at last describes his process in prolix and unintelligible terms.

"℞ of living gold one part, and three parts of quick mercury, not of the vulgar, but the philosophical everywhere to be found without charges or labour." He recommends, but not as essential, the addition to the gold of an equal part of silver. "The mixture of male and female will yield a greater variety of colours, and who knoweth the power of the cordial union of gold and silver?" These metals being mixed in a philosophical vessel will be dissolved by the mercury in a quarter of an hour, acquiring a purple colour. Heating for half an hour, this will be changed to a green. The compound is to be dissolved in water of dew, the solution filtered and abstracted in a glass alembic three times until the greenness turns to a black like ink, "stinking like a carcase."

After standing for forty hours the blackness and stink will depart, leaving a milky white solution. This is to be dried to a white mass, which will change into divers colours, ultimately becoming a finer green than formerly. That green gold is to be dissolved in spirit of wine, to which it will impart a quintessence, red as blood, which is the quickening tincture, a superfluous ashy body being left. After some more distillations and abstractions a strong red solution will be obtained which is capable of being diluted with any liquid and may be kept as a panacea for the most desperate diseases. Next to "the stone" this is the best of all medicines.

The author cautions his readers against the yellow or red waters sold by distillers of wine at a great price as potable gold. Further he explains that the solution of gold made with aqua regia or spirit of salt is of little or no medicinal value, because the Archeus cannot digest it, but can only separate the gold and discharge it in the excrements.

In the "Secrets of Alexis" (John Wight's translation) a recipe for a potable liquor of gold is given which "conserveth the youth and health of man, and will heal every disease that is thought incurable in the space of seven doses at the furthest." Gold leaf, lemon juice, honey, common salt, and spirit of wine were to be frequently distilled. "The oftener it is distilled the better it be."

Kenelm Digby made a tincture of gold thus:—Gold calcined with three salts and ground with flowers of sulphur; burnt in a reverberatory furnace twelve times, and then digested with spirit of wine.

Lemery gives a formula for potable gold, or tincture of gold, or diaphoretic sulphur of gold:—Dissolve any quantity of gold you like in aqua regia; evaporate to dryness, and make a paste of the residue with essence of cannella. Then digest it in spirit. He adds, sarcastically I suppose, "This tincture is a good cordial because of the essence of cannella and the spirit of wine."

About 1540 Antoine Lecoque, a physician of Paris, acquired considerable reputation for his cures of syphilis by gold. Fallopius, Hoffmann, and Dr. Pitcairn, of Edinburgh, more or less fully adopted his treatment, but the theory gradually dropped out of medical practice. It was revived early in the nineteenth century by Dr. Chrestien, of Montpellier, a physician of considerable reputation, and his ardent advocacy had for a time considerable effect. But subsequent trials in the French hospitals gave negative results.

There were, no doubt, many honest attempts to make aurum potabile, and certainly there were a multitude of frauds palmed off on to a public who had come to believe in the miraculous remedial powers of the precious metal. The following is one of the simplest formulas for extracting the virtue of gold. It is given in "Lewis's Dispensatory," 1785, but not with any suggestion of its medicinal value:—One drachm of fine gold was dissolved in 2 ounces of aqua regia. To the solution 1 ounce of essential oil of rosemary was added, and the mixture well shaken. The yellow colour of the acid solution was transferred to the oil, which was decanted off, and diluted with 5 ounces of spirit of wine. The mixture was digested for a month, and then acquired a purple colour. Lewis explains that the oil takes up some of the gold, which, however, is deposited on the sides of the glass, or floats on the surface in the form of a slight film.

AURUM FULMINANS

was described in the works attributed to Basil Valentine, and later by Oswald Crollius. It is sometimes termed Volatile Gold. Valentine explains very clearly the process of making it, that is, by dissolving gold leaf in aqua regia and precipitating the fulminating gold by salt of tartar. By treatment with vinegar or sulphur its explosive properties were to be reduced. It was supposed to possess the medicinal value of gold in a special degree, and was particularly recommended as a diaphoretic. It appears from reports that it occasioned violent diarrhœas, and was, no doubt, often fatal. The so-called Mosaic Gold, which was given as a remedy for convulsions in children, was an amalgam of mercury with tin, ground with sulphur and sal ammoniac.

Hahnemann insisted that gold had great curative powers, and several homœopathic physicians of our time have highly extolled it. Dr. J. C. Burnett, in "Gold as a Remedy," recommended triturations of gold leaf, one in a million, as a marvellous heart tonic, especially in cases of difficult breathing in old age.

IRON.

Iron was not regarded as of special medicinal value by the ancients. The alleged administration of the rust of iron by Melampus was apparently looked upon as a miracle, and though this instance is often quoted as the earliest record of ferruginous treatment, it does not appear to have been copied. Classical allusions, such as that of the rust of the spear of Telephus being employed to heal the wounds which the weapon had inflicted, which is referred to by Homer, can hardly be treated as evidences of the surgical skill of that period. Iron is not mentioned as a remedial agent by Hippocrates, but Dioscorides refers to its astringent property, and on this account recommends it in uterine hæmorrhage. He states that it will prevent conception; it subsequently acquired the opposite reputation. The same authority, as well as Celsus, Pliny, and others, allude to a practice of quenching a red-hot iron in wine or water in order to produce a remedy for dysentery, weak stomachs, or enlargement of the spleen.

The later Latin physicians made very little use of iron or its compounds. Oribasius and Aetius write of the uses of its oxide outwardly in the treatment of ulcers, and Alexander of Tralles prescribes both an infusion and the metal in substance for a scirrhus of the spleen. He was probably the earliest physician who discovered its value as a deobstruent. Rhazes, the Arab, gave it in substance, and in several combined forms, but Avicenna regarded iron as a dangerous drug, and suggested that, if any had been accidentally taken, some loadstone should be administered to counteract any evil consequences.

Vitriol (sulphate of iron and sulphate of copper) was the iron medicine most in use up to the sixteenth century; but it was not given with the special intention of giving iron. Paracelsus had great faith in the Arcanum Vitrioli, which, indeed, appears to have been sulphur. He also introduced the use of the magnet, but only externally. It was in the century after him that the salts of Mars came into general medical use. In the course of the seventeenth and eighteenth centuries the preparations of iron became very numerous. Iron filings brought into an alcohol, that is very finely powdered, were much employed, sometimes alone and sometimes saccharated, or combined with sugar candy. Crocus martis was the sesquioxide, æthiops martial was the black oxide, and flores martis, made by subliming iron filings and sal ammoniac, yielding an ammoniated chloride of iron, was included in the several British pharmacopœias of the eighteenth century.

The association of iron with Mars probably influenced the early chemical physicians in their adoption of iron salts in anæmic complaints, and as general tonics. The undoubted effect of iron remedies in chlorotic disease was naturally observed, and the reputation of the metal was established for the treatment of this condition long before it was discovered that iron is an invariable constituent of the human body. When this physiological fact came to be recognised it was supposed that the action of iron salts was explained; but, in fact, the investigations of the last century have only tended to make this theory doubtful.

It is known that in health the proportion of iron in the body is fairly constant. An average man's blood contains about 38 grains, almost all of which is contained in the hæmoglobin. He requires from one to two grains every day to make up for waste, and this he gets in the meat and vegetable food which he absorbs. The vegetables obtain iron from the soil, and animals acquire it from the corn, roots, or grasses which they eat. So far as is known it is from these sources only that human beings assimilate the iron they require. It is very doubtful whether a particle of the iron administered in any of the multitudinous forms which pharmacy provides is retained. A noted modern physiologist, Kletzinsky, says "From all the hundredweights of iron given to anæmics and chlorotics during centuries not a single blood corpuscle has been formed." For all that there is no medical practitioner of any considerable experience who has not found directly beneficial results follow the administration of these medicines in such cases.

To Sydenham and Willis, two of the most famous physicians of the seventeenth century, the general employment of iron as a medicine may be traced. Sydenham, in his treatise on hysteric diseases, which, he says, are occasioned by the animal spirits being not rightly disposed, and not as some supposed by the corruption of the blood with the menstrual fluid, points out that the treatment must be directed to the strengthening of the blood, for that is the fountain and origin of the spirits. In cachexies, loss of appetite, chlorosis, and in all diseases which we describe as anæmic, he recommends that if the patient is strong enough recourse should be had first to bleeding, this to be followed by a thirty days' course of chalybeate medicine. Then he describes, much the same as modern treatises do, how rapidly iron quickens the pulses, and freshens the pale countenances. In his experience he has found that it is better to give it in substance than in any of the preparations, "for busy chemists make this as well as other excellent medicines worse rather than better by their perverse and over officious diligence" (Pechey's translation). He advises 8 grains of steel filings made into two pills with extract of wormwood to be taken early in the morning and at 5 p.m. for thirty days; a draught of wormwood wine to follow each dose. "Next to the steel in substance," he adds, "I choose the syrup of it prepared with filings of steel or iron infused in cold Rhenish wine till the wine is sufficiently impregnated, and afterwards strained and boiled to the consistence of a syrup with a sufficient quantity of sugar."

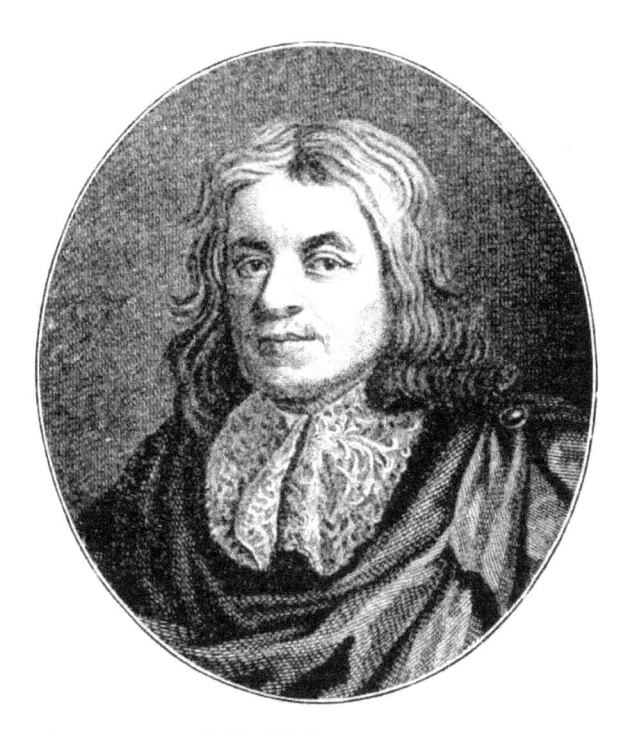

DR. THOMAS SYDENHAM. 1624–1689.

(Originator of Sydenham's Laudanum.)

Dr. Willis had a secret preparation of iron of which Dr. Walter Harris, physician in ordinary to Charles II, in "Pharmacologia Anti-Empirica" (1683), writes:—"The best preparation of any that iron can yield us is a secret of Dr. Willis. It has hitherto been a great secret and sold at a great price. It was known as Dr. Willis's Preparation of Steel." Dr. Harris thinks it will not be an unacceptable service to the public to communicate this masterpiece of that eminent and ever famous man. "It was no strained stately magistery, no sublimation or salification, no calcined crocus, and no chemical mystery; but an easy and a natural way of opening this hard body that it may open ours." It was given particularly for the removal of obstructions. The formula was equal parts of iron filings and crude tartar powdered and mixed with water in a damp mass in a glazed earthen vessel. This was to be dried over a slow fire or in the sun; wetted and dried again; and this process repeated four or five times. It might be given in white wine, or made into a syrup, or into pills, electuary, or lozenges. Dr. Willis preferred the crude tartar because the cream of tartar sold by the druggists was generally a cheat, often combined with alum. The crude could be bought at 6d. to 8d. per lb. In the apothecaries' shops cream of tartar was sold at 3s. to 3s. 6d. per lb.

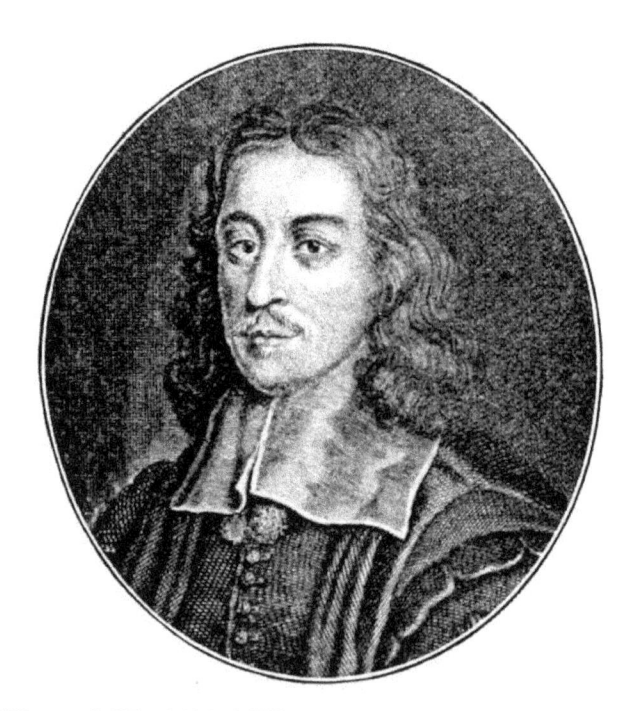

THOMAS WILLIS, M.D. 1621–1675.

Quincy (1724), who frequently offers explanations of the exact way in which medicines exercise their remedial power, thus scientifically describes the action of iron in removing obstructions:—"Mechanics teach nothing more plainly than that the momenta of all percussions are as the rectangles under the gravities and celerities of the moving bodies. By how much more gravity then a metalline particle has more than any other particle in the Blood, if their celerities are equal, by so much the greater will the stroke of the metalline particle be against everything that stands in its way than of any other not so heavy; and therefore will any Obstruction in the Glands and Capillaries be sooner removed by such particles than by those which are lighter. This is a way of reasoning that is plain to the meanest Capacity."

Tartarised iron has always been a favourite form for its administration. The Balls of Mars (boules de Mars, or boules de Nancy), still a popular medicine in France, are a tartarised iron prepared by a complicated process. First, a decoction of vulnerary species is made from 12 parts of water and 2 of the species. This is strained and poured on 12 parts of pure iron filings in powder. The mixture is evaporated to dryness and powdered. On this powder another decoction, 18 of water and 3 of species, is poured, and 12 parts of red tartar added. This compound is evaporated to the consistence of a firm paste, and a third decoction, 35 water and 5 species, is added to 25 of the paste and 25 of red tartar. This is evaporated to the proper consistence to make balls, which are usually about 1 oz. or 2 oz. in weight. They are kept to dry and then wrapped in wrapper. They are taken in doses of 4 to 5 grains much as Blaud's pills are taken here. Sometimes the balls are dipped in water until a brown colour is imparted to the liquid. This water is also used as an application to bruises.

Mistura Ferri Composita was adopted in the P.L., 1809, from the formula of his anti-hectic mixture which Dr. Moses Griffith, of Colchester, had published thirty or forty years previously. Paris quotes it as a successful instance of a medical combination which could not receive the sanction of chemical law; and he testifies to the opposition offered on that ground to its official acceptance, but adds that subsequent inquiry had proved that the chemical decompositions which constituted the objections to its use were in fact the causes of its utility. It yields a protocarbonate of iron in suspension, and a sulphate of potash in solution. The compound of iron is in the state in which it is most active.

As evidence of the faith in ferruginous waters as tonics of the generative system, Phillips quotes from the thesis of Dr. Jacques, of Paris, a curious marriage contract said to have been common at one time among the burghers of Frankfort to the effect that their wives should not visit the iron springs of Schwalbach more than twice in their lives for fear of being too fruitful. The story looks suspiciously like an advertisement of Schwalbach.

Tincture of perchloride of iron acquired its reputation in the 18th century from the secret medicines known as La Mothe's "gouttes d'or," and Bestucheff's Nerve Tincture (see page 321). The formula of the latter, published by the Academy of Medicine of St. Petersburg, was corrected by Klaproth, and under various names and in different forms found its way into all the pharmacopœias. Klaproth's process was to dissolve powdered iron in a mixture of muriatic acid 3, and nitric acid 1; evaporate to dryness, and then leave the mass to deliquesce to a brown liquor. Mix this with twice its weight of sulphuric ether. The saturated ethereal solution to be mixed with twice its volume of spirit of wine, and kept in small bottles exposed to light until the liquid acquired the proper golden tint. A similar preparation is retained in the French Codex under the title of ethereal-alcoholic tincture of muriate of iron.

Reduced Iron, or Iron reduced by hydrogen, was first prepared by Theodore Quevenne, chief pharmacist of the Hôpital de la Charité, about the year 1854. Pharmacological experiments were made with it by himself in association with Dr. Miquelard. It was believed at first that the metallic iron obtained by the process described, which was to heat the hydrated oxide of iron in a porcelain tube to dull red, and then to pass a current of hydrogen through the tube, was absolutely pure, and from experiments on dogs they came to the conclusion that the metal in this form was more assimilable than any of its salts. It had besides the advantage of being almost tasteless. Quevenne's treatise describing the process and the experiments was published in 1854 under the title of "Action physiologique et therapeutique des ferrugineux." Later investigations, while supporting the original opinion to a great extent as to the assimilability of the reduced iron, established that the product is not and cannot be pure. Dusart showed in 1884 that the proportion of actual iron could not exceed 87 per cent., and was not likely to be more than 84 per cent. Oxides, and carbonates of iron were inevitable, while sulphur, arsenic, phosphorus, and silicon were probable contaminations from the gas.

Citrate of Iron in scales was introduced by Beral, of Paris, in 1831. His formula is given in the *Pharm. Jnl.*, vol. I, p. 594.

Syrup of Phosphate of Iron was introduced in a paper read to the Medical Society of London in 1851 by Dr. Routh, and Mr. Greenish subsequently described to the Pharmaceutical Society the process by which it was prepared. The formula was afterwards improved by Mr. Gale, and his process was adopted in the B.P. It has since been modified.

A solution of iodide of iron was first employed in medicine in this country by Dr. A. T. Thomson some time in the '30's of the nineteenth century. It was introduced into the London and Edinburgh Pharmacopœias in the form of a solid salt, and in the latter also in the form of a solution. Neither of those preparations could be preserved from decomposition, and the first suggestion of a syrup appears to have been made in Buchner's Repertorium in 1839, and soon after by other experimenters. Dr. Thomson gave a formula for a syrup of iodide of iron to one of the earliest meetings of the Pharmaceutical Society in 1841, reported in the first volume of the *Pharm. Jnl.*

LEAD.

Lead is one of the ancient metals and was associated in classical writings with Saturn. The lead compounds used by the ancients in medicine were white lead or ceruse (carbonate and hydrate), and litharge (oxide). Ceruse is supposed to owe its name to cera, and to mean waxy; litharge is from Greek, and means silver stone; it was regarded as the scum of silver. Red lead or minium was also used to some extent in the form of an ointment.

Although not much used now as a medicine for internal administration, lead in various forms has been tried and advocated by doctors, usually as a sedative. The Pil. Plumbi c. Opio is what remains in our Pharmacopœia of these recommendations. Galen mentions lead as a remedy in leprosy and plague, and little bullets of lead were at one time given in cases of twisted bowels. The sedative property of lead salts has caused them to be prescribed for neuralgia, hysteria, and convulsive coughs; Goulard, recognising the anticatarrhal and astringent effects of the acetate, recommended it in urethritis; and on the theory that lead poisoning and phthisis were incompatible French practitioners at one time hoped to find in lead a remedy for tuberculosis.

Litharge was the basis of most of the popular plasters, and a century or two ago there were about a hundred of these either official or in demand. Litharge was called lithargyrum auri or lithargyrum argenti, according to its colour; but the deeper tint was only the result of a stronger fire in preparing the oxide. White lead was an ingredient in several well-known old ointments, the unguentum tripharmacum of Mesuë, which was the ceratum lithargyri of Galen, the unguentum nutritum, the unguentum diapomphologos, in which it was associated with pompholyx or oxide of zinc, and others. To a large extent these ointments were superseded after Goulard's time by the unguentum Saturninum which he introduced. The ointment of Rhazes was composed of white lead, wax, and camphor dissolved in oil of roses. He also ordered the addition of the white of an egg to every half-pound, but this came to be omitted as it caused the ointment to become odorous. The Mother's Ointment (onguent de la Mère) has long been a favourite ointment in France for promoting suppuration, and it is included in the Codex. It was made empirically by a nun at the Hotel Dieu, named La Mère Thecle, and as it became much sought after she furnished the formula. It is made by heating together mutton suet, lard, and butter, and when vapours are being exhaled, finely powdered litharge is sifted into the fats, causing a violent effervescence. Some wax and pure black pitch are afterwards added. The process has been studied by several pharmacists, and the conclusion come to is that the fats are decomposed and a number of fatty acids with some acroleine are produced. The operation is a rather dangerous one, especially if there is any naked light in the vicinity.

Magistery of Saturn was a white lead precipitated from a solution of the acetate by carbonate of potash. This was the principal ingredient in the Powder of Saturn devised by Mynsicht. The other components of this powder, which was recommended in phthisis and asthma especially, were magistery of sulphur (lac sulphuris), squine root, flowers of sulphur, pearls, coral, oatmeal, Armenian bole, flowers of benzoin, olibanum, sugar candy, saffron, and cassia.

The chief apostle of lead in medical practice was Goulard, whose name has become inseparably associated with the solution of the acetate. Some account of the bearer of this familiar name, and of his medicinal preparations of lead will be found in the section on Masters in Pharmacy.

QUICKSILVER
BOTTLE (present style)

QUICKSILVER
BOTTLE (Old Style)

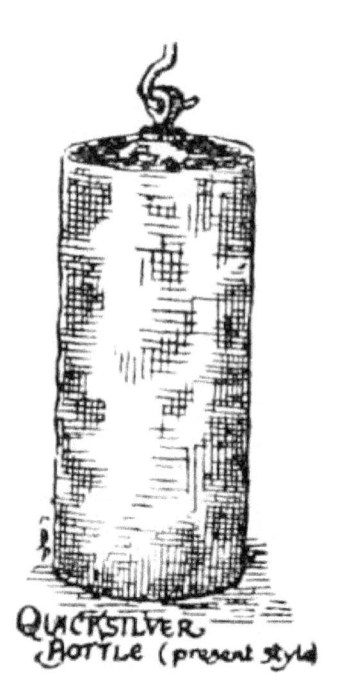

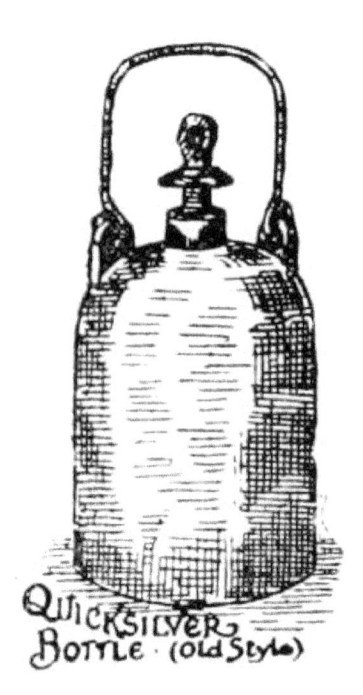

QUICKSILVER

is first alluded to in Greek writings by Theophrastus, about 315 B.C., but it was certainly known and used medicinally by the Chinese and in India long before. Apparently, too, it was known by the Egyptians. Dioscorides invented the name hydrargyrum, or fluid silver, for it. Pliny treats it as a dangerous poison. Galen adopted the opinion that the metal is poisonous, but states that he had no personal knowledge of its effects. With these authors argentum vivum was the term generally used to mean the native quicksilver, while hydrargyrum was more usually employed to describe the quicksilver obtained from the sulphide, cinnabar. Ancient writers appear to have regarded the two substances as distinct. Dioscorides points out that cinnabar was often confused with minium (red lead). The name Mercury, and the association of the metal (or demi-metal, as it was often regarded) with the planet and with its sign, formerly associated with tin, dates from the middle ages. It is mentioned first in this connection in a list of metals by Stephanus of Alexandria, in the seventh century.

ARABS USED MERCURY MEDICINALLY.

The Arabs, who inherited the medical lore of the Greeks, and probably added to this in the case of mercury knowledge acquired from India, were much interested in mercury. In the chemical works attributed to Geber not only the metal itself, but its compounds, red precipitate and corrosive sublimate, are described. Much use of mercury was made by the Arabs in the form of ointments for skin diseases, for which Mesuë recommended it, and Avicenna was probably the first physician to express doubt in regard to the poisonous nature of the metal. He observed that many persons had swallowed it without any bad effect, and he noted that it passed through the body unchanged.

MERCURY PRESCRIBED INTERNALLY.

Fallopius (1523–1562) remarks that in his time shepherds gave quicksilver to sheep and cattle to kill worms, and Brassavolus (1500–1554) states that he had given it to children in doses of from 2 to 20 grains, and had expelled worms by that means. Matthiolus (died 1577) relates that he had known women take a pound of it at a dose with the object of procuring abortion, and says it had not produced any bad result.

FRICTIONS AND FUMIGATIONS.

Sprengel fixes the year 1497 as that in which mercury was first employed externally for the cure of syphilis. Frictions, fumigations, and plasters were the earliest forms in which it was employed. Berenger de Carpi, a famous surgeon and anatomist of Bologna, who practised in the early part of the sixteenth century, is said to have made an immense fortune by inventing and prescribing frictions with mercurial ointment for syphilis. John de Vigo was a strong partisan of fumigations in obstinate cases. His fumigations were made from cinnabar and storax. It is not quite clear whether this physician gave red precipitate internally in syphilis. He expressly indicates its internal use in plague.

MERCURY A REMEDY FOR SYPHILIS.

Peter Andrew Matthiolus, born at Sienna in 1500, died at Trent in 1577, latterly the first physician to the Archduke Ferdinand of Austria, a botanist and author of "Commentaries on Dioscorides," was, according to Sprengel, the first who is known for certain to have administered mercury internally. Paracelsus, however, was without doubt the practitioner who popularised its use. He gave red precipitate, corrosive sublimate, and nitrate of mercury, and describes how each of these was made. Sprengel credits him also with acquaintance with calomel, but other authors do not recognise this in any of his writings.

VIGO'S PLASTER.

The Emplastrum Vigonium was a highly complicated compound, which was held in great veneration and is the subject of innumerable comments in the pharmaceutical writings of the sixteenth, seventeenth, and eighteenth centuries. Charas, Lemery, Baumé, and others modified and simplified it.

John de Vigo was a native of Naples, where he was born about 1460, and he became the first physician of Pope Julius II. His plaster still figures in the French Codex, and contains 600 parts of mercury by weight in 3,550 parts. This made into a liquid with olive oil and spread on calico makes the sparadrap of Vigo, in which form it is most frequently used, as an application to syphilitic eruptions.

Ambrose Paré gives the earliest formula for Vigo's plaster, which was then called Emplastrum Vigonium seu de Ranis. It was looked upon as a masterpiece of combination. First 3½ oz. of earthworms were washed in water, and afterwards in wine. Then they and twenty-six live frogs were macerated in 2 lb. of odoriferous wine, and the whole was boiled down to two-thirds of its volume. A decoction of camel's hay (andropogon schœnanthus), French lavender, and matricaria (chamomilla) was then mixed with this wine. Meanwhile 1 lb. of golden litharge had been "nourished" for twelve hours with oils of chamomile, dill, lilies, and saffron; these were melted down with 1 lb. each of the fat of the pig, calf, and viper. Human fat might be used instead of that of vipers. Juices of elder root and of elecampane with euphorbium, frankincense, and oil of spike were then worked in and the whole melted with white wax. Lastly, quicksilver extinguished by turpentine, styrax, oil of bitter almonds, and oil of bay, were added. In Lemery's time the minimum proportion of mercury was 1 drachm to 1 oz. of the plaster. There was also a simple Vigo's plaster made without mercury. In the Codex formula the worms, the frogs, the fats, the herbs, roots, and oils have all gone, but some more aromatic resins are added.

THE FIRST MERCURIAL PILLS.

The first formula for mercurial pills was one which Barbarossa II, a famous pirate and king of Algiers, and admiral of the Turkish Fleet under Soliman, Sultan of Turkey, sent to Francis I, king of France, some time in the second quarter of the sixteenth century. The recipe was published (says Dr. Etienne Michelon, of Tours, in his "Histoire Pharmacotechnique de Mercure") in 1537 by Petrus de Bayro, physician to the Duke of Savoy. He does not give the exact formula, but Lemery quotes it as follows:—

"Best aloes, and quicksilver extinguished by rose juice, aa 6 drachms;

"Trochises of agaric, ½ oz.; selected rhubarb, 2 drachms;

"Canella, myrrh, mastic, aa 1 drachm; musk, amber, aa 1 scruple;

"Make a mass with Venice turpentine."

Lemery says you cannot kill the mercury with rose juice, but must use some of the Venice turpentine.

These pills were largely used in syphilis, but they were practically superseded later by the pills of Belloste, which are still official in the French Codex. These were very similar. Belloste was a French Army surgeon, and his formula was devised about the year 1700. A formula for them was published in the Pharmacopœia of Renaudot during Belloste's lifetime, but after the death of Belloste in 1730 his son tried to make a mystery of the pills and sold them as a proprietary product, which probably had the effect of making them popular. The formula of Renaudot, which is also that of the Codex, was: Mercury, 24 (killed with honey); aloes, 24; rhubarb, 12; scammony, 8; black pepper, 4. Made into pills, each of which should contain 5 centigrams of mercury.

THE TREATMENT OF SYPHILIS.

It was at the close of the fifteenth century that syphilis began to spread through Europe. There are doubtful evidences of its existence in both Europe and Asia long previously, but the theory is generally accepted that it was brought from America by the sailors of the earliest expeditions, while its rapid spread throughout the old world in the decade from 1490 to 1500 has often been attributed to the Spanish Jews in the first place, and also particularly to the siege of Naples by the French in 1495. That large numbers of the French soldiers then engaged contracted it in the course of that war is undoubted, and as they were largely instrumental in spreading the contagion the disease soon came to be known as the French disease, or morbus Gallicus, though it has been questioned whether the adjective was not originally a reference to the skin diseases known under the name of "gale" or "itch." The opinion that syphilis came from the west is not universally adopted. It has been pointed out that Columbus only reached Lisbon on March 6, 1493, on his return from his first voyage of discovery; and there are several more or less authentic allusions to the French disease before that date.

The rapidity with which this epidemic seized on all the countries of Europe, and the virulence of its symptoms, alarmed all classes and staggered the medical men of the day. Special hospitals were opened and Parliamentary edicts were promulgated in some of the French and German cities, ordering all persons contaminated to at once leave the neighbourhoods. Mercury was one of the first remedies to suggest itself to practitioners. It had been employed by the Arabs in the form of ointments and fumigations for skin diseases, and quacks and alchemists had long experimented with it in the hope of extracting a panacea from it. Before Paracelsus had begun to administer it, Torrella, physician to the Borgias, had prescribed mercurial lotions made from corrosive sublimate, and Jean de Vigo, of Naples, had compounded his mercurial plaster, and mercurial ointment, and had even given red precipitate in pills.

At the time when syphilis was causing excitement through Europe sarsaparilla and guaiacum were much praised as sudorifics, and wonderful cures of syphilis by them were reported. The poet and reformer Ulrich von Hutten wrote a book, De Morbo Gallico, in which he related his own years of suffering from the disease, and his complete cure by means of guaiacum in 30 days. "You may swallow these woods up to the tomb," said Paracelsus. He had not much more respect for fumigations with cinnabar, which he regarded as a quack treatment by which it was impossible to measure the dose of the mercury, though he recognised that it cured sometimes. Red precipitate with theriacum made into pills with cherry juice was his favourite remedy, and was one of his laudanums. His Catholicon, or universal panacea, was a preparation of gold and corrosive sublimate, which was largely used by his followers under the name of Aurum Vitæ.

Corrosive sublimate was the great quack remedy for syphilis for more than a century, and the so-called vegetable remedies, syrups and decoctions of guaiacum, sarsaparilla, and sassafras, maintained their reputation largely in consequence of the perchloride of mercury, which was so often added to them. Aqua Phagadænica, 1 drachm of corrosive sublimate in 1 pint of lime water, was a very noted lotion for venereal ulcers. It began from a formula by Jean Fernel, a Paris medical professor and Galenist (1497–1558), who dissolved 6 grains of sublimate in 3 oz. of plaintain water. This was known as the Eau Divine de Fernel. By the time when Moses Charas published his Pharmacopœia this lotion had acquired the name by which it was so long known, and was made from ½ oz. of sublimate in 3 lb. of lime water, and ½ lb. of spirit of wine. It yielded a precipitate which varied in colour from yellow to red.

A curious controversy prevailed for a long time among the chemical and medical authorities in France in regard to a popular proprietary remedy for syphilis known as Rob Boyveau-Laffecteur. It was sold as a non-mercurial compound. It was first prepared or advertised in 1780 by a war office official named Laffecteur, whose position enabled him to get it largely used in the army. Subsequently a Paris doctor named Boyveau bought a share in the business, but in time the partners separated, and both sold the Rob. Boyveau wrote a bulky volume on the treatment of syphilis, and in that he strongly praised the Rob. After the deaths of Laffecteur and Boyveau the business came into the hands of a Dr. Giraudeau, of St. Gervais. This was about the year 1829. In 1780 the Academie de Medicine had examined this preparation, and had apparently, though not formally, tolerated its sale. Their chemist, Bucquet, had been instructed specially to examine the syrup for sublimate. He reported that he could not find any, but he was by no means sure that there was none there, for he stated that he had himself added 2 grains to a bottle, and could not afterwards detect its presence. Between that time and 1829 several chemists studied the subject, and came to the conclusion that if corrosive sublimate had been added to the syrup the vegetable extractive or the molasses with which it was made so concealed it or decomposed it into calomel that it could not be detected. In 1829 Giraudeau was prosecuted for selling secret medicines, and for this offence was fined 600 francs. But the interesting feature of this trial was the testimony of Pelletier, Chevallier, and Orfila that the Rob contained no mercurial. They reported that the formula given by the maker might be the correct one, but that in that case the mixture would contain too small a quantity of active substances to possess the energetic properties claimed for it. Guaiacum and sarsaparilla were the principal ingredients, but there were also lobelia, astragalus root, several other herbs, and a little opium. The history of this discussion is related at some length in Dr. Michelon's "Histoire Pharmacotechnique et Pharmacologique du Mercure" (1908).

RED PRECIPITATE.

Red precipitate was one of the first preparations of mercury known. It is traced to Geber, but when the works attributed to that chemist were written is doubtful. Avicenna in the tenth century was acquainted with it. In his writings he says of the metal mercury that "warmed in a closed vessel it loses its humidity, that is to say its liquid state, and is changed into the nature of fire and becomes vermilion." Being obtained direct from mercury acted on by the air, it became known to the early chemical experimenters as "precipitatus per se." Paracelsus obtained it by acting on mercury with aqua regia and heating the solution until he got the red precipitate. Then he reduced it to the necessary mildness for medicinal purposes by distilling spirit of wine from it six or seven times. Charas described a method of obtaining the precipitate by nitric acid but by a complicated process, and to the product he gave the name of arcana corallina. Boyle obtained the red oxide by boiling mercury in a bottle fitted with a stopper which was provided with a narrow tube by which air was admitted. The product was called Boyle's Hell, because it was believed that it caused the metal to suffer extreme agonies.

OTHER MERCURIAL PRECIPITATES.

The multitude of experiments with mercury yielded many products, and often the same product by a different process which acquired a distinct name.

Turbith mineral was a secret preparation with Oswald Crollius who gave it this name, probably, it is supposed, on account of its resemblance in colour to the Turbethum (Convolvulus) roots which were in his time much used in medicine. It is a subsulphate, made by treating mercury with oil of vitriol and precipitating with water.

The precipitation of mercury by sal ammoniac was first described by Beguin in 1632. For a time it was given as a purgative and in venereal diseases. A double chloride of mercury and ammonium was also made by the alchemists and was highly esteemed by them, especially as it was soluble. It was called Sal Alembroth and also Sal Sapientiæ. The origin of the first name is unknown, but it has been alleged to be of Chaldean birth and to signify the key of knowledge.

A green precipitate was obtained by dissolving mercury and copper in nitric acid, and precipitating by vinegar. This was also used in syphilis.

Homberg put a little mercury into a bottle and attached it to the wheel of a mill. The metal was thereby transformed into a black powder (the protoxide.)

By a careful and very gradual precipitation of a solution of nitrate of mercury by ammonia Hahnemann obtained what he called soluble mercury. Soubeiran proved that this precipitate was a mixture in variable proportions of sub-nitrate and ammonio-proto-nitrate of mercury.

Calomel.

Calomel was introduced into practice by Sir Theodore Turquet de Mayerne about the year 1608. It has been said that he was the inventor of the product, but as it was described and, perhaps, to some extent used by other medical authorities, Crollius among these, who lived and died before Turquet was born, this was evidently impossible. Theodore Turquet de Mayerne had been a favourite physician to Henri IV, but he had been compelled to leave Paris on account of the jealousies of his medical contemporaries. His employment of mineral medicines, antimony and mercury especially, was the occasion of bitter attacks, but his professional heresy was perhaps actually less heinous than his firm Protestantism. Both James I and Charles I accepted his services and placed great confidence in his skill. He was instrumental, as explained in another section, in the independent incorporation of the apothecaries, and was also one of the most active promoters of the publication of the "London Pharmacopœia."

It appears likely that Turquet invented the name by which this milder form of mercurial has come to be most usually known. The alchemical writers of the time called it Aquila Alba or Draco Mitigatus. A notorious Paracelsian of Paris, Joseph Duchesne, but better known by his Latinised surname of Quercetanus, who shared with Turquet the animosity of Gui Patin and his medical confederates, and for similar reasons, also made calomel and administered it, probably sold it, under the designation of the mineral Panchymagogon, purger of all humours. Panacea mercurialis, manna metallorum, and sublimatum dulce, were among the other fanciful names given. It was believed by the old medical chemists that the more frequently it was resublimed the more dulcified it became. In fact, resublimation was likely to decompose it, and thus to produce corrosive sublimate.

What the name "calomel" was derived from has been the subject of much conjecture. "Kalos melas," beautiful black, is the obvious-looking source, but it does not seem possible to fit any sense to this suggested origin. A fanciful story of a black servant in the employ of de Mayerne manufacturing a beautiful white medicine is told by Pereira with the introduction of "as some say." A good remedy for black bile is another far-fetched etymology, and another conceives the metal and the sublimate in the crucible as blackish becoming a fair white. Some thirty years ago, in a correspondence published in the "Chemist and Druggist," Mr. T. B. Groves, of Weymouth, and "W. R." of Maidstone, both independently broached the idea that "kalos" and "meli" (honey) were the constituents of the word, forming a sort of rough translation of the recognised term, dulcified mercury; a not unreasonable supposition, though this leaves the "kalos" not very well accounted for. In Hooper's "Medical Dictionary" it is plausibly guessed that the name may have been originally applied to Ethiops Mineral, and got transferred to the white product; and Paris quotes from Mr. Gray the opinion that a mixture of calomel and scammony which was called the calomel of Rivierus may have been the first application of the term, meaning a mixture of a white and dark substance.

Beguin (1608) is generally credited with having been the first European writer to describe calomel. He gave it the name of "Draco mitigatus" (corrosive sublimate being the dragon). But Berthelot, in his "Chemistry of the Middle Ages," has shown that the protochloride of mercury was prepared as far back as Democritus, and that it is described in certain Arab chemical writings. It is also alleged to have been prepared in China, Thibet, and India many centuries before it became known in Europe.

QUICKSILVER GIRDLES,

made by applying to a cotton girdle mercury which had been beaten up with the white of egg, were used in the treatment of itch before the true character of that complaint was understood.

BASILIC POWDER

was the old Earl of Warwick's powder or Cornachino's powder (equal parts of scammony, diaphoretic antimony, and cream of tartar), to which calomel, equal in weight to each of the other ingredients, was added. But I have not succeeded in tracing why or when the name of basilic (royal) was given to the compound.

Corrosive Sublimate.

Van Swieten's solution of corrosive sublimate was introduced in the middle of the eighteenth century as a remedy for syphilis, and for a long time was highly esteemed. Its author, Baron von Swieten, was of Dutch birth, and was a pupil of Boerhaave. He was invited to Vienna by the Empress Maria Theresa, and exercised an almost despotic authority in medical treatment. His original formula was 24 grains of corrosive sublimate dissolved in two quarts of whisky, a tablespoonful to be taken night and morning, followed by a long draught of barley-water.

Corrosive sublimate was the recognised cure for syphilis, at least in Vienna, at that time. Maximilian Locher, another noted physician of the same school, claimed to have cured 4,880 cases in eight years with the drug. This was in 1762.

Cinnabar.

The bisulphide of mercury (cinnabar) was also used in many nostrums. Paris says it was the active ingredient in Chamberlain's restorative pills, "the most certain cure for the scrophula, king's evil, fistula, scurvy, and all impurities of the blood."

"Killing" Mercury.

The art of extinguishing or "killing" mercury has been discussed and experimented on from the fifteenth century until the present day. The modern use of steam machinery in the manufacture of mercurial ointment, mercurial pills, and mercury with chalk has put a check on the ingenuity of patient pharmacists, who were constantly discovering some new method for accelerating the long labour of triturating, which many operators still living can remember. Venice turpentine, or oil of turpentine, various essential oils, sulphur, the saliva of a person fasting, and rancid fat were among the earlier expedients adopted and subsequently discarded. The turpentines made the ointment irritating, the sulphur formed a compound, and the rancid fat was found to be worse than the turpentines. Nitrate of potash, sulphate of potash, stearic acid, oil of almonds and balsam of Peru, the precipitation of the mercury from its solution in nitric acid, spermaceti, glycerin, and oleate of mercury have been more modern aids.

It would be outside the purpose of this sketch to deal with the questions which the numerous processes suggested have raised. Apparently it is not completely settled now whether the pill, the powder, and the ointment depend for their efficiency on any chemical action such as the oxidation of the metal in the cases of the two former, or on a solution in the fat in the case of the ointment. These theories have been held, and do not seem unlikely; but there also seems good reason to believe that mercury in a state of minute division has definite physiological effects by itself. At any rate, it is well established that the more perfectly the quicksilver is "killed" the more efficient is the resulting compound.

SILVER.

The moon was universally admitted under the theory of the macrocosm and the microcosm to rule the head, and as silver was the recognised representative of Luna among the metals the deduction was obvious that silver was the suitable remedy for all diseases affecting the brain, as apoplexy, epilepsy, melancholia, vertigo, and failure of memory. Tachenius relates that a certain silversmith had the gift of being able to repeat word for word anything that he heard, and this power he attributed to his absorption of particles of silver in the course of his work. It does not appear, however, that all silversmiths were similarly endowed.

The Greek and Latin doctors make no allusion to silver as a medicine, and the earliest evidence of its actual employment as a remedy is found in the writings of Avicenna, who gave it in the metallic state "in tremore cordis, in fœtore oris." He is also believed to have introduced the practice of silvering pills with the intention of thereby adding to their efficacy. To John Damascenus, a Christian saint who lived among the Arabs before Avicenna, is attributed the remark concerning silver, "Remedium adhibitum est, et in omnibus itaque capitis morbis, ob Lunæ, Argenti, et Cerebri sympathicam trinitatem." This association of the moon, silver, and the brain was believed in firmly by the chemical doctors of the sixteenth century, and for a long time a tincture of the moon, tinctura Lunæ, was the most famous remedy in epilepsy and melancholia. A great many high authorities, among them Boyle, Boerhaave, and Hoffmann in the eighteenth century, continued to prescribe this tincture or the lunar pills, but silver gradually dropped out of fashion. A great number of medical investigators since have from time to time recommended the nitrate or the chloride of silver in various diseases, but without succeeding in securing for silver a permanent reputation as an internal medicine.

The Pilulæ Lunares were generally composed of nitrate of silver combined with opium, musk, and camphor. Nitrate of silver was given in doses varying from a twentieth to a tenth of a grain. The tincture of the moon was a solution of nitrate of silver with some copper, which gave it a blue tint and probably was the active medicinal ingredient. Fused nitrate of silver or lunar caustic seems to have succeeded to the reputation of fused caustic potash as a cautery, and also to have acquired the name of lapis infernalis (sometimes translated "hell-stone" in old books) originally applied to the fused potash.

The only reason assigned for this title is the keen pain caused by the application of the caustic, though probably it was first adopted to contrast it with the lapis divinus, which was a combination of sulphate of copper and alum used as an application to the eyes.

Christopher Glaser, pharmacien at the court of Louis XIV, who subsequently had to leave France on suspicion of being implicated in the Brinvilliers poisonings, was the first to make nitrate of silver in sticks.

TIN.

Tin came into medical use in the middle ages, and acquired its position particularly as a vermifuge. For this purpose tin had a reputation only second to mercury. Several compounds of this metal were popular as medicines both official and as nostrums in the seventeenth and eighteenth centuries, and tin did not drop out of medicinal employment until early in the nineteenth century.

The beautiful mosaic gold (aurum musivum), a pet product with many alchemists, was probably the first tin compound to be used in medicine. It was made by first combining tin and mercury into an amalgam, and then distilling this substance with sulphur and sal ammoniac. It is now known to be a bisulphide of tin. The mercury only facilitates the combination of the tin and the sulphur, and the sal ammoniac has the effect of regularising the temperature in the process. The product is a beautiful golden metal of crystalline structure and brilliant lustre. It was given in doses of from 4 to 20 grains; was sudorific and purgative; and was recommended in fevers, hysterical complaints, and venereal disorders. The subsequent preparations of tin which came to be used principally as vermifuges were the Calx Jovis (the binoxide), the sal Jovis (sometimes the nitrate and sometimes the chloride), and the Amalgama Jovis. These, however, were all ultimately superseded by the simple powder of tin given either with chalk, sugar, crabs' eyes, or combined with honey or some conserve. The dose was very various with different practitioners. Some prescribed only a few grains, others gave up to a drachm, and Dr. Alston, an eminent Edinburgh physician in the eighteenth century, said its success depended on being administered in much larger doses. He recommended an ounce with 4 ounces of treacle to be given on an empty stomach. To be followed next day with ½ oz., and another ½ oz. the day after; the course to be wound up by a cathartic.

The Anti-hecticum Poterii was a combination of tin with iron and antimony, to which nitrate of potash was added. It was sudorific and was thought to be especially useful in the sweats of consumption and blood spitting. Flake's Anti-hæmorrhoidal Ointment was an amalgam of tin made into an ointment with rose ointment, to which some red precipitate was added. Brugnatelli's Poudre Vermifuge was a sulphide of tin. Spielman's Vermifuge Electuary was simply tin filings and honey.

Oxide of tin is the basis of certain applications for the finger nails. As supplied by perfumers the pure oxide is coloured with carmine and perfumed with lavender. Piesse says pure oxide of tin is similarly used to polish tortoiseshell.

ZINC.

The earliest known description of zinc as a metal is found in the treatise on minerals by Paracelsus, and it is he who first designates the metal by the name familiar to us. Paracelsus says:

"There is another metal, zinc, which is in general unknown. It is a distinct metal of a different origin, though adulterated with many other metals. It can be melted, for it consists of three fluid principles, but it is not malleable. In its colour it is unlike all others, and does not grow in the same manner; but with its *ultima materia* I am as yet unacquainted, for it is almost as strange in its properties as argentum vivum."

The alloy of zinc with copper which we call brass was known and much prized by the Roman metal workers, and they also knew the zinc earth, calamine, and used this in the production of brass. Who first separated the metal from the earth is unknown; so too is the original inventor of white vitriol (sulphate of zinc). Beckmann quotes authorities who ascribe this to Julius, Duke of Brunswick, about 1570. Beckmann says white vitriol was at first known as erzalaum, brass-alum, and later as gallitzenstein, a name which he thinks may have been derived from galls, as the vitriol and galls were for a long time the principal articles used for making ink and for dyeing. Green vitriol, he adds, was called green gallitzenstein. The true nature of several vitriols was not understood until 1728, when Geoffrey studied and explained them.

The ideas entertained of zinc by the chemists who studied it were curious. Albertus Magnus held that it was a compound with iron; Paracelsus leaned to the idea that it was copper in an altered form; Kunckel fancied it was congealed mercury; Schluttn thought it was tin rendered fragile by combination with some sulphur; Lemery supposed it was a form of bismuth; Stahl held that brass was a combination of copper with an earth and phlogiston; Libavius (1597) described zinc as a peculiar kind of tin. The metal he examined came from India.

The white oxide of zinc was originally known as pompholyx, which is Greek for a bubble or blister, nihil album, lana philosophica, and flores zinci. The unguentum diapompholygos, which was found in the pharmacopœias of the eighteenth century, and was a legacy from Myrepsus, was a compound of white lead and oxide of zinc in an ointment which contained also the juice of nightshade berries and frankincense. It was deemed to be a valuable application for malignant ulcers.

Oxide of zinc as an internal medicine was introduced by Gaubius, who was Professor of Medicine at Amsterdam about the middle of the eighteenth century. It had been known and used under the name of flowers of zinc from Glauber's time. A shoemaker at Amsterdam, named Ludemann, sold a medicine for epilepsy which he called Luna fixata, for which he acquired some fame. Gaubius was interested in it and analysed it. He found it to be simply oxide of zinc, and though he did not endorse the particular medical claim put forward on its behalf he found it useful for spasms and to promote digestion.

END OF VOL. I

FOOTNOTES:

[1] Schelenz in "Geschichte der Pharmacie," 1904, has collected a remarkable number of facts and documents illustrative of the development of pharmacy in Germany. He quotes a Nuremberg ordinance of 1350 which forbids physicians to be interested in the business of an apothecary, and requires apothecaries to be satisfied with moderate profits.

[2] Dr. Monk gives a copy of the Latin minute in the books of the College referring to this curious recantation. The actual words which Geynes signed were these:—"Ego, Johannes Geynes, fateor Galenum in iis, quae proposui contra eum, non errasse."

[3] "Free Phosphorus in Medicine," 1874.

www.ingramcontent.com/pod-product-compliance
Ingram Content Group UK Ltd.
Pitfield, Milton Keynes, MK11 3LW, UK
UKHW040814280325
456847UK00003B/400